....
Immunopathogenetic Aspects of Disease Induced by Helminth Parasites

....

Chemical Immunology

Vol. 66

Series Editors   *Luciano Adorini,* Milan
                      Ken-ichi Arai, Tokyo
                      Claudia Berek, Berlin
                      J. Donald Capra, Dallas, Tex.
                      Anne-Marie Schmitt-Verhulst, Marseille
                      Byron H. Waksman, New York, N.Y.

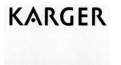

Basel · Freiburg · Paris · London · New York ·
New Delhi · Bangkok · Singapore · Tokyo · Sydney

....

Immunopathogenetic Aspects of Disease Induced by Helminth Parasites

Volume Editor   *David O. Freedman,* Birmingham, Ala.

37 figures and 5 tables, 1997

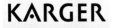
KARGER   Basel · Freiburg · Paris · London · New York ·
New Delhi · Bangkok · Singapore · Tokyo · Sydney

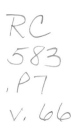

....

Chemical Immunology

Formerly published as 'Progress in Allergy'
Founded 1939 by Paul Kallòs

Library of Congress Cataloging-in-Publication Data
Immunopathogenetic aspects of disease induced by Helminth parasites / volume editor,
David O. Freedman.
(Chemical immunology; vol. 66)
Includes bibliographical references and index.   1. Helminthiasis – Immunological aspects.
I. Freedman, David O.   II. Series.
[DNLM: 1. Helminthiasis – immunology.   2. Helminthiasis – pathology.
W1 CH 25G v.66 1997/ WC 800 I33 1997]
RC 119.7.I458 1997
616.9′ 62–dc21
ISBN 3–8055–6400–7 (hard cover: alk. paper)

Bibliographic Indices. This publication is listed in bibliographic services, including Currents Contents® and Index Medicus.

Drug Dosage. The authors and the publisher have exerted every effort to ensure that drug selection and dosage set forth in this text are in accord with current recommendations and practice at the time of publication. However, in view of ongoing research, changes in government regulations, and the constant flow of information relating to drug therapy and drug reactions, the reader is urged to check the package insert for each drug for any change in indications and dosage and for added warnings and precautions. This is particularly important when the recommended agent is a new and/or infrequently employed drug.

© Copyright 1997 by S. Karger AG, P.O. Box, CH–4009 Basel (Switzerland)
Printed in Switzerland on acid-free paper by Thür AG Offsetdruck, Pratteln
ISBN 3–8055–6400–7

....
Contents

The Basis of IgE Responses to Specific Antigenic Determinants in Helminthiasis

Immunopathology of Onchocerciasis: A Role for Eosinophils in Onchocercal Dermatitis and Keratitis

Enteric Helminth Infection: Immunopathology and Resistance during Intestinal Nematode Infection

Pathogenesis of Human Hookworm Infection: Insights from a 'New' Zoonosis

Human Toxocariasis and the Visceral Larva Migrans Syndrome: Correlative Immunopathology

Lymphatic Filariasis

Contents

Immunopathology of Echinococcosis

Taenia solium Cysticercosis: Host-Parasite Interactions and the Immune Response

Preface

Just at the time when the magnitude of the growth and developmental problems attributable to human helminthiasis are being fully realized, we are in recent years able for the first time to describe defined immune responses responsible for the pathological lesions seen. This has to a large extent developed from the concept that, based on the different sets of cytokines produced by CD4+ T cells in response to an invading organism, immune responses can be classified as Th1, Th2, or Th0. Deleterious inflammatory responses to metazoan parasites appear to be for the most part associated with a polarized Th2 cytokine profile. Thus, host-parasite models involving a number of enteric and tissue helminths have provided seminal information on immunoregulatory and immunopathogenetic responses that is parasite specific yet at the same time is generalizable to a more complete understanding of the entire Th1/Th2 paradigm. The ready infection and manipulation of helminthic organisms in cytokine gene knockout mice have proved to be an especially powerful tool.

The importance of particular cytokines by themselves in the pathogenesis of disease in helminthic infection remains to be completely defined. An appropriate emphasis is placed in several of the articles in this volume on describing emerging molecular mechanisms utilized by cytokine-sensitive effector cells such as eosinophils, basophils, and mast cells in mediating immunopathology and resistance during nematode infection. For example, the ability to study in detail the eosinophilic response to *O. volvulus* larvae in the murine cornea, as described in the article by Pearlman, now provides us with an easily manipulated in vivo incubation chamber for the study of this relatively poorly understood effector cell.

The significance of the markedly elevated levels of IgE found during helminthic infection in mediating either protection or pathology has been poorly understood. Insights into many of the immunoregulatory aspects of the control of IgE production have evolved in recent years during studies of both atopic and parasitized individuals. However, an understanding of the basis of responses to specific IgE inducing antigenic determinants on parasitic nematodes will be necessary before postulates regarding the etiologic role of IgE in helminthic infection can be formulated. The paper by Lobos describes innovative work on IgE responses to a molecularly characterized filarial allergen in patients with tropical pulmonary eosinophilia and postulates the induction of autoimmunity by molecular mimicry of a key parasite enzyme, γ-glutamyl transpeptidase.

The first three articles in the volume present, respectively, a generalized overview of recent advances in the understanding of the induction of IgE, eosinophilic, and cytokine regulatory responses to helminthic infection. Subsequent articles comprehensively review recent developments for a specific metazoan organism, while at the same time providing authoritative emphasis within the text on key directions and priorities. While many chapters are necessarily heavily weighted with work on animal models of infection, conclusions are set in the context of human disease wherever possible. An interesting bridge between animal and human models of helminthic infection is provided in the chapter by Prociv reviewing work demonstrating that the canine nematode *Ancylostoma caninum* is a human enteric pathogen causing eosinophilic enteritis. The comparison of human and canine hookworm in the human host provides a cautionary tale with regard to development of anti-helminth vaccines for human use which may exacerbate subsequent inflammatory encounters with animal nematodes.

David O. Freedman

Freedman DO (ed): Immunopathogenetic Aspects of Disease Induced by Helminth Parasites.
Chem Immunol. Basel, Karger, 1997, vol 66, pp 1–25

....

The Basis of IgE Responses to Specific Antigenic Determinants in Helminthiasis

Edgar Lobos

Swiss Tropical Institute, Basel, Switzerland

Parasitic helminth nematodes, either gut or tissue-dwelling, show extremely diverse life cycles and numerous developmental stages. However, despite the diversity in their morphology, physiology and host specificity, infection with helminths has long been recognized to be characterized by a selective upregulation of IgE antibody levels, together with induction of peripheral and tissue eosinophilia and mucosal mastocytosis [1–5]. Production of IgE antibody is known to trigger the mechanisms involved in allergic diseases, but their role in parasitic diseases is still controversial as allergic manifestations in helminth infections are rare. Hence, from this observation a dual role of IgE in the induction of pathology and protective immunity has been proposed [4].

The IgE antibody class usually constitutes only a minuscule fraction of total antibody in human serum (50–300 ng/ml versus 7–12 mg/ml of IgG). The amplification of the immune responses involving IgE antibody is due to its interaction with specific receptors: the high-affinity (type I) Fcε receptor (FcεRI) present on the surface of effectors cells. The low-affinity receptor (FcεRII) is found on subsets of leukocytes and platelets. Allergen-specific IgE-induced cross-linking of FcεRI receptors mediates the subsequent release of potent chemotactic and vasoactive factors and cytokines involved in the allergic reaction [6]. Infection with helminths selectively upregulates nonspecific and specific IgE antibody levels, with up to a hundredfold increase of IgE levels. Remarkable progress has been made in identifying the factors and mechanisms that initiate and control IgE responses; however, we still have a fragmentary understanding of the specific factors that initially induce the hypersensitivity responses in helminthic infections and allergy.

Regulation of IgE Immune Responses in Helminthic Infection

The regulation of IgE antibody responses and eosinophilia as a result of infection with helminth parasites was shown to be primarily T cell dependent both in humans and in animal models [5, 7]. Understanding of the polarized pattern of immune responses induced by helminth parasites only came with the important discovery that infection with different pathogens results in the development of distinct subsets of CD4+ T cells defined by the production of characteristic cytokine profiles [8, 9]. Intracellular parasitism is generally associated with induction of type 1 T helper cells (Th1) producing interferon-γ (IFN-γ), interleukin 2 (IL-2) and tumor necrosis factor-β (TNF-β), whereas infection with helminths induces type 2 T helper cells (Th2) producing IL-4, IL-5, IL-6, IL-9, IL-10, IL-13. Th1 responses are implicated in cell-mediated cytotoxic and inflammatory reactions and are in general more protective against intracellular parasites, while Th2 responses promote antibody production, especially IgE, and promote and maintain eosinophilia. A less differentiated CD4+ T cell subset with an intermediate cytokine pattern (Th0) arises when no clear polarizing signals are present [10–13]. In addition, T cells provide cognate and noncognate signals to B cells that favor the secretion of cytokines promoting IgE synthesis [14].

The Th1 and Th2 patterns of response are maintained and balanced by a complex network of cytokines and other factors. IL-4 is the dominant factor in the induction of Th2 responses [15], while IL-12 is the most potent cytokine driving Th1 development [16, 17].

Studies in both murine and human sytems indicated that IL-4 is essential for IgE synthesis by B cells previously primed with mitogens, antigens or helminth-derived products. IL-4 induces isotype switching from IgM to IgE and IgG1 in the mouse or IgG4 in humans. The effects of IL-4 can be antagonized by the addition of rIFN-γ [18–21]. The cytokine IL-12 mainly produced by antigen-presenting cells (APC) and monocytes is one of most important factors counterregulating Th2 immune responses. IL-12 has the intrinsic capacity to drive Th1 responses and the observed suppression of Th2 responses is more a by-product of its capacity to stimulate the production of IFN-γ which in turn downregulates Th2 responses [17].

Administration of anti-IL-4 or anti-IL-4 receptor monoclonal antibody (mAb) in mice infected with the helminths *Nippostrongylus brasiliensis, Heligmosoides polygyrus* or *Schistosoma mansoni*, known to be potent inducers of IgE and IgG1, completely suppressed IgE antibody production [19], and mice lacking a functional IL-4 gene showed significantly impaired IgE antibody responses to the intestinal nematode *N. brasiliensis* [22].

The presence of exogenous cytokines secreted by APC and/or other cell types at the sites at which T cells are initially activated crucially influences the pattern of differentiation. Thus, early production of IL-4 is an important factor in the differentiation of naive T cells into Th2 cells. In mouse models, CD4+ T cells are not the only source of IL-4 and other cells types including mast cells, basophils, non-B non-T FcεRI+ cells and NK1.1 CD4+ T cells were shown to produce IL-4 and thus may contribute to the polarized Th2 responses observed in helminthic infection [reviewed in ref. 16]. There is still an open question as to which of the former cell types may have the primacy in the production of IL-4 for the skewing into Th2 responses.

Recently, intraepithelial T lymphocytes (γδ T cells) were shown to differentially produce IFN-γ in response to an intracellular pathogen *(Listeria monocytogenes)* or IL-4 in response to a helminth *(N. brasiliensis)*. This showed that γδ T cells responded early during infection in a biased manner to different pathogens and that activation of γδ T cells by unknown signals from helminths or from activated APC resulted in the immediate production of intracellular IL-4 before antigen processing. This mechanism might be a first line of defense against pathogens and perhaps a crucial step for priming the milieu with cytokines for further differentiation [23]. This implies the existence of unknown factors with a potential of inducing IL-4 or other unknown factors skewing towards Th2 responses. The adaptive CD4+ responses to infectious agents including helminths might be determined by this early contact reflecting an ancient nonspecific immune mechanism [23].

In addition to cytokines, other modulatory factors underlying the polarization towards Th2 responses may be involved: the genetic background of the host, the amount of the priming antigen, the type of APC, the site of antigen presentation, and the nature of the antigen. Excellent reviews that analyze the factors influencing the initiation and maintenance of Th1 and Th2 responses in infectious diseases have recently been published, and the reader is referred to them for further details [11, 16, 25, 26].

Role of IgE Antibodies in Animal Models of Helminthic Infections

The role of the parasite-specific IgE antibodies in protection against helminthic infection has been the subject of intense studies and controversies, especially because involvement in protective immunity is dependent on the parasite and on the murine animal model used. Using the rat model, passive transfer of *S. mansoni*-specific monoclonal IgE antibodies was shown to mediate protection, and transfer of cells from immune animals bearing surface IgE induced significant levels of protection in naive rats indicating that parasite-specific IgE on the effector cells play a central role [27]. Several cell types known to bear Fcε receptors including mast cells, eosinophils, macrophages, monocytes and platelets were able to interact with parasite-specific IgE to effectively kill schistosomula in vitro [27].

Protection in *Trichinella spiralis*-infected rats was mediated by transfusion of IgE antibodies [28] and in experimental filariasis, rats infected with *Brugia pahangi* which did not develop microfilaremia consistently developed elevated filarial-specific IgE antibodies [29]. A potential involvement of IgE antibodies in protection was obtained in cats infected with *B. pahangi;* animals that were able to kill adult worms consistently developed high levels of parasite-specific IgE antibodies whereas animals in which adult filariae were able to survive did not [30].

Antibody-dependent cell-mediated cytotoxicity involving several isotypes of antimicrofilarial antibodies, including IgE has been implicated in resistance to microfilariae in vitro but their contribution to the in vivo clearance of microfilariae remains to be established [31, 32]. Furthermore, evidence from experimental studies utilizing the feline model of lymphatic filariasis indicates that amicrofilaremic cats that kept high levels of immediate hypersensitivity reactions developed lymphangitis. Clearance of microfilariae after repeated reinfections was associated with the development of lymphatic pathology, but it is unclear whether the killing of microfilariae predisposes to pathology or whether it is the consequence of immune-mediated killing of adults with collateral lymphatic pathology [33].

In contrast to the studies cited above, depletion of IgE antibodies failed to alter resistance in *S. Mansoni*-infected mice [34] and similarly, injection with anti-IgE mAb of *H. polygyrus*-infected mice did not influence protective immunity to secondary infection. However, injection with IL-4 or IL-4R mAb completely blocked protective immunity and the capacity to expel the parasite from the host [35]. Therefore the mechanism of action of IL-4 in limiting nematode infections is not only derived from its potential to induce IgE but it might directly affect the parasite or influence the host's gut to make it inhospitable for the parasite [36]. In a mouse model of filarial infection, resistance was not dependent on Th2 responses as infection of IL-4 deficient mice with *B. malayi* did not influence the survival of the different parasite stages [37]. However, resistance to reinfection was shown to be dependent on Th2 responses being effective against infective larvae [38].

Taken together, the results from the different murine animal models of helmintic infections do not rule out an involvement of IgE antibodies and its effector cells in protective immunity. Such effector mechanisms may act against certain helminths, or only contribute partially or in combination with other mechanisms in parasite attrition in other models.

Role of IgE Antibodies in Humans Infected with Helminths

In humans, analysis of the immune responses of resistant and susceptible individuals in epidemiological studies in areas endemic for schistosomiasis support the idea that IgE plays a major protective role against schistosomes. Resistance to reinfection was associated with the development of antischistosome IgE antibodies, and individuals with high levels of specific IgE antibodies were ten times less likely to become reinfected than individuals with low specific IgE antibody levels, and reinfection was observed when patients produced high levels of competing IgG4 antibodies [39]. Similar studies in other endemic areas of Brazil and Kenya revealed a correlation between high levels of IgE immune responses and resistance to reinfection [40, 41]. There was an age-related correlation in the development of schistosome-specific IgE antibodies; the balance of the specific IgE/IgG4 antibodies was demonstrated to be predictive of the severity of the infection [42].

Further evidence in favor of a protective role for parasite-specific IgE was provided by the observation that children infected with *Ascaris* were significantly less likely to become reinfected after chemotherapy if they possesed high levels of *Ascaris*-specific IgE. In contrast, children with higher levels of total IgE before chemotherapy were significantly more frequently reinfected. The levels of total or specific IgE did not correlate with the degree of exposure, and genetic factors were suggested to influence the observed variability of immune responses [43]. Immunoepidemiological studies of gastrointestinal nematodes that examined the relationship between levels of specific IgE and the weight of *Necator americanus* revealed that levels of specific IgE against excretory/secretory products may be associated with immunity to adult hookworms [44].

In filariasis, high levels of specific IgE antibodies have been documented, but, as in human schistosomiasis, allergic manifestations are rarely seen. The ratio of IgG4:IgE antibodies is related to the clinical outcome of infection [45, 46]. In areas endemic for *Wuchereria bancrofti* and Brugian filariasis, elevated filarial specific IgE antibodies are found in amicrofilaremic patients and in endemic controls, suggesting a regulatory mechanism for specific IgE antibodies in filarial infection, but their role in the pathogenesis of elephantiasis is uncertain [32].

The elevated nonspecific IgE synthesis in helminthic infections might be beneficial to both the host and the parasite, since saturation of Fcε receptors on mast cells can inhibit allergic reactions and/or helminth specific-IgE synthesis reducing parasite attrition [47, 48]. Thus, the nonspecific IgE antibodies might be beneficial to both the host and the parasite as it may limit the amount of allergic reactions in the host and killing of the parasite. It is likely that several mechanisms are involved in limiting IgE-mediated allergic reactions, including high levels of nonspecific IgE antibodies, blocking IgG4 antibodies and nonanaphylactogenic anti-idiotypic IgE antibodies, whose existence and relevance in helminthiasis are largely unknown. Studies on *N. americanus*-infected individuals from Papua New Guinea demonstrated significant IgG auto-IgE antibodies in hookworm-infected patients, but a lack of correlation between anti-IgE antibodies and the degree of infection was observed, suggesting that auto-IgE antibodies are more beneficial for the host [49].

IgE-Binding Antigens from Helminths

In contrast to the field of allergy, there is an extreme paucity of knowledge about the nature and biological properties of nematode allergens. Many IgE-binding proteins from helminths have been described by immunoblotting but for the majority no information is available on their biochemical, structural or functional properties. Some of the allergens from helminths described here are glycoproteins of low molecular weight (MW) with acidic isoelectric points conforming to the suggested consensus for allergens, others are polyproteins proteolytically processed to smaller units [50].

Enhanced IgE antibody responses are detected in murine models not only as a consequence of experimental infection with nematodes, but also following immunization with nematode products or accidental inhalant exposure of humans to nematode products [5, 51]. A preferential expansion of Th2-like CD4+ lymphocytes is observed when cells from an individual are stimulated with nematode products. In contrast, when cells of the same individual are stimulated with tetanus toxoid antigen a preferential expansion of Th-1 like CD4+ lymphocytes occurs [21]. How the immune system translates the initial antigen recognition into the appropriate signals is one of the major unknown questions in our understanding of the polarized Th2 responses observed both in atopic and helminth-infected individuals.

In this chapter, I will review and discuss some of the best characterized helminth allergens and present data on a newly characterized filarial allergen homolog of the crucial enzyme γ-glutamyl transpeptidase (γ-GT) , a key enzyme in the γ-glutamyl cycle and the relevance of this finding to our understanding of the immunopathogenesis of infection with helminths.

The Nematode Polyprotein Allergens/Antigens

Many nematode species produce a protein of approximately 15 kD, present at all life stages and in excretory/secretory products. It is synthesized as a large precursor and posttranslationally processed by proteases to 15-kD unit or to a ladder of descending MW polypeptides. Due to this characteristic synthesis and mode of processing, ABA-1 and its homologs in other nematodes have been termed the 'nematode polyprotein allergens/antigens' (NPA) protein family [52]. Members of this family of proteins include: the ABA-1 allergen from *Ascaris suum* and *Ascaris lumbricoides*, and the polyproteins gp15/400 and the Dva-1 from lymphatic filariae and bovine lung worm *Dictyocaulus viviparus*, respectively.

The ABA-1 IgE-binding allergen initially isolated from *A. suum*, but shown to be present in helminths belonging to the genus *Ascaris*, is one of the few helminthic allergens for which information on its immunochemical properties, biochemistry, structure, as well as its biological function are available. ABA-1 is the most abundant protein in the pseudocelomic fluid of adult parasites and is secreted during in vitro cultivation of larval and lung stages [53, 54]. It is probably the same protein as an earlier characterized *Ascaris* allergen with similar MW and allergenicity, isolated from the body fluid and the culture supernatants of larval *Ascaris* [55, 56].

The first 41 amino acids from the N-terminus of isolated ABA-1 proteins from *A. suum* of pigs and *A. lumbricoides* of humans are 100% identical. Purification of ABA-1 by immunoaffinity chromatography from *Ascaris* body fluid allowed estimation of its MW at 14.6 kD, and ABA-1 homologs are present in the ascarid nematodes *Anisakis simplex* and the canine nematode *Toxocara canis* (TBA-1) [57, 58].

Molecular cloning of cDNAs and genomic clones encoding the ABA-1 gene revealed an unusual structure consisting of 20 ABA-1-encoding units in head to tail array. The ABA-1 gene is translated as a large polyprotein which is then processed into multiple copies by endoproteolytic cleavage [59]. The proteolytic cleavage site consists of a cluster of four basic residues (arginines). Such putative peptidase cleavage sites are recognized by the subtilisin family of serine endoproteases. The calculated MW of ABA-1 as determined by mass spectroscopy (14.6 kD) corresponds to the MW of 129 amino acids left after removal of the four arginines. Although the first ABA-1 deduced amino acid sequence indicated striking homology between the tandemly repeat units, further analysis demonstrated a significant amino acid sequence diversity (up to 49%) of adjacent repeat units of ABA-1 in *Ascaris*. The sequence diversity does not appear to affect the predicted four-helix structure but it is still an open question whether all units have the same function [52, 59]. In contrast to other polyprotein allergens of the NPA family, the 14.6-kD *Ascaris* allergen ABA-1 does not contain any glycosylation sites. ABA-1 has high binding affinity for fatty acids, retinol and retinoic acid [60].

Early studies using rodent animal models showed significant differences in the antibody responses to experimental infection with *Ascaris* [61]. Involvement of the major histocompatibility complex (MHC) in the control of antibody responses to ABA-1 was investigated using H-2 congenic mice on BALB and B10 backgrounds. It was established that both IgG and IgE antibody responses to ABA-1 were restricted to mice bearing the H-2^s haplotype of the MHC and to rats with the RT^u haplotype [61–63]. Furthermore, the antibody response to ABA-1 was shown to be under conventional class II-associated Ir gene control. MHC restriction of the antibody responses to ABA-1 operated only in the context of infection and broke down under adjuvant-assisted immunization using purified ABA-1 protein [64, 65].

Humans infected with *A. lumbricoides* show considerable variability in their immune response to ABA-1 with only a small percentage of the infected individuals having detectable antibody responses to ABA-1. It is likely that the IgG and IgE antibody responses to ABA-1 might be HLA-restricted as in the murine models. An association between host age and the intensity of precipitating anti-ABA-1 antibodies was found, indicating that factors such as the intensity of exposure may also influence the development of the immune response [66, 67]. IgE-mediated immediate hypersensitivity responses to *Ascaris* larvae migrating through the lungs might play a role in the lung pathology that ranges from mild respiratory distress to life-threatening immune responses (Loeffler syndrome). The analysis of the cellular and immunological responses to ABA-1 in *Ascaris*-infected patients showing pulmonary pathology should clarify its suggested potential in the pathology.

Previous studies on the characterization of surface-associated proteins from *B. malayi* and *B. pahangi* identified a soluble protein complex termed the 'gp15/400' antigens. The protein complex immunoprecipitated as a 'protein ladder' with MWs between 15 and 400 kD (with increasing size in approximately 15-kD increments). The proteins are glycosylated and treatment with trypsin results in a loss of the ladder except for the smallest subunit [68]. cDNAs from *Dirofilaria immitis*, the filaria causing feline heartworm disease, encode proteins with characteristics similar to gp15/400. The *D. immitis* precursor proteins were composed of tandemly repeated units of approximately 15 kD with tetrabasic amino acid sequences presumed to be the processing sites of the precursor polypeptide by trypsin-like proteases [69, 70]. The deduced amino acid sequences showed significant similarity to the partial amino acid sequence reported for the ABA-1 allergen. Molecular cloning of cDNAs encoding the gp15/400 protein complex from *B. malayi, B. pahangi* and *W. bancrofti* revealed an identical molecular organization [71, 72].

In *Brugia* spp., the endoproteolytic cleavage of gp15/400 is not complete and the processing results in a 'ladder' of descending molecular mass as opposed to the processing of the ABA-1 allergen. The repeat unit of gp15/400 also showed a significant 45% identity to the ABA-1 unit. It became evident that ABA-1 and the filarial polyproteins belong to the same family of proteins [52]. gp15/400 from *B. malayi* binds fatty acid and retinoid binding proteins with high affinity. Whether binding of such ligands to native ABA-1 or other NPAs alters their antigenicity/allergenicity is not yet known [73].

The NPA homolog from the bovine lung worm *D. viviparus* (DvA-1) is the only member of this family of proteins for which a full-length cDNA is available. Its deduced amino acid sequence revealed unique characteristics such as a hydrophobic N-terminal leader sequence, extensive diversity in the 12 units, diversity and the lack of consensus cleavage sites and the existence of a small unit. Due to the strong phylogenetic conservation of the NPAs in nematodes, some of the noted structural characteristics may apply to the rest of the NPAs. Analysis of immune responses against Dva-1 in the bovine host should give more insights into its allergenicity during natural infection [74].

Studies in different mouse strains have shown that the gp15/400-specific antibody responses are controlled by factors both within and outside the MHC complex, as only one mouse strain (BALB/c) with d alleles in the A region of the H-2 gene produced an IgG antibody response [75]. Furthermore, analysis of the fine specificity of the genetically determined B and T cell responses to both native and recombinant gp15/400 demonstrated that the restriction in immune responses was only directed to the native molecule, and that in analogy to the responses induced by ABA-1, this restriction can be circumvented when mice are immunized with recombinant gp15/400. In BALB/c mice, contrasting poor antibody recognition of linear gp15/400 fragments were detected when compared to the whole native gp15/400 molecule, suggesting that conformational determinants on gp15/400 induce stronger immune responses.

Comparison of T cell responses against either synthetic peptides, native or recombinant gp15/400 indicated that T cell responses were influenced by post-translational modifications or structural constraints absent in the recombinant gp15/400. These results highlight the importance of studying and comparing the immune responses to native and recombinant antigen/allergens in the context of infection and immunization [76].

The presence of gp15/400-specific IgE antibodies was demonstrated in patients with different clinical manifestation of lymphatic filariasis due to infection with *B. malayi*. Patients with elephantiasis had elevated titers of specific IgE (mean 3.2 ng specific IgE ml^{-1}) when compared to microfilaremics (mean 0.045 ng specific IgE ml^{-1}) or asymptomatic microfilaremics (mean 1.2 ng specific IgE ml^{-1}) [72]. The elevated levels of filarial-specific IgE antibodies in asymptomatic microfilaremic and in patients with elephantiasis suggest an involvement of such antibodies in protection but also a potential in immune-mediated pathology.

Proteases Preferentially Inducing IgE Immune Responses

Helminthic parasites have different pathways of invasion and migration through the skin or intestinal lumen of their mammalian hosts. Penetration and migration are mediated by proteases secreted by the parasite that digest the different structures of the skin, including connective tissue, basement membranes and extracellular matrix [77, 78]. Besides their known functional biological activities of catalyzing the hydrolysis of peptide bonds, proteolytic enzymes have been implicated in the modulation of immune responses towards a Th2 phenotype [20].

In schistosomiasis, serine proteases present in schistosomula-released products were shown early to potentiate IgE synthesis in rat and human cells. Inhibition of serine protease activity in the Schistosomula-released products totally blocked the IgE-potentiating effect, relating the protease activity to the in vitro synthesis of IgE antibodies. The potentiating effect on immunoglobulin synthesis was exclusively related to the IgE isotype as production of IgG or IgM was unaffected. Labeling of schistosomula-released products from *S. mansoni* with [^{3}H]di-isopropyl phosphofluoridate, a general inhibitor of serine proteases, revealed two enzymes with an MW of 27.5 and 29 kD. The same binding pattern was observed when schistosomulum and cercarial surfaces or homogenates were analyzed, confirming previous results that newly transformed cercariae and schistosomula had similar enzymatic activities. The specificity of the enzymes was studied using different substrates suggesting a similarity with trypsin. In addition, serine proteases upregulated the expression of FcɛRII expression on rat cells in vitro. These studies were the first to identify and describe the potentiating effect of parasite-derived proteases on IgE antibody production and FcɛRII expression [79, 80].

A cysteine protease present in adult *S. mansoni* worms with an MW of 32 kD (Smw32) was shown to induce anti-SMw32 IgE antibodies in mice after experimental infection [81]. Likewise, a cysteine protease found in adults and excretory/secretory products from *N. brasiliensis* has been shown to preferentially induce high levels of IgE and IgG1 antibodies in infected rats. The purified proteolytic enzyme has an MW of 16 kD and a pI of 8.5 showing a maximum reactivity at pH 5.5 [82]. A significant number of related proteases have been identified in other parasites including hookworm, *Anisakis, Ascaris, Toxocara, Onchocerca,* and *Brugia* but their potential to induce Th2 responses including induction of IgE/IgG4 (IgG1) antibodies during natural infection in humans or in murine models has not yet been determined. Interestingly, sequence analysis of cDNAs encoding aeroallergens revealed that several of the most potent allergens are proteolytic enzymes: Der p I and Der f I the major allergens of the house dust mites *Dermatophagoides pteronyssinus* and *Dermatophagoides farinae* are cysteine proteases; a recently characterized allergen from *D. farinae,* Der f 3, was identified as a serine protease [83, 84]. Furthermore, exposure to papain, a cysteine protease, is associated with IgE-mediated allergic responses, injection in the footpad of mice with papain induce early production of IL-4 and IgE and IgG1 antibodies [20, 51].

Helminth Protease Inhibitor Homologs Preferentially Induce IgE/IgG4 Antibodies

Infection with filarial parasites characteristically induce high levels of parasite-specific IgE and IgG4 antibodies. Crude filarial antigen has been shown to induce IgE and IgG4 but there is no information about the nature of the antigen inducing such responses. Interestingly, a recent study of 24 recombinant filarial proteins identified two antigens that preferentially induced polyclonal and specific-IgE/IgG4 antibodies as well as secretion of IL-4, IL-5 and IL-10 as opposed to IFN-γ [85]. Both *O. volvulus* antigens were protease inhibitors: OV27 analogue to OV7/cystatin, a cysteine protease inhibitor and OVD5B (analogue to OV33, an aspartyl protease inhibitor) [86, 87].

In this context, it is interesting to note that major grass and plant pollen allergens such as Lol p 11, Ole 1 were recently classified as members of a family of soybean trypsin inhibitor-related proteins although they lack the active site of the inhibitor [88]. A cystatin homolog from the pollen of *Ambrosia artemifolia* (short ragweed), one of the most important aeroallergens in North America, has been recently demonstrated to be an allergen [89].

Serpins is the collective name given to a family of related serine protease inhibitors that function as the natural inactivators of proteases released by phagocytic cells, especially neutrophils. The prototype serpins are the elastase inhibitor α1-antitrypsin and α1-anti-chymotrypsin. One of the few *Schistosoma haematobium* antigens that have been characterized biochemically and immunologically and shown to induce species-specific IgE antibodies is the serine protease inhibitor serpin (SH serpin) [90].

A cDNA encoding *S. haematobium* serpin was characterized, the derived protein has an MW of 46.26 kD. Native *S. haematobium* serpin is found primarily on the surface of schistosomes and is synthesized by adult worms showing an MW of 54–58 kD. The predicted amino acid sequence shows highest homology with inhibitors of thrombin (antithrombin III); the amino acids present in the reactive center suggest activity against chymotrypsin, elastase or cathepsin G-like proteases. Schistosome serpin might therefore prevent clot formation around the parasite, protecting it from neutrophil-induced damage during inflammation. The sequence similarity to human serpins is not very high (22%) but disperse sequence homology concerning short structural blocks is a characteristic of the serpin family. The functional activity of these serpin homologs remains to be determined [91]. A closely related serine protease inhibitor with an MW of 56 kD was identified in *S. mansoni* adult worms (Smpi56) [92].

Native *S. haematobium* serpin is a concanavalin A-binding glycoprotein; the deduced SH serpin amino acid sequence has 7 potential glycosylation sites. Many structural regions responsible for activity in other serpins are present, including the conserved serpin motif Glu-X-Gly-X-Glu in the A4 strand (amino acids 353–357) and conserved Gly residues at interstrand hinges important for secondary structure common to all serpins (positions 172, 317, 355) [90].

Quantitative analysis of the recombinant serine protease inhibitor (rSH serpin) defined it as a prominent target of IgG4 and IgE antibody responses in patients infected with *S. haematobium*. Serpin-specific IgE antibodies showed a striking species-specificity (95%) and sensitivity (100%) when compared to soluble adult worm extract or soluble egg antigen. The presence of specific IgE and IgG4 antibodies to recombinant SH serpin in *S. haematobium*-infected patients defined it as a major allergen. An important finding of this study was that while levels of soluble adult worm extract-specific IgE and IgG4 antibodies in the same patients were correlated, serpin-specific IgE and IgG4 were not. Following chemotherapy, serpin-specific IgE antibody levels rose 50- to 100-fold, while IgG4 antibody production dropped. Furthermore, in vitro analysis of rSH serpin induced antibody production indicated that IgE and IgG4 antibody responses were not coordinately regulated [93].

The increase of IgG4 antibodies that parallels that of IgE in chronic helminthic infections like schistosomiasis has been proposed to be a key element in the regulation of the hypersensitivity responses by blocking the access of allergens to IgE-specific coated mast cells. The balance of both isotypes is probably important for the clinical outcome of infection [94, 95]. The dual recognition of parasite proteins by IgE and IgG4 antibodies as determined by Western blot analysis using total parasite protein extracts suggested a parallel regulation of both immunoglobulin isotypes. However, analysis using recombinant serpin suggests that the mechanisms for generating IgE and IgG4 in response to certain antigens may be different. The formation of complexes of parasite-derived protease inhibitors and proteases from the host may interfere with antigen processing and/or antigen presentation, but how this effect translates into signals skewing towards Th2 responses remains unknown.

Structural Proteins of Helminths as Targets of IgE Antibody Responses

Structural proteins of helminthic parasites like paramyosin, a major myofibrillar protein of invertebrate muscles, have been reported to be targets of IgE immune responses. They have been proposed as potential vaccine candidates from studies in murine schistosomiasis [96]. Surprisingly, *S. mansoni* paramyosin (Sm97) was immunolocalized in the tegument in the form of membrane-bound elongated bodies and it has been proposed that this localization facilitates and induces protective immune responses. In mice infected with *S. japonicum*, the target molecule recognized by a protective IgE antibody was identified as paramyosin (Sj97). The Sj97 deduced amino acid sequence was 96% identical with *S. mansoni* paramyosin. Ultrastructural localization in *S. japonicum* indicated its presence in the tegument, muscles and in the postacetabular glands of certain larvae, suggesting that paramyosin may be an excretory protein that is incorporated into the tegument [97]. A role for Sj97 in the induction of pulmonary responses during experimental infection was proposed, but has not been elucidated yet.

Paramyosins from the filarial parasites *D. immitis* and *O. volvulus* are 99% identical [98] and isotypic and epitope analysis of *D. immitis* paramyosin in patients with onchocerciasis from Ghana and Guatemala demonstrated antiparamyosin IgE antibodies that were inversely correlated to their microfilarial load [99]. Similarly, major allergens involved in allergy to shrimps and other crustaceans as well as aeroallergens from the house dust mite *D. farinae* were identified as tropomyosins [100]. In contrast, tropomyosins from mammalian species do not react.

Filarial Allergens: Involvement in the Immunopathogenesis of Tropical Pulmonary Eosinophilia Syndrome

The tropical pulmonary eosinophilia syndrome (TPE) results from infection with the lymphatic filarial parasites *W. bancrofti* or *B. malayi*. Extensive studies have shown that this disease is induced by hypersensitivity reactions to microfilariae. TPE occurs in many filarial endemic areas including India, South-East Asia and Brazil. The clinical picture of acute TPE is typified by persistent pulmonary symptoms that may include cough, dyspnea accompanied by attacks of paroxysmal nocturnal asthma and systemic signs such as malaise, fever and weight loss [101, 102]. Characteristically, TPE is accompanied by striking increases of total IgE and marked increases of parasite-specific antibodies (IgE and IgG) together with high-grade peripheral and lung eosinophilia ($>3,000/$ mm^3). Microfilariae are absent in the blood, with clearance taking place mainly in the lungs [103, 104]. The accumulation and activation of eosinophils in the lungs is thought to play a central role in the pathology of TPE [105, 106]. Previous studies demonstrated a striking increase in total and filarial specific IgE in the bronchoalveolar lavage fluid (BAL) of patients with TPE along with high levels of parasite-specific IgG. Importantly, antifilarial IgE and IgG antibodies localized in the lower respiratory tract lining fluid analyzed by Western blotting recognized only a subset of the filarial antigens detected by serum antibodies [107].

Understanding the pathogenesis of the tropical pulmonary eosinophilia syndrome requires the identification of the target filarial antigens inducing humoral and cellular immune responses. Using biochemical and immunological approaches, we identified and characterized Bm2325, a major IgE-inducing filarial antigen of the lymphatic filaria *B. malayi* in patients with TPE. The Bm2325 allergen has an estimated MW of 23–25 kD, is glycosylated, and is expressed in the microfilariae, both in adult male and female worms. Enzymatic deglycosylation of Bm2325 and subsequent Western blot analysis revealed that Bm2325 retained its allergenicity. The Bm2325 filarial allergen is only a minor component of the parasite but it is a major target of immune responses in the lungs of patients with TPE. Bm2325 not only has an striking IgE-binding capacity, but also stimulated IgE production in vitro by peripheral blood mononuclear cells obtained both from patients with TPE and those with lymphatic filariasis. A further important finding was the presence of Bm2325-specific IgE in the lungs of patients with TPE [108].

Using a targeted screening with affinity-purified IgE antibodies to Bm2325 from patients with clinical manifestations of TPE, we identified a corresponding cDNA from a *B. malayi* λgt11 cDNA expression library prepared from mRNA of male *B. malayi*. The full coding sequence of the filarial gene encoding Bm2325 was elucidated. The clone was shown to be 1,939 bp long and included a 85-bp-long 5′ untranslated leader and a single long open reading frame of 1,773 bp encoding a protein of 590 amino acids and an 81-bp 3′ untranslated region without the polyadenylation site or the poly-A tail. The estimated size of the Bm2325 transcript (2.4 kb), as judged by Northern blot, is consistent with this 1.94 kb cDNA representing most of the mRNA. The deduced protein has a calculated MW of 65.44 kD, an isoelectric point (pI) of 6.32 and contains 7 potential sites for N-glycosylation [109]. The deduced MW of the filarial polypeptide encoding Bm2325 was much larger than expected.

The Filarial Allergen Bm2325, a Homolog of γ-Glutamyl Transpeptidase

A homology search in database banks revealed that the cloned gene encodes a protein that is homologous to the membrane-bound enzyme γ-glutamyl transpeptidase (γ-GT, EC2.3.2.2). The reaction catalyzed by γ-GT is of major importance in the γ-glutamyl cycle, a metabolic pathway that accounts for the enzymatic synthesis and degradation of glutathione [110, 111]. γ-GT is a heterodimeric enzyme composed of two polypeptide chains of unequal sizes, the heavy and the light chain subunits. The two subunits originate from a common, single-chain precursor that is cotranslationally inserted in the membrane and glycosylated [112]. The identity of the parasite protein with the human γ-GT is 35% and 43% for the heavy and the light chain, respectively [109, 113]. When conservative amino acid substitutions were taken into account, the similarity to the human heavy and light subunits increased to 57 and 66%, respectively. The homology of the *B. malayi* protein to other γ-GTs from vertebrates is in the same range of similarity as the homology to the human γ-GT (rat 35 and 43%, pig 36 and 42% for the heavy and light chains, respectively) [114, 115]. As expected, there was less homology to the bacterial γ-GT gene from *Escherichia coli* [116] (30 and 37%, respectively). A multiple-sequence alignment of the filarial sequence and some of the known γ-GT amino acid sequences is shown in figure 1.

Interestingly, the best conserved region along the sequences is around the *B. malayi* Asp-438 and Asp-439 corresponding to Asp-422 and Asp-423 in the human sequence. Site-directed mutagenesis of both Asp residues indicated that they play a crucial role in the active center of the enzyme [117]. In addition to the extensive similarity between the filarial and the γ-GT sequences, we found the signature pattern motif common to all described γ-GTs, i.e. TSHVSVLDSMGN-GVSSTSTVNRWFG, at the N-terminus of the mature *B. malayi* light chain. This region matches the known consensus sequence perfectly [109, 116]. Furthermore, γ-GT enzymatic activity in *B. malayi* protein extracts was not only blocked by specific inhibitors of the enzyme, but could be completely abrogated by mouse antibodies against the full precursor of the filarial γ-GT homolog [unpubl. results].

To analyze the structural and immunological characteristics of the *B. malayi* γ-GT homolog, we overexpressed and isolated the full precursor polypeptide and the light-chain homologs. Western blot analysis of *B. malayi* adult protein extracts using mouse antibodies raised against the purified recombinant precursor polypeptide identified both the light-chain (Bm2325) and the heavy-chain subunit of the filarial γ-GT [109]. This result confirmed that the parasite's γ-GT homolog is a heterodimeric protein arising from a single polypeptide precursor. The *B. malayi* deduced amino acid sequence shares structural features with other γ-GTs such as similar hydrophobicity profiles, and the large number of potential glycosylation sites along the parasite sequence indicates that the filarial γ-GT, like the mammalian enzymes, are highly glycosylated proteins [113–115, 118]. This last result agrees with our previous findings that glycosylation of the light chain (Bm2325) may explain the heterogeneity in MW and the multiple isoforms observed in two-dimensional gel immunoblot analysis.

The recombinant full precursor (P) and the light-chain homologs from the filarial protein were subjected to Western blot analysis using sera from patients with clinical manifestation of TPE. Both recombinant proteins were shown to bind significantly specific IgE antibodies (lanes) to varying extents as seen in figure 2. Therefore IgE-binding determinants provided by linear and/or conformational epitopes are localized in both the recombinant precursor and the light chain subunit of the *B. malayi* γ-GT. We are currently analyzing quantitatively the IgE/IgG4 antibody isotypes induced by the filarial allergen in patients with TPE, as well as the more important question concerning the nature of the T cell immune responses activated by the parasite γ-GT.

As a first-priority confirmation that the *B. malayi* γ-GT was shed by *W. bancrofti*, the major lymphatic filarial parasite inducing TPE was sought. Protein

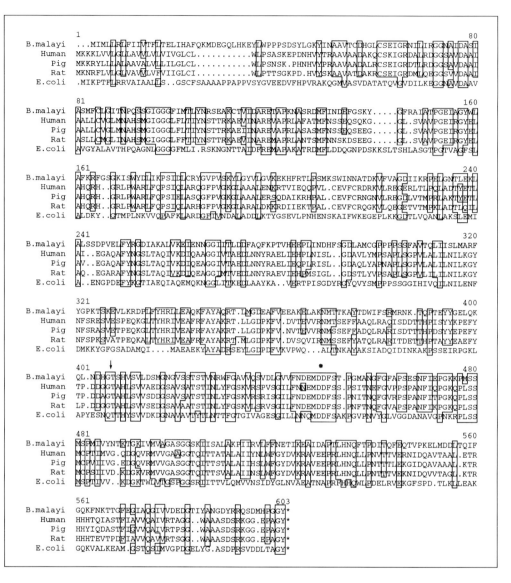

Fig. 1. Multiple alignment of the *B. malayi* γ-GT homolog and γ-GT sequences from human, pig, rat, and *E. coli*. Boxes indicate identical residues; at least 3 residues have to be identical to be included. The arrow indicates the site of the cleavage site by signal peptidase I involved in the processing of the heavy and light chain subunits. The asterisk marks the position of the two crucial Asp residues located at the putative active site of the enzyme.

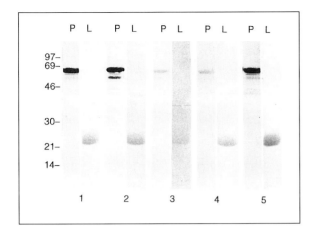

Fig. 2. SDS-PAGE and Western blot analysis of the IgE-binding capacity of the recombinant filarial γ-GT homolog. Immunoblot analysis of purified precursor polypeptide (P) or the mature light-chain (L) homologs (1 μg each), showing the binding of human IgE antibodies from 5 patients with clinical symptoms of TPE [108]. Molecular size standards are indicated on the left.

extracts of *B. malayi* and *W. bancrofti* (a kind gift from Dr. Gerusa Dreyer) were analyzed by Western blot using mouse anti-*B. malayi* γ-GT antibody. As shown in figure 3A, the presence of the γ-GT in *W. bancrofti* was revealed by the cross-reacting antibodies (lane 2). Interestingly, the heavy chain of the *W. bancrofti* enzyme appeared to have a slightly smaller MW. The comparative analysis of *B. pahangi* and *W. bancrofti* homologs is in progress and will reveal whether the basis for the observed differences lies at the molecular level or whether they might be due to differences in post-translational modifications as in other eukaryotic enzymes. Importantly, the allergenicity of the *W. bancrofti* homolog was confirmed using affinity-purified IgE antibodies against the *B. malayi* γ-GT from patients with clinical manifestations of pulmonary eosinophilia. As shown in figure 3B, lane 2, a comparatively strong IgE-binding to the light chain of *W. bancrofti* similar to that observed against *B. malayi* was revealed demonstrating the allergenic potential of *W. bancrofti* γ-GT in patients with TPE.

Induction of Autoimmunity by the Filarial γ-Glutamyl Transpeptidase

The importance of the enzyme γ-GT lies in its key role in the breakdown and synthesis of intracellular and extracellular glutathione (GSH), the metabolism of powerful mediators of physiological function (leukotrienes, hepoxilins and pros-

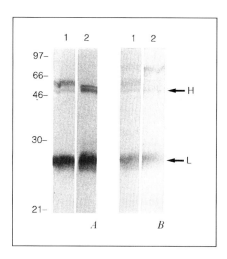

Fig. 3. Detection of the *B. malayi* and *W. bancrofti* γ-GT homologs and analysis of their allergenicity. *B. malayi* (lane 1) or *W. bancrofti* (lane 2) adult protein extracts (15 μg) separated by denaturing SDS-PAGE were transferred to nitrocellulose. *A* Incubation with mouse anti-*B. malayi* γ-GT antibody. *B* Incubation with human IgE antibodies, prepared by affinity purification of serum from patients with clinical manifestations of TPE against the recombinant *B. malayi* γ-GT. The arrows show the positions of the light (L) and the heavy chain subunits (H).

taglandins), cellular detoxification of xenobiotics and carcinogens and cellular processes depending on the oxidation/reduction of glutathione [119]. The enzyme γ-GT is an apical membrane protein of many epithelial cells and in the lungs γ-GT has been found in the airways epithelium from the trachea to the bronchioles, on the apical surface of alveolar epithelium type I and type II cells and of ciliated bronchial cells of rats [120–122].

The extensive homologies found both at the structural and amino acid levels between the filarial γ-GT homolog and the human enzyme, and the fact that γ-GTs are important membrane-bound enzymes of lung epithelial cells prompted us to analyze the existence of immunological cross-reactivity between them. First, mouse antifilarial γ-GTs antibody recognizes the human γ-GT present in bronchial epithelial cells. More importantly, IgG antibodies present in the serum of patients with clinical manifestations of pulmonary eosinophilia but not in the serum of normal human controls recognized the γ-GT present in bronchial epithelial cells from human lungs [109]. Thus, autoimmunity induced by molecular mimicry between the parasite and the host's enzyme likely contributes to the pathogenesis of the TPE syndrome.

Discussion

Studies on the induction and regulation of IgE immune responses induced by helminth parasites have greatly contributed to our understanding of the basic common mechanisms that mediate hypersensitivity responses. The analysis of the parasite targets of IgE antibody responses have defined some biological characteristics thought to be involved in the induction of IgE antibody responses. However, the basic mechanisms of the IgE antibody induction remain to be discovered.

The IgE-binding capacity of the helminth NPA family and structural proteins such as paramyosin have been documented only in the context of infection. When these proteins are isolated and used for adjuvant-assisted immunization they do not elicit IgE antibody responses. The implications of this finding is that such molecules do not have any intrinsic allergenic properties, but rather that in the context of the preferential Th2 responses during nematode infection they become the target of IgE responses. They could as such play a role in IgE-mediated pathology. In contrast, parasite allergens with biological activities such as proteases and inhibitors of protease activity are able to preferentially induce IgE/IgG4(IgG1) immune responses in human and animal models. We identified a potent IgE-inducing antigen from filarial nematodes as the homolog of the crucial enzyme γ-GT.

Previous studies have shown γ-GT to play an important role in the antioxidant defense mechanisms of several pulmonary cells types [123–125]. Cells adapt to oxidative stress by enhancing their capacity to utilize extracellular GSH through upregulation of γ-GT expression and γ-GT activity [126]. Immune reactions against the parasite γ-GT may contribute to the pathogenesis of TPE by autoimmune-mediated damage of the host epithelial cells. Furthermore, inhibition of the human γ-GT may subvert the capacity of the host to deal with oxidative stress directly, which enhances inflammation, because oxidants and other mediators accumulate in the pulmonary tissue. In addition to the known important metabolic functions of γ-GT, we reported for the first time the presence of autoantibodies to human γ-GT in the serum of patients infected by *W. bancrofti* with clinical symptoms of pulmonary eosinophilia. Immune responses against cell surface proteases might also be important, because there are indications of protease involvement in signal transduction. Knowledge of the structure and biological function of parasite antigen targets of specific IgE immune responses in conjunction with studies of the fine specificity of the immune responses and their restriction by the MHC will contribute to further understanding of the immune pathogenesis. This knowledge might lead to the prevention of pathological manifestations and help in the development of immunological control strategies against helminths.

Acknowledgements

This work was supported by a grant from the Swiss National Science Foundation (NF 31-42495.94). I would like to thank Dr. Thomas Bürgin from the Department of Cell Biology of the Biozentrum, University of Basel, Switzerland, for his helpful discussions on the manuscript.

References

1   Ogilvie BM: Reagin-like antibodies in animals immune to helminth parasites. Nature 1964;204: 91–92.
2   Ogilvie BM, Smithers SR, Terry, RJ: Reagin-like antibodies in experimental infection of *Schistosoma mansoni* and the passive transfer of resistance. Nature 1966;209:1221.
3   Askenase PW: Immune inflammatory response to parasites: The role of basophils, mast cells and vasoactive amines. Am J Trop Med Hyg 1977;26:96–107.
4   Capron A, Dessaint J-P: A role for IgE in protective immunity. IRCS J Med Sci 1975;3:477–481.
5   Jarrett EEE, Miller HRP: Production and activities of IgE in helminth infection. Progr Allerg. Basel, Karger, 1982, vol 31, pp 178–233.
6   Sutton BJ, Gould HJ: The human IgE network. Nature 1993;366:421–428.
7   Jarrett EEE, Ferguson A: Effect of T cell depletion on the potentiated reagin response. Nature 1974; 250:420–422.
8   Mosman TR, Cherwinski H, Bond MW, Giedlin MA, Coffman RL: Two types of murine helper T cell clone I. Definition according to profiles of lymphokine activities and secreted proteins. J Immunol 1986;136:2348–2357.
9   Mosmann TR, Coffman RL: TH1 and TH2 cells different patterns of lymphokine secretion lead to different functional properties. Annu Rev Immunol 1989;7:145–173.
10 Romagnani S: Regulation of the development of type 2 T-helper cells in allergy. Curr Opin Immunol 1994;6:838–846.
11 Romagnani S: Atopic allergy and other hypersensitivities. Curr Opin Immunol 1995;7:745–750.
12 Reiner SL, Seder RA: T helper cell differentiation in immune response. Curr Opin Immunol 1995; 7:360–366.
13 Mosman TR, Sad S: The expanding universe of T-cell subsets: Th1, Th2 and more. Immunol Today 1996;17:138–146.
14 Vercelli D: Immunoglobulin E regulation in humans, 1989–1994. Allergy 1995;50(suppl 25):5–8.
15 Finkelman FD, Katona IM, Urban JFJ, Holmes J, Ohara J, Tung AS, Sample JG, Paul WE: Interleukin 4 is required to generate and sustain in vivo IgE responses. J Immunol 1988;141:2335–2341.
16 Jankovic D, Sher A: Initiation and regulation of CD4+ T cell function in host-parasite models; in Romagnani S (ed): Th1 and Th2 Cells in Health and Disease. Chem Immunol. Basel, Karger, 1996, vol. 63, pp 51–62.
17 Manetti R, Gerosa F, Guidici MG, Biagiotti R, Parronchi P, Piccini MP, Sampognaro S, Maggi E, Romagnani S, Trinchieri G: Interleukin-12 induces stable priming for interferon-γ (IFN-γ) production during differentiation of human T helper (Th) cells and transient IFN-γ production in established Th2 clones. J Exp Med 1994;179:1273–1283.
18 Finkelman F, Pearce EJ, Urban JP, Sher A: Regulation and biological function of helminth-induced cytokine responses. Immunol Today 1991;12:A62–A66.
19 Sher A, Coffman RL: Regulation of immunity to parasites by T cells and T cell-derived cytokines. Annu Rev Immunol 1992;10:385–409.
20 Urban JF, Madden KB, Svetic A, Cheever A, Trotta PP, Gause WC, Katona IM, Finkelman FD: The importance of Th2 cytokines in protective immunity to nematodes. Immunol Rev 1992;127: 205–220.

21 Nutman TB: T-cell regulation of immediate hypersensitivity: Lessons from helminth parasites and allergic diseases; in Moqbel R (ed): Allergy and Immunity to Helminths. Common Mechanisms or Divergent Pathways? London, Taylor & Francis, 1992, pp 187–204.

22 Kopf M, Le Gros G, Bachmann M, Lamers MC, Bluthmann H, Kohler G: Disruption of the murine IL-4 gene blocks Th2 cytokine responses. Nature 1993;362:245–248.

23 Ferrick DA, Schrenzel MD, Mulvania T, Hsieh B, Ferlin WG, Lepper H: Differential production of interferon-γ and interleukin-4 in response to Th1- and Th2-stimulating pathogens by γδT cells in vivo. Nature 1995;373:255–257.

24 Garside P, Mowat A McI: Polarization of Th-cell responses. A phylogenetic consequence of non-specific immune defence. Immunol Today 1995;16:220–223.

25 Pearce EJ, Reiner SL: Induction of Th2 responses in infectious diseases. Curr Biol 1995;7:497–504.

26 Daser A, Meissner N, Herz U, Renz H: Role and modulation of T-cell cytokines in allergy. Curr Biol 1995;7:762–770.

27 Capron A, Dessaint JP, Capron M, Ouma JH, Butterworth AE: Immunity to schistosomes: Progress toward vaccine. Science 1987;238:1065–1972.

28 Ahmad A, Wang CH, Bell RG: A role for IgE in intestinal immunity. Expression of rapid expulsion of *Trichinella spiralis* in rats transfused with IgE and thoracic duct lymphocytes. J Immunol 1991; 146:3563–3570.

29 Gusmao R d'A, Stanley AM, Ottesen EA: *Brugia pahangi* immunologic evaluation of the different susceptibility to filarial infection in inbred Lewis rats. Exp Parasitol 1981;52:147–154.

30 Baldwin CI, De Medeiros F, Denham DA: IgE responses in cats infected with *Brugia pahangi*. Parasite Immunol 1993;15:291–296.

31 Kazura JW, Davis RS: Soluble *Brugia malayi* microfilarial antigens protect mice against challenge by an antibody-dependent mechanism. J Immunol 1982;128:1792–1796.

32 Maizels RM, Sartono E, Kurniawan A, Partono F, Selkirk ME, Yazdanbakhsh M: T-cell activation and the balance of antibody isotypes in human lymphatic filariasis. Parasitol Today 1995;11:50–56.

33 Grenfell BT, Michael E, Denham DA: A model for the dynamics of human lymphatic filariasis. Parasitol Today 1991;7:318–323.

34 Sher A, Coffman RL, Hieny S, Cheever AW: Ablation of eosinophils and IgE responses with anti-IL-5 or anti-IL-4 antibodies fails to affect immunity against *Schistosoma mansoni* in the mouse. J Immunol 1990;145:3911–3916.

35 Urban JF, Katona IM, Paul WE, Finkelman FD: IL-4 is important in protective immunity to a gastrointestinal nematode infection in mice. Proc Natl Acad Sci USA 1991;88:5513–5517.

36 Finkelman FD, Gause WC, Urban JF: Cytokine control of protective immunity against nematode infections; in Boothroyd JC, Komuniecki R (eds): Molecular Approaches to Parasitology. New York, Wiley-Liss, 1995, pp 467–476.

37 Lawrence RA, Allen JE, Gregory WF, Kopf M, Maizels RM: Infection of IL-4 deficient mice with the parasitic nematode *Brugia malayi* demonstrates that host resistance is not dependent on a T helper 2-dominated immune response. J Immunol 1995;154:5995–6001.

38 Bancroft AJ, Grencis RK, Else KJ, Devaney E: The role of CD4 cells in protective immunity to *Brugia pahangi*. Parasite Immunol 1994;16:385–387.

39 Hagan P, Blumenthal UJ, Dunne D, Simpson AJG, Wilkins HA: Human IgE, IgG4, and resistance to reinfection with *Schistosoma haematobium*. Nature 1991;349:243–245.

40 Rihet P, Demeure C, Bourgois A, Prata A, Dessein AJ: Evidence for an association between human resistance to Schistsoma mansoni and high anti-larval IgE levels. Eur J Immunol 1991;21:2679–2686.

41 Dunne DW, Butterworth AE, Fulford AJC, Kariuki HC, Langley JG, Ouma JH, Capron A, Pierce RJ, Sturrock RF: Immunity after treatment of human schistosomiasis: Association between IgE antibodies to adult worm antigens and resistance to reinfection. Eur J Immunol 1992;22:1483–1494.

42 Demeure CE, Rihet P, Abel L, Ouattara M, Bourgois A, Dessein AJ: Resistance to *Schistosoma mansoni* in humans: Influence of the IgE/IgG4 balance and IgG2 in immunity to reinfection after chemotherapy. J Infect Dis 1993;168:1000–1008.

43 Hagel I, Lynch NR, DiPrisco MC, Rojas E, Pérez M, Alvarez N: *Ascaris* reinfection of slum children. Relation with the IgE response. Clin Exp Immunol 1993;94:80–83.

44 Pritchard DI, Quinnell RJ, Walsh EA: Immunity in humans to *Necator americanus:* IgE, parasite weight and fecundity. Parasite Immunol 1995;17:71–75.

45 Hussain R, Poindexter RW, Ottesen EA: Control of allergic reactivity in human filariasis: Predominant localization of blocking antibody to the IgG4 subclass. J Immunol 1992;148:2731–2737.

46 Kurniawan A, Yazdanbakhsh M, Vanree R, Aalberse R, Selkirk ME, Partono F, Maizels RM: Differential expression of IgE and IgG4 specific antibody responses in asymptomatic and chronic human filariasis. J Immunol 1993;150:3941–3950.

47 Pritchard DI: Parasites and allergic disease: A review of the field and experimental evidence for a 'cause-and-effect' relationship; in Moqbel R (ed): Allergy and Immunity to Helminths. Common Mechanisms or Divergent Pathways. London, Taylor & Francis, 1992, pp 38–50.

48 Lynch NR: Influence of socio-economic level on helminthic infection and allergic reactivity in tropical countries; in Moqbel R (ed): Allergy and Immunity to Helminths. Common Mechanisms or Divergent Pathways. London, Taylor & Francis, 1992, pp 51–62.

49 Shakib F, Pritchard DI, Walsh EA, Smith SJ, Powell-Richards A, Kumar S, Edmonds P: The detection of autoantibodies to IgE in plasma of individuals infected with hookworm *(Necator americanus)* and the demonstration of a predominant IgG1 anti-IgE autoantibody response. Parasite Immunol 1993;15:47–53.

50 Lind P, Lowenstein H: Characterization of Asthma-Associated Allergens. Baillière's Clinical Immunology and Allergy. London, Baillière-Tindall, 1988, vol 2, pp 67–89.

51 Novey HS, Marchioli LE, Sokol WN, Wells ID: Papain-induced asthma – physiological and immunological features. J Allergy Clin Immunol 1979;63:98–103.

52 McReynolds LA, Kennedy MW, Selkirk ME: The polyprotein allergens of nematodes. Parasitol Today 1993;9:403–406.

53 Kennedy MW, Qureshi F: Stage-specific secreted antigens of the parasitic larval stages of the nematode *Ascaris.* Immunology 1986;58:515–522.

54 Kennedy MW, Qureshi F, Haswell-Elkins M, Elkins DB: Homology and heterology between the secreted antigens of the parasitic larval stages of *Ascaris lumbricoides* and *Ascaris suum.* Clin Exp Immunol 1987;678:20–30.

55 Hussain R, Bradbury SM, Strejan G: Hypersensitivity of *Ascaris* allergens. J Immunol 1973;111:260–268.

56 Ambler J, Miller JN, Johnson P, Orr TSC: Characterisation of an allergen extracted from *Ascaris suum.* Determination of the molecular weight, isoelectric point, amino acid and carbohydrate content of the native allergen. Immunochemistry 1973;10:815–820.

57 Kennedy MW, Tierney J, Ye P, McMonagle FA, McIntosh A, McLaughlin D, Smith JW: The secreted and somatic antigens of the third stage larva of *Anisakis simplex,* and antigenic relationship with *Ascaris suum, Ascaris lumbricoides,* and *Toxocara canis.* Mol Biochem Parasitol 1988;31:35–46.

58 Christie JF, Dunbar B, Kennedy MW: The ABA-1 allergen of the nematode *Ascaris suum:* epitope stability, mass spectrometry, and N-terminal sequence comparison with its homologue in *Toxocara canis.* Clin Exp Immunol 1993;92:125–132.

59 Spence HJ, Moore J, Brass A, Kennedy MW: A cDNA encoding repeating units of the ABA-1 allergen of *Ascaris.* Mol Biochem Parasitol 1993;57:339–344.

60 Kennedy MW, Brass A, McCruden AB, Price NC, Kelly SM, Cooper A: The ABA-1 allergen of the parasitic nematode *Ascaris suum:* Fatty acid and retinoid binding function and structural characterization. Biochemistry 1995;34:6700–6710.

61 Kennedy MW, Gordon AMS, Tomlinson LA, Qureshi F: Genetic (major histocompatibility complex?) control of the antibody repertoire to the secreted antigens of *Ascaris.* Parasite Immunol 1987;9:269–273.

62 Tomlinson LA, Christie JF, Fraser EM, McLaughlin D, McIntosh AE, Kennedy MW: MHC restriction of the antibody repertoire to secretory antigens, and a major allergen, of the nematode parasite *Ascaris.* J Immunol 1989;143:2349–2356.

63   Kennedy MW, Tomlinson LA, Fraser EM, Christie JF: The specificity of the antibody response to internal antigens of *Ascaris:* Heterogeneity in infected humans, and MHC (H-2) control of the repertoire in mice. Clin Exp Immunol 1990;80:219–224.

64   Kennedy MW, Christie J: MHC class II (I-A) region control of the IgE antibody repertoire to the ABA-1 allergen of the nematodes *Ascaris.* Immunology 1991;72:577–579.

65   Christie JF, Fraser EM, Kennedy MW: Comparison between the MHC-restricted antibody repertoire to *Ascaris* antigens in adjuvant-assisted immunization or infection. Parasite Immunol 1992; 14:59–73.

66   Haswell-Elkins MR, Kennedy MW, Maizels RM, Elkins DB, Anderson RM: The antibody recognition profiles of humans naturally infected with *Ascaris lumbricoides.* Parasite Immunol 1989;11: 615–627.

67   Kennedy MW: Genetic control of the antibody responses to parasite allergens; in Moqbel R (ed): Allergy and Immunity to Helminths. Common Mechanisms or Divergent Pathways? London, Taylor & Francis, 1992, pp 63–80.

68   Maizels RM, Gregory WF, Kwan-Lim GE, Selkirk ME: Filarial surface antigens: The major 29 kilodalton glycoprotein and a novel 17–200 kilodalton complex from adult *Brugia malayi* parasites. Mol Biochem Parasitol 1989;32:213–228.

69   Culpepper J, Grieve RB, Friedman L, Mika-Grieve M, Frank GR, Dale B: Molecular characterization of a *Dirofilaria immitis* cDNA encoding a highly immunoreactive antigen. Mol Biochem Parasitol 1992;54:51–62.

70   Poole CB, Grandea AG III, Maina CV, Jenkins RE, Selkirk ME, McReynolds LA: Cloning of a cuticular antigen that contains multiple tandem repeats from the filarial parasite *Dirofilaria immitis.* Proc Natl Acad Sci 1992;89:5986–5990.

71   Tweedie S, Paxton WA, Ingram L, Maizels RM, McReynolds LA, Selkirk ME: *Brugia pahangi* and *Brugia malayi:* A surface-associated glycoprotein (gp 15/400) is composed of multiple tandemly repeated units and processed from a 400-kDa precursor. Exp Parasitol 1993;76:156–164.

72   Paxton WA, Yazdanbakhsh M, Kurniawan A, Partono F, Maizels RM, Selkirk ME: Primary structure and immunoglobulin E response to the repeat subunit of gp15/400 from human lymphatic filarial parasites. Infect Immun 1993;61:2827–2833.

73   Kennedy MW, Allen JE, Wright AS, McCruden AB, Cooper A: The gp15/400 polyprotein antigen of *Brugia malayi* binds fatty acids and retinoids. Mol Biochem Parasitol 1995;71:41–50.

74   Britton C, Moore J, Gilleard J, Kennedy MW: Extensive diversity in repeat unit sequences of the cDNA encoding the polyprotein antigen/allergen from the bovine lungworm *Dictyocaulus viviparus.* Mol Biochem Parasitol 1995;72:77–88.

75   Kwan-Lim G-E, Maizels RM: MHC and non-MHC-restricted recognition of filarial surface antigens in mice transplanted with adult *Brugia malayi* parasites. J Immunol 1990;145:1912–1920.

76   Allen JE, Lawrence RA, Maizels RM: Fine specificity of the genetically controlled immune response to native and recombinant gp15/400 (polyprotein allergen) of *Brugia malayi.* Infect Immun 1995; 63:2892–2898.

77   Dubremetz JF, McKerrow JH: Invasion Mechanisms; in Marr JJ, Müller M (eds): Biochemistry and Molecular Biology of Parasites. New York, Academic Press, 1995, pp 307.

78   McKerrow JH: Parasite Proteases. Exp Parasitol 1989;68:111–115.

79   Damonneville M, Auriault C, Verwaerde C, Delanoye A, Pierce R, Capron A: Protection against experimental *Schistosoma mansoni* schistosomiasis achieved by immunization with schistosomula released products antigens (SRP-A): Role of IgE antibodies. Clin Exp Immunol 1986;65:244–252.

80   Verwaerde C, Auriault C, Neyrinck JL, Capron A: Properties of serine protease of *Schistosoma mansoni* schistosomula involved in the regulation of IgE synthesis. Scand J Immunol 1988;27: 17–24.

81   Chappel CL, Kalter DC, Dresden MH: The hypersensitivity response to the adult worm protease, SMw32, in *Schistosoma mansoni* infected mice. Am J Trop Med Hyg 1988;39:463–468.

82   Kamata I, Yamada M, Uchikawa R, Matsuda S, Arizono N: Cysteine protease of the nematode *Nippostrongylus brasiliensis* preferentially evokes an IgE/IgG1 antibody response in rats. Clin Exp Immunol 1995;102:71–77.

83 Chua KY, Stewart GA, Thomas WR, Simpson RJ, Dilworth RJ, Ploza TM, Turner KJ: Sequence analysis of cDNA coding for a major house dust mite allergen Der p 1. Homology with cysteine protease. J Exp Med 1988;167:175.

84 Nishiyama C, Yasuhara T, Yuuki T, Okumura Y: Cloning and expression in *Escherichia coli* of cDNA encoding house dust mite allergen Der f 3, serine protease from *Dermatophagoides farinae.* FEBS Lett 1995;377:62–66.

85 Garraud O, Nkenfou C, Bradley JE, Perler FB, Nutman TB: Identification of recombinant filarial proteins capable of inducing polyclonal and antigen-specific IgE and IgG4 antibodies. J Immunol 1995;155:1316–1325.

86 Lustigman S, Brotman B, Huima T, Prince AM: Characterization of an *Onchocerca volvulus* cDNA clone encoding a genus specific antigen present in infective larvae and adult worms. Mol Biochem Parasitol 1991;45:65–76.

87 Lucius R, Erodu N, Kern A, Donelson JE: Molecular cloning of an immunodominant antigen of *Onchocerca volvulus.* J Exp Med 1988;168:1199–1204.

88 v Ree R, Hoffman DR, v Dijk W, Brodard V, Mahieu K, Koeleman CAM, Grande M, v Leeuwen WA, Aalberse RC: Lol p XI, a new major grass pollen allergen, is a member of a family of soybean trypsin inhibitor-related proteins. J Allergy Clin Immunol 1995;95:970–978.

89 Rogers BL, Pollock J, Klapper DG, Griffith IJ: Sequence of the proteinase-inhibitor cystatin homologue from the pollen of *Ambrosia artemisiifolia* (short ragweed). Gene 1993;133:219–221.

90 Blanton RE, Licate LS, Aman RA: Characterization of a native and recombinant *Schistosoma haematobium* serine protease inhibitor gene product. Mol Biochem Parasitol 1994;63:1–11.

91 Modha J, Roberts MC, Kusel JR: Schistosomes and Serpins: A complex business. Parasitol Today 1996;12:119–121.

92 Ghendler Y, Arnon R, Fishelson Z: *Schistosoma mansoni:* Isolation and characterization of Smpi56, a novel serine protease inhibitor. Exp Parasitol 1994;78:121–131.

93 Li Z, King CL, Ogundipe JO, Licate LS, Blanton RE: Preferential recognition by human IgE and IgG4 of a species-specific *Schistosoma haematobium* serine protease inhibitor. J Inf Dis 1995;171:416–422.

94 Hussain R, Poindexter RW, Ottesen EA: Control of allergic reactivity in human filariasis: Predominant localization of blocking antibody to the IgG4 subclass. J Immunol 1992;148:2731–2737.

95 Kurniawan A, Yazdanbakhsh M, Vanree R, Aalberse R, Selkirk ME, Partono F, Maizels RM: Differential expression of IgE and IgG4 specific antibody responses in asymptomatic and chronic human filariasis. J Immunol 1993;150:3941–3950.

96 Dunne DW, Hagan P, Abath FG : Prospects for immunological controls of schistosomiasis. Lancet 1995;345:1488–1491.

97 Nara T, Matsumoto N, Janecharut T, Matsuda H, Yamamoto K, Irimura T, Nakamura K, Aikawa M, Oswald I, Sher A, Kita K, Kojima S: Demonstration of the target molecule of a protective IgE antibody in secretory glands of *Schistosoma japonicum* larvac. Int Immunol 1994;6:963–971.

98 Limberger RJ, McReynolds LA:Filarial paramyosin: cDNA sequences from *Dirofilaria immitis* and *Onchocerca volvulus.* Mol Biochem Parasitol 1990;38:271–280.

99 Steel C, Limberger RJ, McReynolds LA, Ottesen EA, Nutman TB: Isotypic analysis and epitope mapping of filarial paramyosin in patients with onchocerciasis. J Immunol 1990;145:3917–3923.

100 Daul CB, Slattery M, Reese G, Lehrer SB: Identification of the major brown shrimp *(Penaeus aztecus)* allergen as the muscle protein tropomyosin. Int Arch Allergy Immunol 1994;105:49–55.

101 Neva FA, EA Ottesen: Tropical (filarial) eosinophilia. N Engl J Med 1978;298:1129–1131.

102 Ottesen EA: Immunological aspects of lymphatic filariasis. Trans R Soc Trop Med Hyg 1984;73(suppl):9–18.

103 Spry CJF, Kumaraswami V: Tropical eosinophilia. Semin Hematol 1982;19:101–115.

104 Ottesen EA, Nutman TB: Tropical pulmonary eosinophilia. Annu Rev Med 1992;43:417–424.

105 Rom WN, Vijayan VK, Cornelius MJ, Kumaraswami V, Phrabakar R, Ottesen EA, Crystal RG: Persistent lower respiratory tract inflammation associated with interstitial lung disease in patients with tropical pulmonary eosinophilia following conventional treatment with diethylcarbamazine. Am Rev Respir Dis 1990;142:1088–1092.

106 Pinkston P, Vijayan VK, Nutman TB, O' Donell KM, Cornelius MJ, Kumaraswami V, Ferrans WJ, Takemura T, Yenokida G, Thiruvengadam KV, Tripathy SP, Ottesen EA, Crystal RG: Tropical pulmonary eosinophilia: Characterization of the lower respiratory tract inflammation and its response to therapy. J Clin Invest 1987;80:216–225.

107 Nutman TB, Vijayan VK, Pinkston P, Kumaraswami V, Steel C, Crystal RG, Ottesen EA: Tropical pulmonary eosinophilia: Analysis of antifilarial antibody localized to the lung. J Infect Dis 1989; 160:1042–1050.

108 Lobos E, Ondo A, Ottesen EA, Nutman TB: Biochemical and immunological characterization of a major IgE-inducing filarial antigen of *Brugia malayi* and implications for the pathogenesis of tropical pulmonary eosinophilia. J Immunol 1992;149:3029–3034.

109 Lobos E, Zahn R, Weiss N, Nutman TB: A major allergen of lymphatic filarial nematodes is a parasite homolog of the γ-glutamyl transpeptidase. Mol Med 1996;2:712–724.

110 Meister A, Tate SS, Ross LL: Membrane bound γ-glutamyl transpeptidase; in Martinosi A (ed): The Enzymes of the Biological Membranes. New York, Plenum, 1976, vol 3, pp 315–347.

111 Meister A: Metabolism and function of glutathione; in Dolphin D, Poulson R, Avramovic O (eds): Glutathione: Chemical, Biochemical and Medical Aspects. New York, Wiley, 1989, pp 367–476.

112 Finidori J, Laperche Y, Haguenauer-Tsapis R, Barouki R, Güellan G, Hanoune J: In vitro biosynthesis and membrane insertion of γ-glutamyl transpeptidase. J Biol Chem 1984;259:4687–4690.

113 Rajperts-De Meyts E, Heisterkamp N, Groffen J: Cloning and nucleotide sequence of human γ-glutamyl transpeptidase. Proc Natl Acad Sci USA 1988;85:8840–8844.

114 Laperche Y, Bulle F, Aissani T, Aissani T, Chobert M-J, Aggerbeck M, Hanoune J, Guellaen: Molecular cloning and nucleotide sequence of rat kidney γ-glutamyl transpeptidase cDNA. Proc Natl Acad Sci USA 1986;83:937–941.

115 Papandrikopoulou A, Frey A, Gassen H: Cloning and expression of γ-glutamyl transpeptidase from isolated porcine brain capilaries. Eur J Biochem 1989;183:693–698.

116 Suzuki H, Kumagai H, Echigo T, Tochikura T: DNA sequence of the *Escherichia coli* K-12 γ-glutamyl transpeptidase gene, ggt. J Bacteriol 1989;171:5169–5172.

117 Ikeda Y, Fujii J, Taniguchi N, Meister A: Human γ-glutamyl transpeptidase mutants involving conserved aspartate residues and the unique cysteine residue of the light subunit. J Biol Chem 1995; 270:12471–12475.

118 Tate SS, Khadse V, Wellner D: Renal γ-glutamyl transpeptidases: Structural and immunological studies. Arch Biochem Biophys 1988;262:397–408

119 Liebermann MW, Barrios R, Carter BZ, Habib GM, Lebowitz RM, Rajagopalan S, Sepulveda AR, Shi Z, Wan D: γ-Glutamyl transpeptidase: What does the organization and expression of a multi-promoter gene tell us about its functions? Am J Pathol 1995;147:1175–1185.

120 Dinsdale D, Green JA, Manson MM, Lee MJ: The structural localization of γ-glutamyl transpeptidase in rat lung: Correlation with the histochemical demonstration of enzyme activity. Histochem J 1992;24:144–152.

121 Yamaya M, Sekizawa K, Yamauchi K, Hoshi H, Sawai T, Sasaki H: Epithelial modulation of leukotriene-C$_4$-induced human tracheal smooth muscle contraction. Am J Respir Crit Care Med 1995; 151:892–894.

122 Ingbar D, Hepler K, Dowin R, Jacobsen E, Dunitz JM, Jamieson JD: γ-Glutamyl transpeptidase is a polarized alveolar epithelial membrane protein. Am J Physiol 1995;269:L261–L271.

123 Forman HJ, Skelton DC: Protection of alveolar macrophages from hyperoxia by gamma-glutamyl transpeptidase. Am J Physiol 1990;259:102–107.

124 Chang M, Shi M, Forman HJ: Exogenous glutathione protects endothelial cells from menadione toxicity. Am J Physiol 1992;6:L637–L643.

125 Shi M, Gozal E, Choy A, Forman HJ: Extracellular glutathione and gamma-glutamyl transpeptidase prevent H$_2$O$_2$-induced injury by 2,3-dimethoxy-1,4-naphthoquinone. Free Radic Biol Med 1993; 15:57–67.

126 Kugelman A, Choy HA, Liu R, Ming Shi M, Gozal E, Forman HJ: γ-Glutamyl transpeptidase is increased by oxidative stress in rat alveolar L2 epithelial cells. Am J Physiol 1995;11:586–592.

Dr. Edgar Lobos, Swiss Tropical Institute, Socinstrasse 57, CH–4002 Basel (Switzerland)

Freedman DO (ed): Immunopathogenetic Aspects of Disease Induced by Helminth Parasites.
Chem Immunol. Basel, Karger, 1997, vol 66, pp 26–40

....

Immunopathology of Onchocerciasis: A Role for Eosinophils in Onchocercal Dermatitis and Keratitis

Eric Pearlman

Division of Geographic Medicine, CWRU School of Medicine,
Cleveland, Ohio, USA

Introduction

Onchocerciasis (river blindness) is a leading cause of infectious blindness and visual impairment world-wide. *Onchocerca volvulus*, the causative organism of river blindness, is a filarial nematode that infects approximately 17.7 million people in Africa, the Eastern Mediterranean and the Americas. A recent report from the World Health Organization [1] estimates that 270,000 people are blinded from onchocerciasis and 500,000 are severely visually impaired. In some villages in hyperendemic areas of Africa, up to 10% of the inhabitants have serious vision impairment as a result of onchocerciasis. Although corneal inflammation (keratitis) accounts for most cases of blindness, the parasites can also induce damage to posterior sections of the eye, including the choroid, retina and optic nerve [2, 3]. Dermatitis caused by infections with this parasite leads to severe pruritus, depigmentation and loss of skin elasticity [1, 4]. Other manifestations of the disease include development of subcutaneous nodules around adult worms and inflammation in the lymphatics (lymphadenitis) leading to severe disfigurement [5].

Most of the pathology of onchocerciasis is caused by the first-stage larvae, termed microfilariae (Mf), as they migrate through the dermal and ocular tissue (fig. 1). Although Mf contain proteolytic enzymes that facilitate their migration and may damage tissue directly, it is likely that most of the tissue damage occurs as a result of the host immune response to parasite antigens which are either secreted or released after parasite death. The life span of adult worms can be up to 16 years, and Mf survive in the skin for about 14 months [1, 6]. In heavily infected

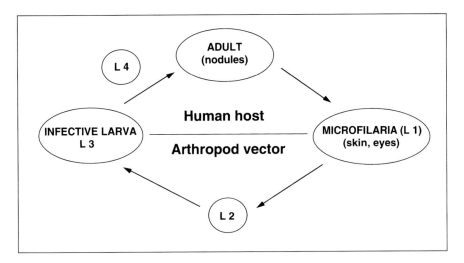

Fig. 1. Life cycle of *O. volvulus.* Infection is initiated when a Simulium blackfly inoculates infective larvae into the skin during a blood meal. The larvae migrate to the subcutaneous tissues, molt twice and develop into mature male and female adults in about 12 months. Adults mate and produce live larvae, termed microfilariae (Mf) which migrate through the skin. The life cycle is completed when Mf are ingested by a blackfly and develop into infectious stage larvae in the salivary glands. Note that it is the Mf that cause onchocercal keratitis and dermatitis.

individuals, it has been estimated that Mf die at a rate of up to 500,000 per day [6], resulting in the host exposure to very high antigen load. A characteristic feature which individuals in endemic areas acquire is parasite-specific anergy, where infected individuals have significantly diminished cellular responses to parasite antigens relative to uninfected persons and consequently modulate the inflammatory response [7–9]. Within a population, there are individuals with observed pathology, which is considered to be a hyperreactive response to parasite antigens, and distinct clinical groups have been defined based on the extent of pathology [9]. In general, the cellular proliferative response and levels of parasite specific IgE and IgG are higher in individuals with more severe pathological manifestations and no Mf in the skin than in persons with high numbers of Mf in the skin and no pathology [9]. (A similar dichotomy in responses has been reported in endemic populations of lymphatic filariasis [10]). A third group of endemic normal, or putatively immune, individuals has also been described [9, 11, 12]. These individuals are resident in endemic areas, but have no detectable Mf and no pathology. A recent review by Ottesen [9] discusses the cellular and humoral responses of these clinical groups in relation to possible mechanisms of immunity.

The current review will focus on the role of eosinophils in dermal and corneal pathology, as these cells are a prominent feature of the immunopathological response to this parasite.

Eosinophils as Cytotoxic Cells

Eosinophils are a hallmark feature of helminth infection. The cytotoxic properties of these cells are derived primarily from the granules which contain several preformed cytotoxic proteins, including eosinophil major basic protein (MBP), eosinophil cationic protein, eosinophil-derived neurotoxin (EDN) and eosinophil peroxidase. MBP is a highly cationic protein which forms the crystalline core of the eosinophil granule. The likely mode of cytotoxicity is through a nonspecific interaction with the anionically charged lipid membrane [13], causing disruption of the cell membrane and lysis. In addition to direct cellular cytotoxicity, MBP induces platelet, mast cell and eosinophil degranulation, thereby exacerbating the inflammatory response [14, 15]. Release of mast cell granule products in the dermis is likely to contribute directly to pruritis. For reviews on eosinophils, see Gleich et al. [16] and Weller [17].

The Role of IL-5 in Eosinophil Production

Several reports indicate an essential role for IL-5 in eosinophil development: (1) IL-5 transgenic mice have significantly elevated serum IL-5 levels and produce 65–265 times more eosinophils than control mice in peripheral blood and in tissues such as the lung and spleen [18]; (2) in vivo depletion of IL-5 inhibits eosinophil production in response to helminth infection [19], and (3) IL-5 gene knockout mice do not develop blood and tissue eosinophilia after helminth infection [20]. Interestingly, IL-5 gene knockout mice have normal baseline levels of eosinophils in the bone marrow and blood, and these cells have normal granules and morphology. The presence of this IL-5-independent population of eosinophils is thought to be due to IL-3 and GM-CSF [20]. However, individuals infected with filarial helminths have elevated IL-5 mRNA and protein compared to uninfected persons, whereas there was no effect on IL-3 or GM-CSF [21].

Eosinophils in Onchocercal Dermatitis

Mf are present in the upper dermis and cause no apparent distress while alive. However, an inflammatory response ensues when Mf die either as a result of natural attrition or after treatment with diethylcarbamazine (DEC) which

---

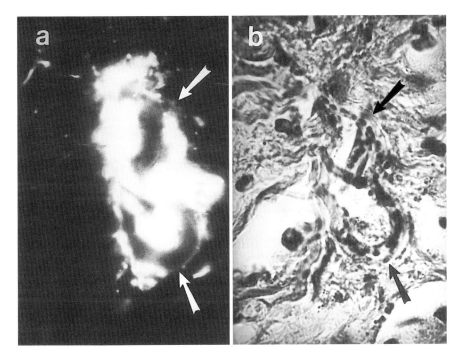

Fig. 2. Extracellular deposition of MBP onto degenerating Mf in the skin of an infected individual 24 h after treatment with DEC. Skin section stained for MBP by immunofluorescence (*a*) and the identical field counterstained with HE (*b*). × 850. *a* Extensive extracellular fluorescent staining for MBP surrounding a degenerating Mf. MBP is present on and around the cuticular surface of the Mf (arrows). Reproduced with permission from Ackerman et al. [24].

causes rapid Mf death [4, 5, 22]. Degeneration and release of parasite antigens into the surrounding tissue also lead to accumulation of eosinophils, which degranulate around degenerating Mf and deposit MBP and presumably other granule proteins onto the cuticle of the parasite [22, 23]. Figure 2 shows the deposition of MBP around degenerating Mf in the skin of a DEC-treated individual. In a temporal study of infected individuals after DEC treatment, Mf counts in the skin decreased to 22% of pretreatment levels by 24 h and to less than 5% of pretreatment levels by 48 h [24]. Mf death correlated with eosinophil degranulation and release of MBP as early as 1.5 h after DEC treatment. After an initial decrease in eosinophil numbers (possibly due to degranulation), the number of eosinophils in the skin increased and led to development of microabscesses around degenerating Mf [24]. Blood eosinophil levels also rose dramatically above the pretreatment value, reaching a maximum of 2.5-fold higher levels

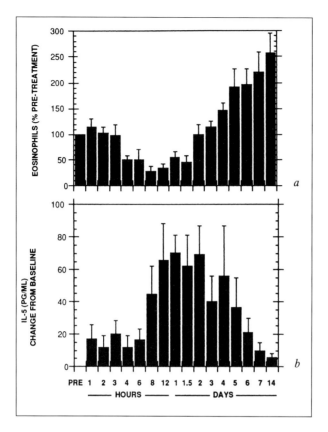

Fig. 3. Post-DEC treatment changes of serum IL-5 and blood eosinophil numbers in 10 patients with onchocerciasis. Mean eosinophil level (*a*) expressed as a percent of the pretreatment eosinophil level, and mean serum IL-5 levels (*b*) expressed as an absolute concentration above pretreatment baseline values. Reproduced with permission from Limaye et al. [25].

14 days after treatment, and MBP and EDN in blood plasma were also significantly elevated, as detected by immunoassay [24]. In a separate study, serum levels of IL-5 were elevated in patients treated with DEC and showed a temporal relationship with blood eosinophilia [25]. As shown in figure 3, serum IL-5 levels in 10 patients increased from undetectable levels to >150 pg/ml 12 h after treatment, and subsequently declined to baseline levels. The number of blood eosinophils decreased initially after treatment, presumably as a result of extravasation, and then gradually increased to >250% of pretreatment values (>2,500 cells/μl). These observations are consistent with a role for IL-5 in eosinophil production after DEC-mediated parasite death. I n this study, neither GM-CSF nor IL-3 were

detected, indicating that these cytokines were not mediating the eosinophil response [25]. A similar response is seen after DEC treatment of individuals infected with the related filarial helminth, *Wuchereria bancrofti* [26].

Role of IL-5 and Eosinophils in Onchocercal Keratitis

Corneal pathology is thought to occur when *O. volvulus* Mf enter the cornea after migrating through the periorbital skin and conjunctiva. As with dermal onchocerciasis, the Mf elicit little or no inflammatory response as long as they remain alive. Motile worms can be detected in the cornea by slitlamp examination. However, when the Mf die, parasite antigens are released into the microenvironment of the corneal stroma and trigger a local inflammatory response. In individuals who have been sensitized by chronic exposure to the parasites, the immediate inflammatory response is characterized by discrete areas of corneal inflammation (seen as opaque areas in the otherwise transparent cornea) termed punctate keratitis [4, 27]. DEC treatment also results in exacerbated corneal pathology, although Ivermectin, which is now used routinely, has no such side effects [1]. Histological examination of punctate keratitis shows local edema with infiltrating lymphocytes and eosinophils [28]. These lesions resolve spontaneously with minimal visual impairment [28]. In contrast, in heavily infected individuals with prolonged invasion of the cornea by large numbers of Mf, the inflammatory response results in sclerosing keratitis, which is characterized by scarring and severe visual impairment [5]. In these patients, the cornea appears opaque and is vascularized. Although it is likely that punctate lesions progress to sclerosing keratitis, this has not been clearly demonstrated by longitudinal studies.

Investigation of immune mechanisms underlying onchocercal keratitis (either punctate or sclerosing) has been hampered by the difficulty in obtaining corneas from infected individuals. Many of the corneal samples are from end stage disease, when the corneas are mostly fibrotic. Studies have therefore used adjacent conjunctival tissue and demonstrated abscesses comprising dead Mf with eosinophils and lymphocytes [27]. Animal models of onchocercal keratitis have been developed which utilize either intraconjunctival or intrastromal (corneal) injection of live Mf, or intrastromal injection of a soluble antigen extract of *O. volvulus* (OvAg) [reviewed in Pearlman, 29]. Eosinophils are a prominent component of cellular infiltrate of rabbits injected subconjunctivally with live *O. volvulus* Mf [30], guinea pigs injected subconjunctivally or intrastromally with live Mf of the cattle parasite *Onchocerca lienalis* [31, 32], and mice injected intrastromally with OvAg [33]. In animal models in which corneas are injected directly with OvAg, the experimental protocol requires prior systemic immunization, which is intended to reproduce a level of sensitization induced by chronic infection [33–

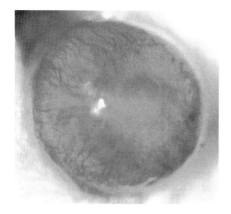

Fig. 4. Slitlamp appearance of murine onchocercal keratitis. BALB/c mice were immunized subcutaneously and injected intracorneally with soluble OvAg as described in Pearlman et al. [33]. Note the corneal opacification and neovascularization 7 days after intracorneal injection. × 18.

Table 1. Proposed sequence of events leading to eosinophil-mediated corneal and dermal immunopathology during onchocerciasis

---

Chronic exposure to helminth antigens induces a Th2 response resulting in IL-4 and IL-5 secretion which stimulates IgE and eosinophil production, respectively

Microfilarial death and release of parasite antigen into the dermis and corneal stroma triggers production of proinflammatory cytokines, chemokines and cellular adhesion molecules ICAM-1 and VCAM-1

Circulating eosinophils expressing the counter-receptors LFA-1 and VLA-4 bind to vascular endothelial cells and migrate into the tissue, following a chemokine gradient to the site of parasite degradation

IgE and other isotypes on the surface of eosinophils are cross-linked by parasite antigen, and eosinophils degranulate

MBP and other granule proteins are released into the surrounding tissue

Clinical signs of dermatitis and keratitis ensue

Chronic antigen stimulation leads to fibrosis

35]. Following intrastromal injection, slitlamp examination reveals that the cornea is opaque and that new blood vessels have grown from the periphery to the central cornea (neovascularization; fig. 4).

Although the presence of eosinophils in the cornea has been reported by several investigators, identification is based primarily on light microscopy, and identification of cell types is hampered by their physical distortion between the collagen fibrils of the corneal stroma. Ultrastructural analysis of onchocercal keratitis reveals that many of the eosinophils appear elongated, but show the characteristic bilobed nucleus and distinctive eosinophil granules. At higher magnification,

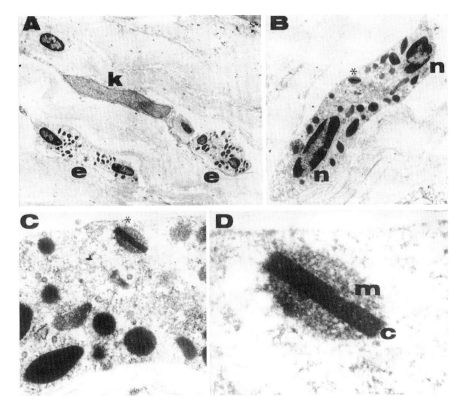

Fig. 5. Ultrastructural characteristics of eosinophils during onchocercal keratitis. Corneal stroma from an OvAg-immunized, stroma-injected mouse. *A* Eosinophils (e) in the same field as a corneal fibroblast (keratocyte, k) and an unidentified mononuclear cell. × 1,900. *B* A single distended eosinophil showing two lobes of the nucleus (n) and characteristic granules. The electron-dense core can be clearly seen in one granule (indicated by *). × 7,000. *C, D* Same granule at higher magnification. *C* × 13,000. *D* × 130,000. The granule core (c) and matrix (m) are indicated.

granule core and matrix can be clearly identified (fig. 5). At lower magnification (× 2,000), eosinophils are observed to be among the prominent cells of the infiltrate (not shown), thereby supporting the conclusions made by light microscopic analysis. Further examination shows that eosinophils in the corneal stroma are highly pleomorphic [36].

Given the evidence for the role of eosinophils in immunopathology of onchocerciasis, it is worthwhile considering a possible series of events leading to eosinophil-mediated disease. A proposed sequence of events is outlined in table 1, and the evidence supporting each step is presented below.

Onchocerca Antigens Preferentially Induce Th2 Responses which Are Associated with Immunopathology

Human Disease

In vitro stimulation of peripheral lymphocytes from *O. volvulus*-infected individuals induces IL-4 and IL-5 production, although the responses vary depending on the clinical status of the individual [11, 12, 37, 38]. A comparison between long-term residents of an endemic area (chronically infected) and returning Peace Corps workers (acutely infected) showed that chronically infected individuals had elevated IL-4 and IL-5 levels (and elevated peripheral IgE and eosinophils) compared with the nonendemic group, indicating that chronic infection was necessary to induce a Th2 response [38]. Furthermore, only individuals in the endemic group showed ocular manifestations of the disease, whereas symptoms of onchocercal dermatitis were evident in both groups [38]. These observations suggest a correlation between Th2 responses and development of ocular pathology.

This notion is supported by a more recent study which examined parasite antigen-driven cytokine responses in individuals with ocular Mf and determined the relationship with corneal pathology [39]. IL-5 and IL-10 cytokine production and IL-4, IL-5 and IL-10 mRNA expression were elevated in individuals with ocular disease compared with those with no apparent ocular disease [39]. Together, these observations implicate Th2 responses in the immunopathology of this disease.

Due to the difficulty in obtaining human ocular specimens, there is only a single report examining the Th response near the site of inflammation [40]. In 7 of 10 patients with ocular tissue, IL-4 mRNA expression was elevated, although no correlation was found with disease status [40].

Animal Models

Murine models of keratitis were used to examine more directly the Th response induced by parasite antigens both systemically and at the site of inflammation. Mice were immunized with irradiated *O. volvulus* or *O. lienalis* larvae or with soluble OvAg antigens, and cytokines were measured in response to in vitro stimulation with parasite antigens. Spleen cells and lymph node cells draining the site of injection selectively produced IL-4 and IL-5 in response to onchocerca antigens, and CD4+ T cells were found to be the source [33, 41, 42]. Prior sensitization or adoptive transfer of spleen cells from sensitized animals is required before keratitis can be induced [8, 31–33, 35, 43], thereby demonstrating a role for T cells in keratitis. CD4 and CD8 cells are also detected in the corneal stroma of mice developing keratitis after intracorneal injection with onchocerca antigens [33, 43]. The role for Th2 responses in onchocercal keratitis was demonstrated by

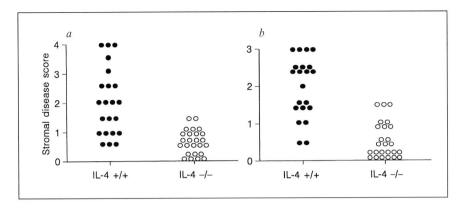

Fig. 6. IL-4 is required for the development of onchocercal keratitis. Opacification (*a*) and neovascularization (*b*) scores of 22 IL-4+/+ and 25 IL-4–/– mice from 4 separate experiments are shown. All mice were immunized and injected intrastromally with 10 µg OvAg as described in the legend to figure 1. Scores are from day 7 after intrastromal injection. Reproduced with permission from Pearlman et al. [33].

the following observations: (1) IL-4 and IL-5 gene expression is selectively upregulated in corneas injected with parasite antigen and which have a severe inflammatory response [33, 44], and (2) in contrast to immunocompetent mice, IL-4 gene knockout mice do not develop keratitis (fig. 6). Although the mechanism by which IL-4 mediates keratitis has yet to be determined, IL-4 gene knockout mice had no detectable IgE and few inflammatory cells (including eosinophils) in the corneal stroma [33].

Eosinophil Chemotaxis, Extravasation and Degranulation

The molecular basis for eosinophil chemotaxis to the site of Mf degradation has yet to be determined. Several eosinophil chemotactic factors have been described, including IL-5, platelet-activating factor, leukotriene B_4 and several chemotactic cytokines (chemokines), including RANTES, MIP1-α, MCP-1 and eotaxin [45, 46]. Chemokines are a superfamily of low-molecular-weight (8–10 kD) cytokines that are highly chemotactic for selected leukocytes (reviewed in Bagglioni et al., 45]. Eotaxin is a recently described chemokine which has a selective chemotactic activity for injected eosinophils when administered directly into the skin or lungs of naive guinea pigs [47, 48]. The selective activity of eotaxin is due to the presence of a high-affinity receptor on the eosinophil surface [49]. A synergistic effect with IL-5 on eosinophil recruitment was shown by intravenous injection of IL-5 followed by intradermal injection of eotaxin [50]. From this study, it was proposed that IL-5 stimulates eosinophil maturation and differentiation and that eotaxin is important in eosinophil recruitment. Eotaxin protein expression has been detected in fibroblasts, epithelial cells and in eosinophils [49]. In onchocerca-mediated immunopathology, it is likely that the source of eotaxin and other chemoattractants will initially be resident epithelial and fibroblast cells (keratocytes and keratinocytes), whereas inflammatory cells, including eosinophils, are likely to be the major source of chemokines at later stages. Gene expression for chemokines with activity for lymphocytes and eosinophils is present in corneas isolated from mice with severe onchocercal keratitis [44].

In addition to receptors for chemokines, eosinophils express the integrins LFA-1 ($\alpha1/\beta2$) and VLA-4 ($\alpha4/\beta1$) on the cell surface [51]. Extravasation of circulating eosinophils requires initial low-affinity binding selectin molecules to carbohydrate ligands followed by high-affinity interactions between integrins and vascular adhesion molecules of the immunoglobulin supergene family (including ICAM-1, ICAM-2 and VCAM-1) on vascular endothelial cells. As VCAM-1 expression and eosinophil transmigration are upregulated by IL-4 [52, 53], it is possible that IL-4 controls eosinophil transmigration into the sites of Mf degradation.

Eosinophil Degranulation and Release of Toxic Mediators

In addition to the effect of IL-4 on VCAM-1 expression, this cytokine is required for B cell isotype switching to IgE [54], and IgE has been shown to trigger eosinophil degranulation [55]. IL-4 also upregulates low-affinity IgE receptor (CD23) expression on eosinophils and triggers activation in the presence of IgE [56]. An additional or alternative mechanism for the diminished inflammatory response in IL-4 gene knockout mice may therefore be decreased IgE and CD23 expression. Once present at the site of inflammation, it is likely that eosinophil degranulaton requires cross-linking of surface Fc receptors. As eosinophils have receptors for IgG, IgA and IgE [16, 17], it is likely that degranulation will depend on which antigen-specific antibody isotypes are present at this site. IgE levels are extremely high in human onchocerciasis: 12,000–40,000 ng/ml compared with 300 ng/ml for uninfected individuals [57]. In addition, IgE is elevated in the sera and anterior chambers of mice and guinea pigs with onchocercal keratitis [33, 58, 59]. In the latter study, elevated IgE levels induced by immunization or after treatment with DEC correlated with increased severity of corneal inflammation [58, 59]. Cross-linking of IgE on the surface of eosinophils may therefore be a requirement for degranulation and resulting cytopathology that occurs during onchocercal keratitis. Another factor that may affect the extent of local damage relates to the observation that cross-linking of IgG, IgA and IgE receptors stimulates differential release of eosinophil granule proteins [60]. For example, anti-IgE stimulate release of eosinophil peroxidase but not eosinophil cateonic protein from eosinophils from atopic patients, whereas anti-IgG stimulation had the converse effect [60].

Consequences of Eosinophil Granulation on Corneal Clarity

Transparency of the mammalian cornea is dependent on the orderly arrangement of collagen fibrils in the corneal stroma, which permits light to penetrate without diffraction, and on a critical level of hydration in the corneal stroma which is controlled by an ATPase-dependent pump in the corneal endothelial cells [61]. During acute keratitis, it is likely that release of eosinophil granule proteins disrupts the normal level of hydration, resulting in corneal edema and rearrangement of collagen fibrils. Penetrating light would then be diffracted, resulting in the cornea having an opaque appearance. Eosinophil granule proteins are also likely to modulate the activity of resident fibroblasts (keratocytes) which produce the collagen and the proteoglycans that separate the collagen fibrils. The result may be direct cytotoxicity, which would affect maintenance of corneal integrity, or stimulation to produce proinflammatory cytokines or chemokines. Aberrant collagen production in chronically inflamed corneas may then cause the fibrosis which is characteristic of sclerosing keratitis. Although the cytotoxic effect of eosinophil granule proteins on corneal endothelial cells or keratocytes has not been reported, addition of MBP to corneal organ culture inhibits corneal epithelial cell migration after wounding, demonstrating that MBP affects the function of these cells [62].

Summary and Conclusions

This review has sought to demonstrate that eosinophils have an important role in the immunopathology of onchocercal dermatitis and keratitis. The most compelling evidence is the consistent presence of eosinophils and eosinophil granule proteins at the site of tissue damage, either after parasite death or direct injection of parasite antigens. A more definitive role for eosinophils in onchocercal keratitis will be determined using IL-5 gene knockout mice (an animal model of onchocercal dermatitis has yet to be established). Identification of chemoattractants and adhesion molecules necessary for eosinophil recruitment will indicate possible approaches to immune intervention.

Acknowledgements

The author gratefully acknowledges the collaboration of Dr. David Bardenstein in the production of the transmission electron micrographs and the continued collaboration of Drs. James Kazura and Jonathan Lass. The technical support of Eugenia Diaconu, Fred Hazlett, Jamie Albright and Alan Higgins is also acknowledged. Permission to use the work of Drs. Steven Ackerman and Thomas Nutman is also greatly appreciated. Support is from National Institutes of Health grants AI35938 and EY10320 and the Research to Prevent Blindness Foundation.

References

1   Onchocerciasis and its control. World Health Organ Tech Rep Ser 1995;852.
2   Murphy RP, Taylor H, Greene BM: Chorioretinal damage in onchocerciasis. Am J Ophthalmol 1984;98:519–521.
3   Taylor H: Onchocerciasis; in Duane T (ed): Clinical Ophthalmology. Philadelphia, Harper & Row, 1984, pp 1–12.
4   World Health Organization Expert Committee on Onchocerciasis. Third Report. World Health Organ Tech Rep Ser 1987;752.
5   Mackenzie CD, Williams JF, Sisley BM, Steward MW, O'Day J: Variations in host response and the pathogenesis of human onchocerciasis. Rev Infect Dis 1985;7:802–808.
6   Duke B: The population dynamics of *Onchocerca volvulus* in the human host. Trop Med Parasitol 1993;44:61–68.
7   Greene BM, Gbakima AA, Albiez EJ, Taylor HR: Humoral and cellular immune responses to *Onchocerca volvulus* infection in humans. Rev Infect Dis 1985;7:789–795.
8   Gallin M, Edmonds K, Ellner JJ, Erttmann KD, White AT, Newland HS, Taylor HR, Greene BM: Cell-mediated immune responses in human infection with *Onchocerca volvulus*. J Immunol 1988; 140:1999–2007.
9   Ottesen EA: Immune responsiveness and the pathogenesis of human onchocerciasis. J Infect Dis 1995;171:659–671.
10   Ottesen EA: The Wellcome Trust Lecture: Infection and disease in lymphatic filariasis: An immunological perspective. Parasitology 1992;104:s71–79.
11   Elson LH, Calvopina M, Paredes W, Araujo E, Bradley JE, Guderian RH, Nutman TB: Immunity to onchocerciasis: Putative immune persons produce a Th1-like response to *Onchocerca volvulus*. J Infect Dis 1995;171:652–658.
12   Steel, C, Nutman TB: Regulation of IL-5 in onchocerciasis. A critical role for IL-2. J Immunol 1993; 150:5511–5518.
13   Abu GR, Gleich GJ, Prendergast FG: Interaction of eosinophil granule major basic protein with synthetic lipid bilayers: A mechanism for toxicity. J Membr Biol 1992;128:153–164.
14   Kita H, Abu GR, Sur S, Gleich GJ: Eosinophil major basic protein induces degranulation and IL-8 production by human eosinophils. J Immunol 1995;154:4749–4758.
15   Rohrbach MS, Wheatley CL, Slifman NR, Gleich GJ: Activation of platelets by eosinophil granule proteins. J Exp Med 1990;172:1271–1274.
16   Gleich GJ, Adolphson CR, Leiferman KM: The biology of the eosinophilic leukocyte. Annu Rev Med 1993;44:85–101.
17   Weller PF: The immunobiology of eosinophils. N Engl J Med 1991;324:1110–1118.
18   Dent LA, Strath M, Mellor AL, Sanderson CJ: Eosinophilia in transgenic mice expressing interleukin 5. J Exp Med 1990;172:1425–1431.
19   Coffman RL, Seymour BW, Hudak S, Jackson J, Rennick D: Antibody to interleukin-5 inhibits helminth-induced eosinophilia in mice. Science 1989;245:308–310.
20   Kopf M: IL-5-deficient mice have a developmental defect in CD5+ B-1 cells and lack eosinphilia but have normal antibody and cytotoxic T cell responses. Immunity 1996;4:1–20.

21 Limaye AP, Abrams JS, Silver JE, Ottesen EA, Nutman TB: Regulation of parasite-induced eosino-philia: Selectively increased interleukin 5 production in helminth-infected patients. J Exp Med 1990;172:399–402.

22 Connor DH, George GH, Gibson D: Pathologic changes of human onchocerciasis: Implications for future research. Rev Infect Dis 1985;7:809–819.

23 Kephart GM, Gleich GJ, Connor DH, Gibson DW, Ackerman SJ: Deposition of eosinophil granule major basic protein onto microfilariae of *Onchocerca volvulus* in the skin of patients treated with diethylcarbamazine. Lab Invest 1984;50:51–61.

24 Ackerman SJ, Kephart GM, Francis H, Awadzi K, Gleich GJ, Ottesen EA: Eosinophil degranula-tion. An immunologic determinant in the pathogenesis of the Mazzotti reaction in human oncho-cerciasis. J Immunol 1990;144:3961–3969.

25 Limaye AP, Abrams JS, Silver JE, Awadzi K, Francis HF, Ottesen EA, Nutman TB: Interleukin-5 and the posttreatment eosinophilia in patients with onchocerciasis. J Clin Invest 1991;88:1418–1421.

26 Limaye AP, Ottesen EA, Kumaraswami V, Abrams JS, Regunathan J, Vijayasekaran V, Jayaraman K, Nutman TB: Kinetics of serum and cellular interleukin-5 in posttreatment eosinophilia of patients with lymphatic filariasis. J Infect Dis 1993;167:1396–1400.

27 Garner A: Pathology of ocular onchocerciasis: Human and experimental. Trans R Soc Trop Med Hyg 1976;70:374–377.

28 Rodger F: Pathogenesis and pathology of ocular onchocerciasis. Am J Ophthalmol 1960;49:560–594.

29 Pearlman E: Experimental onchocercal keratitis. Parasitol Today 1996;12:261–267.

30 Garner A, Duke BO, Anderson J: A comparison of the lesions produced in the cornea of the rabbit eye by microfilariae of the forest and Sudan-savanna strains of *Onchocerca volvulus* from Came-roon. II. The pathology. Z Tropenmed Parasitol 1973;24:385–396.

31 Donnelly JJ, Rockey JH, Bianco AE, Soulsby EJL: Ocular immunopathologic findings of experi-mental onchocerciasis. Arch Ophthalmol 1984;102:628–634.

32 Sakla AA, Donnelly JJ, Lok JB, Khatami M, Rockey JH: Punctate keratitis induced by subconjunc-tivally injected microfilariae of *Onchocerca lienalis*. Arch Ophthalmol 1986;104:894–898.

33 Pearlman E, Lass JH, Bardenstein DS, Kopf M, Hazlett Jr FE, Diaconu E, Kazura JW: Interleukin 4 and T helper type 2 cells are required for development of experimental onchocercal keratitis (river blindness). J Exp Med 1995;182:931–940.

34 Gallin MY, Murray D, Lass JH, Grossniklaus HE, Greene BM: Experimental interstitial keratitis induced by *Onchocerca volvulus* antigens. Arch Ophthalmol 1988;106:1447–1452.

35 Chakravarti B, Lass JH, Diaconu E, Bardenstein DS, Roy CE, Herring TA, Chakravarti DN, Greene BM: Immune-mediated *Onchocerca volvulus* sclerosing keratitis in the mouse. Exp Eye Res 1993;57:21–27.

36 Bardenstein D, Lass J, Kazura J, Pearlman E: Pleomorphism of stromal eosinophils in murine experimental onchocercal keratitis. Cornea, in press.

37 Mahanty S, King CL, Kumaraswami V, Regunathan J, Maya A, Jayaraman K, Abrams JS, Ottesen EA, Nutman TB: IL-4- and IL-5-secreting lymphocyte populations are preferentially stimulated by parasite-derived antigens in human tissue invasive nematode infections. J Immunol 1993;151:3704–3711.

38 McCarthy JS, Ottesen EA, Nutman TB: Onchocerciasis in endemic and nonendemic populations: Differences in clinical presentation and immunologic findings. J Infect Dis 1994;170:736–741.

39 Plier DA, Awadzi K, Freedman DO: Immunoregulation in Onchocerciasis: Persons with ocular inflammatory disease produce a Th2-like response to *Onchocerca volvulus*-antigen. J Infect Dis 1996;174:380–386.

40 Chan CC, Li Q, Brezin AP, Whitcup SM, Egwuagu C, Ottesen EA, Nussenblatt RB: Immunopa-thology of ocular onchocerciasis. III. Th-2 helper cells in the conjunctiva. Ocular Immunol 1993;1:71–77.

41 Lange A, Yutanawiboonchai W, Scott P, Abraham D: IL-4 and IL-5 dependent protective immuni-ty to *Onchocerca volvulus* infective larvae in BALB/cBYJ mice. J Immunol 1994;153:205–211.

42 Taylor MJ, van Es RP, Shay K, Folkard SG, Townson S, Bianco AE: Protective immunity against *Onchocerca volvulus* and *O. lienalis* infective larvae in mice. Trop Med Parasitol 1994;45:17–23.

43 Chakravarti B, Herring TA, Lass JH, Parker JS, Bucy RP, Diaconu E, Tseng J, Whitfield DR, Greene BM, Chakravarti DN: Infiltration of CD4+ T cells into cornea during development of

Onchocerca volvulus-induced experimental sclerosing keratitis in mice. Cell Immunol 1994;159: 306–314.

44   Pearlman E, Lass J, Bardenstein D, Diaconu E, Hazlett F, Albright J, Higgins A, Kazura J: IL-12 exacerbates helminth-mediated corneal pathology by augmenting inflammatory cell recruitment and chemokine expression. J Immunol 1996, in press.

45   Baggiolini M, Dewald B, Moser B: Interleukin-8 and related chemotactic cytokines-CXC and CC chemokines. Adv Immunol 1994;55:97–179.

46   Resnick MB, Weller PF: Mechanisms of eosinophil recruitment. Am J Respir Cell Mol Biol 1993;8: 349–355.

47   Griffiths JD, Collins PD, Rossi AG, Jose PJ, Williams TJ: The chemokine, eotaxin, activates guinea-pig eosinophils in vitro and causes their accumulation into the lung in vivo. Biochem Biophys Res Commun 1993;197:1167–1172.

48   Jose PJ, Griffiths JD, Collins PD, Walsh DT, Moqbel R, Totty NF, Truong O, Hsuan JJ, Williams TJ: Eotaxin: A potent eosinophil chemoattractant cytokine detected in a guinea pig model of allergic airways inflammation. J Exp Med 1994;179:881–887.

49   Ponath P, Qin S, Ringler D, Clark-Lewis I, Wang J, Kassam N, Smith H, Shi X, Gonzalo J, Newman W, Guitierrez-Ramos J, Mackay C: Cloning of the human eosinophil chemoattractant, eotaxin. Expression, receptor binding, and functional properties suggest a mechanism for the selective recruitment of eosinophils. J Clin Invest 1996;97:604–612.

50   Collins PD, Marleau S, Griffiths JD, Jose PJ, Williams TJ: Cooperation between interleukin-5 and the chemokine eotaxin to induce eosinophil accumulation in vivo. J Exp Med 1995;182:1169–1174.

51   Weller PF, Rand TH, Goelz SE, Chi-Rosso G, Lobb RL: Human eosinophil adherence to vascular endothelium mediated by binding to vascular cell adhesion molecule-1 and endothelial leukocyte adhesion molecule-1. Proc Natl Acad Sci USA 1991;88:7430–7433.

52   Moser R, Fehr J, Bruijnzeel PL: IL-4 controls the selective endothelium-driven transmigration of eosinophils from allergic individuals. J Immunol 1992;149:1432–1438.

53   Moser R, Groscurth P, Carballido JM, Bruijnzeel PL, Blaser K, Heusser CH, Fehr J: Interleukin-4 induces tissue eosinophilia in mice: Correlation with its in vitro capacity to stimulate the endothelial cell-dependent selective transmigration of human eosinophils. J Lab Clin Med 1993;122:567–575.

54   Snapper CM, Finkelman FD, Paul WE: Regulation of IgG1 and IgE production by interleukin 4. Immunol Rev 1988;102:51–75.

55   Gounni AS, Lamkhioued B, Ochiai K, Tanaka Y, Delaporte E, Capron A, Kinet JP, Capron M: High-affinity IgE receptor on eosinophils is involved in defence against parasites. Nature 1994;367: 183–186.

56   Arock M, Le Goff L, Becherel PA, Dugas B, Debre P, Mossalayi MD: Involvement of Fc epsilon RII/CD23 and L-arginine dependent pathway in IgE-mediated activation of human eosinophils. Biochem Biophys Res Commun 1994;203:265–271.

57   Ottesen EA: Immediate hypersensitivity responses in the immunopathogenesis of human onchocerciasis. Rev Infect Dis 1985;7:796–801.

58   Donnelly JJ, Rockey JH, Bianco AE, Soulsby EJ: Aqueous humor and serum IgE antibody in experimental ocular Onchocerca infection of guinea pigs. Ophthalmic Res 1983;15:61–67.

59   Donnelly JJ, Rockey JH, Taylor HR, Soulsby EJ: Onchocerciasis: Experimental models of ocular disease. Rev Infect Dis 1985;7:820–825.

60   Tomassini M, Tsicopoulos A, Tai PC, Gruart V, Tonnel AB, Prin L, Capron A, Capron M: Release of granule proteins by eosinophils from allergic and nonallergic patients with eosinophilia on immunoglobulin-dependent activation. J Allergy Clin Immunol 1991;88:365–375.

61   Kenyon K: Morphology and pathologic responses of the cornea to disease; in Smolin G, Thoft RA (eds): The Cornea. Scientific Foundations and Clinical Practice. Boston, Little, Brown and Company, 1987, pp 63–99.

62   Trocmé SD, Gleich GJ, Kephart GM, Zieske JD: Eosinophil granule major basic protein inhibition of corneal epithelial wound healing. Invest Ophthalmol Vis Sci 1994;35:3051–3056.

Eric Pearlman, Division of Geographic Medicine, CWRU School of Medicine, 2109 Adelbert Rd., Cleveland, OH 44106-4983 (USA)

Freedman DO (ed): Immunopathogenetic Aspects of Disease Induced by Helminth Parasites.
Chem Immunol. Basel, Karger, 1997, vol 66, pp 41–61

....

Enteric Helminth Infection: Immunopathology and Resistance during Intestinal Nematode Infection

R.K. Grencis

School of Biological Sciences, University of Manchester, Manchester, UK

Introduction

Enteric helminth infections of both animals and man are some of the most ubiquitous parasite infections globally. This is particularly true for intestinal nematodes and in man these infections are estimated to cause developmental problems in several tens of millions of children [1]. Such estimates are far greater than previously supposed and serve to illustrate the enormous impact which these parasites have on infected communities. The detailed mechanisms whereby morbidity is generated is much less well defined but is likely to be related to the pathological and immunopathological changes which accompany infection. Whilst there is some descriptive information on the pathological changes which are associated with helminth infection in man and domestic animals, our knowledge of the mechanisms which regulate these changes is scarce.

This is in the main related to the problems of working in field situations where invasive techniques of analysis are severely limited. As a consequence most of our current information on the immunological and pathological changes which are generated during infection by gastrointestinal dwelling helminths have come from studies of a number of well defined laboratory systems, especially nematodes in the mouse host. This review will, therefore, concentrate on the data generated from these studies and will attempt to present an overview of our current understanding of the immunological control of pathological changes induced by these infections highlighting areas of special interest. It is hoped that the review will provide a sound base for comparison with studies in humans and domestic animals and other metazoan infections.

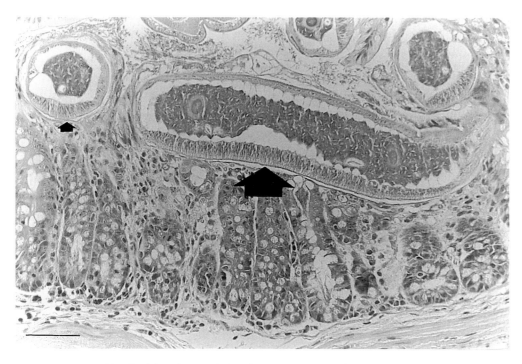

Fig. 1. Light micrograph showing patent *T. muris* infection in susceptible AKR mice (day 35 after infection). The anterior portion of the worm lies embedded in a syncitial tunnel of enterocytes of the caecum with the posterior portion of the worm hanging free in the lumen to facilitate mating and egg laying (small arrow, transverse section; large arrow, longitudinal section). Scale bar: 70 µm.

Gastrointestinal Nematode Infections of Rodents

Infection by gastrointestinal nematodes occurs in a number of ways. This is dependent upon species of nematode and includes skin penetration followed by a tissue migratory phase preceding residence of adult parasites in the gut (e.g. *Nippostrongylus brasiliensis, Strongyloides venezuelensis*) or proceeds following ingestion of eggs or larvae followed by growth and maturation to adult parasites in the intestine (e.g. *Heligmosomoides polygyrus, Trichinella spiralis, Trichuris muris*).

There are also variations in the niche within the intestine in which the parasites live. *N. brasiliensis* and *S. venezuelensis* live within the lumen of the small intestine whereas *T. muris* and *T. spiralis* live within the epithelial layer of the intestine forming a syncitial tunnel of enterocytes (fig. 1). *H. polygyrus* spends early larval stages within the mucosa of the gut before emerging into the lumen and developing into adult worms. The different niches occupied by the worms will influence pathology generated by these infections in the gut through both mechanical damage and activation of the immune system although few studies have been designed to examine these changes.

Intestinal Pathology Associated with Infection

A number of studies with gastrointestinal nematodes have shown that infection is associated with intestinal pathology. The most commonly described changes are villus atrophy and crypt hyperplasia [2–4]. These changes have many of the hallmarks of the pathological changes apparent during other intestinal diseases including coeliac disease, Crohn's disease and graft versus host disease all of which have an immune mediated component [5]. Following helminth infections there has been conflicting evidence to support a role for immune mediated control of the associated gut pathology often observed. This is due to the difficulty in making the discrimination between purely mechanical changes induced by invasive stages of parasites (or through production of destructive secretions such as helminth proteases) and changes induced through specific recognition of parasite antigens and generation of immunopathology.

Some studies have attempted to do this by following intestinal nematode infections in immunodeficient animals such as athymic rodents [4] or in animals which have been chemically immunosuppressed [6]. With regard to the latter an interesting study was done in which intestinal changes were monitored in mice infected with *T. spiralis* and treated with the broadly acting immunosuppressant cyclosporin A (CsA). It was suggested from these data that the considerable pathological changes induced by *T. spiralis* infection were predominantly controlled by T lymphocytes although some mechanically induced changes in villus architecture were likely to be involved in the overall pathology observed. Definitive experiments remain to be done, however, and detailed examination of such pathology in other systems is still lacking.

Parasite excretions and secretions are potent sources of molecules which could induce changes in gut pathology through non-immunological mechanisms. A number of such molecules have been well defined in terms of their molecular weight and for some of them their in vitro functional capabilities have been described. For example, molecules secreted by hookworm species include acetylcholinesterases, glutathione transferases, superoxide dismutases, neutrophil inhibitory factor, anti-haemostatic molecules (fibrinogenolytic proteases) and IgA proteases [reviewed in ref. 7]. All of these have been suggested to play anti-inflammatory roles, with some of them having definite tissue-destructive properties (e.g. superoxide dismutase).

Recently, a 47-kD molecule secreted by the human whipworm *(T. trichiura)* has been identified as a pore-forming molecule and was suggested to be one way in which the parasite facilitates its movement through the intestinal epithelium [8]. Secretion of such a molecule would undoubtedly damage gut enterocytes and disturb normal homeostatic regulation of the intestinal epithelium. Again a major complicating problem in discriminating between immunological and non-immunological induced effects of these molecules is that many of them also act as potent antigens. This is exemplified with regard to the pore-forming molecule of *T. trichiura.* This is one of the dominant molecules recognised immunologically by sera from infected people [9].

Immunologically Mediated Intestinal Pathology

Early work into the immunological control of intestinal nematode infections centred upon the lymphocyte populations controlling resistance and were predominantly done with *N. brasiliensis* in its natural host (the rat), with *T. spiralis* in the mouse and rat and *T. muris* in the mouse. Many of these studies used adoptive transfer of immunity with lymphocytes from infected animals to demonstrate a major role for T lymphocytes in mediating both protective immunity and pathological changes associated with resistance. This was done both with T lymphocytes freshly isolated from lymph nodes draining the intestine, thoracic duct lymphocytes or enriched populations of antigen-specific CD4+ T cells (Th cells) taken after extended in vitro culture [10–17].

Moreover, experiments in the rat with *T. spiralis* used a blocking monoclonal antibody to a mucosal homing receptor (α4 integrin) in vivo to demonstrate that such Th cells need to move to the gut tissue to mediate expulsion of the parasite [18]. Taken together, all these experiments showed that Th cells mediate expulsion of the worms from the intestine and control the production of a number of inflammatory changes including intestinal mastocytosis, eosinophilia, goblet cell hyperplasia and raise levels of serum IgE levels through the secretion of cytokines.

The application of molecular techniques to the cloning and the identification of a variety of cytokines (especially in the mouse) paved the way for the detailed investigation of the role of these molecules in regulating immune responses to intestinal nematodes in the mouse. This also enabled a deeper insight into the involvement of CD4+ Th cells in controlling the types of pathology induced during intestinal nematode infection and came from the description of of distinct Th cell subsets in the mouse (based upon differential cytokine secretion) by Mosmann and Coffman [19] and subsequent studies of their importance in regulating protozoan parasite infections most notably *Leishmania* [20, 21].

T Helper Cell Control of Nematode Infection

With regard to intestinal nematodes there has been a wealth of subsequent studies that demonstrate that the Th2 cell subset is the predominant T cell population activated following helminth infection. Initially these studies centred around experiments measuring cytokine production throughout infection. Data from experiments with *N. brasiliensis, T.spiralis, H. polygyrus* and *T.muris* in the mouse all demonstrated the production of cytokines by T cell such as interleukin 3 (IL-3), IL-4, IL-5, IL-6, IL-9 and IL-10 in the relative absence of interferon gamma (IFN-γ, a Th1 cytokine) [22–25].

Based upon the functional characterisation of particular cytokines in controlling particular immune responses, these data fitted well with the previously described observations of immunopathological changes characteristic of intestinal helminth infections such as eosinophilia, intestinal mastocytosis and elevated serum IgE levels. The critical importance of particular cytokines in both host-protective immunity and the immunopathological changes, however, remain to be comprehensively defined although a number of studies have shown a number of important findings.

Cytokine Control of Protective Immunity

The majority of early studies investigating immunity to intestinal nematodes were performed in systems in which infections were acute in nature, i.e. parasites established in the intestine and were subsequently expelled (the so-called self-cure phenomenon). It became clear from adoptive transfer of host protection with T cells in both rats and mice and from studies from infections in athymic animals that Th cells mediated protection (see above) although passive transfer of immunity with sera from previously infected animals implied that at least in some parasite/host systems antibody may play a role [26–29].

Correlations between Th2 cytokine production and worm expulsion further implied an important role for Th2 cytokines in resistance. The pivotal role of certain Th2 cytokines was most convincingly shown by experiments in which the activity of cytokines was blocked in vivo in infected animals using neutralising monoclonal antibodies. This was first shown for the challenge infection model of *H. polygyrus* using anti-IL-4 monoclonal antibodies [30] and subsequently for *T. muris* using anti-IL-4 receptor monoclonal antibodies [31].

In this latter infection, neutralisation of IL-4 allowed the generation of Th1-dominated response and the establishment of a chronic infection in animals which normally expelled their parasites from the intestine. In mouse strains which naturally harbour a chronic infection of *T. muris* a dominant Th1 response becomes established, and administration of anti-IFN-γ monoclonal antibodies allowed a Th2 response to dominate and worms were expelled from the intestine [reviewed in ref. 32].

The importance of Th2 responses in resistance was strengthened by experiments in which IL-12 was administered to helminth-infected mice. IL-12 promotes a Th1 response and hence downregulates a Th2 response. *N. brasiliensis* infections in mice treated in this way harboured worms in their intestines for an extended period of time in comparison to control animals, which was co-incident with the downregulation of a Th2 response against the parasite [33]. Similar experiments in mice resistant to *T. muris* induced down-regulation of the normally dominant Th2 response and development of a Th1 response and a chronic infection [Bancroft, Sypek and Else, pers. commun.].

Th2 Control of Immunopathological Changes

The kinds of study described above also allowed analysis of Th2-mediated inflammatory responses to be defined and their importance assessed in relation to host-protective immunity. A continuing theme that has run throughout the years with regard to expulsion of intestinal helminth infection has been that expulsion is mediated by an IgE-mediated immediate hypersensitivity-type reaction involving intestinal mast cells [reviewed in Wakelin, 34]. It has been difficult to come to a consensus concerning the importance of these two components in resistance to intestinal nematodes per se because of the differences between the model systems studied and whether the observations made were following primary or secondary infections.

IgE, Immunity and Pathology

With regard to IgE, there is little evidence to support a role for IgE in protective immunity to intestinal nematodes despite the consistently elevated levels of both parasite-specific and non-specific IgE observed following infection. *N. brasiliensis* infections are expelled normally in animals treated with anti-IgE antibodies [35] and more recently there has been a work in mice with a disrupted IL-4 gene in which expulsion again proceeds normally in the absence of IgE [36].

There are, however, some data that does suggest that IgE may be involved in the rapid expulsion response to secondary *T. spiralis* infections in the rat. Rapid expulsion is a mechanism in which a challenge infection is expelled within 24 h and indeed the majority of parasites are removed within the first 4 h. Studies have shown that passive transfer of sera from previously infected rats (with a high IgE titre) into recipients induces expulsion [37]. The response is absent if the IgE is previously removed from the sera by heating. Whether this response is entirely mediated by IgE is not certain as other antibody classes (e.g. IgG) can also mediate the rapid expulsion response [38]. The involvement of mast cells in this process is not known although there are data showing the release of leukotrienes during the rapid expulsion response, with the likely source being mast cells [39].

In mice there are some data to suggest that expulsion of a primary infection of *T. spiralis* does not require any interaction between IgE and mast cells in the expulsion response. Mice with a disruption in the Fcγ chain (which have no high-affinity IgE receptors) expel their parasites efficiently and mount a strong intestinal mastocytosis [Grencis and Ravetch, unpubl data]. It is difficult to assess the importance of such an interaction in a rapid expulsion response following a challenge infection as it is unclear whether mice can mount a response similar to rats [40].

Mast Cells, Immunity and Pathology

The importance of mast cells in expulsion of intestinal nematodes can also present a confused picture. Mucosal mast cell production is under the production of a number of growth factors – predominantly the T-cell-derived cytokines IL-3, IL-4, IL-9 and IL-10 [41–44] although non-lymphocyte factors also play an important role (see below). Mucosal mast cells differ from connective tissue in a number of respects with major differences observed in the granule proteases found [reviewed in ref. 45].

The majority of data concerning control of the growth of mucosal mast cells has come from studies of in-vitro-generated cells grown from bone marrow. Initially, IL-3 was identified as the major growth factor controlling their production [46]. Subsequently, IL-4, IL-9 and IL-10 were shown to act synergistically with IL-3 [47–49] and more recently a non-T-cell derived cytokine stem cell factor (SCF, mast cell growth factor, *kit* ligand, steel factor) was shown to play a major role [54–56]. These cytokines can have pleiotropic effects including effects on growth, proliferation, homing and induction of distinct protease genes [50, 51].

The relationship between bone-marrow-derived mast cells and in vivo mucosal mast cells still remains unclear as studies phenotyping bone-marrow-derived cells on the basis of protease production demonstrate a heterogeneous population of cells [52]. This may reflect the conditions under which they were grown – a comprehensive analysis of combinations of growth factors known to have mast-cell-promoting effects has not been carried out. Nevertheless it appears likely that T cells play a major role as a source of many of these factors for the production of mucosal mast cells in vivo.

Recent work using an immature v-abl-transformed mast cell line has shown that following injection into mice these precursors develop into the mature phenotype dependent upon the site at which they localise. For example, cells located in the lamina propria of the intestine express MMCP1 and MMCP2 in the relative absence of MMCP3, MMCP4, MMCP5, MMCP6 and MMCP7 [53]. Whilst this is not directly analogous to the situation when mast cell hyperplasia follows helminth infection, as mast cells are predominately found in the epithelia, analysis of protease expression in the gut of helminth-infected mice does show that MMCP1 and MMCP2 are found in the relative absence of MMCP3, 4, 5, 6 and 7 [51]. Overall these data support the hypothesis that it is local tissue environmental factors which influence the maturation process of mucosal mast cells. Thus it is likely that T-cell-derived cytokines influence the development of mast cells within the gut tissue.

Recent data from studies of cytokine control of mast cell differentiation of precursors in bone marrow or MLNC from *N. brasiliensis*-infected mice suggested that SCF could influence mast cell development but only in the context of T-cell-derived cytokines such as IL-3 [54]. These data strengthen the idea of both T-cell-derived and non-T-cell-derived factors acting in concert to control mucosal mast cell production.

Mast cells are also known to produce a wide variety of cytokines [55], and it is a distinct possibility that they are able to potentiate their own survival and production through secretion of factors such as IL-3, IL-4, IL-9. It is also likely that a degree of functional redundancy exists within the array of mast-cell-promoting cytokines. As mentioned above, IL-3 is a cytokine believed to play a major role in the production of mucosal mast cells. IL-3, however, may not be essential for intestinal mast cell production. *T. spiralis* infection of mice with a disruption in the IL-3 gene expel their parasites effectively and mount a strong intestinal mast cell response [Grencis and Tybulewicz, unpubl. data]

The preceding discussion has centred around control of mast cells by cytokines produced by T cells. This is not to say that non-T-cell-derived factors do not play an important role also. Indeed, one non-T-cell-derived factor which has been suggested to play *the* major role in controlling mast cell production is SCF [56].

Recently experiments were conducted in which SCF activity has been blocked in vivo in *T. spiralis*-infected mice using monoclonal antibodies specific for SCF or SCF receptor. Such treatment completely suppressed the intestinal mastocytosis (fig. 2) normally observed following infection and was correlated with a delayed worm expulsion [57, 58]. Interestingly, Th cell response in terms of cytokine production and antibody istotype production appeared not to be changed in monoclonal-treated animals. It is also known that treatment of mice with an established mucosal mast cell response with an anti-SCF receptor mono-

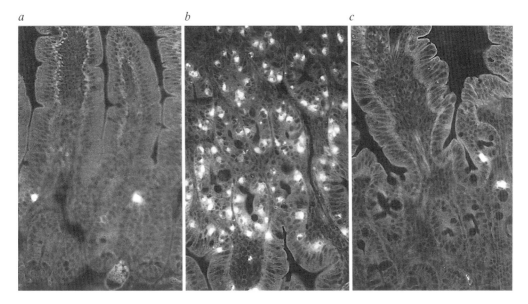

Fig. 2. Intestinal mast cell hyperplasia during infection with *T. spiralis* in mice. Sections were stained with anti-mucosal mast cell protease 1 polyclonal antisera. *a* Small intestine of normal uninfected mice. *b* Small intestine of *T. spiralis* infected mice 10 days after infection. Note extensive intestinal mastocytosis. *c* Small intestine of *T. spiralis*-infected mice 10 days after infection and following treatment with anti-SCF receptor monoclonal antibody in vivo. Notice profound reduction in intestinal mastocytosis as compared to *b*.

clonal antibody markedly depresses mast cell numbers in the gut [Faulkner, pers. commun.] which implies that SCF may also be important for survival of functionally mature cells (see below).

The discovery of SCF in 1990 [59–62] and its description as a ligand for c-*kit* also allowed a rational interpretation of earlier observations of mutant W/W^v mice which are deficient in the receptor for SCF (c-*kit*) and deficient in mast cells [63, 64]. Expulsion of *T. spiralis* from W/W^v mice is very delayed [65] and this observation when taken in the light of the more recent work is compelling evidence for an important role for mucosal mast cells in resistance to *T. spiralis* in mice and emphasises the importance of the myeloid component in overall resistance mechanisms.

Development of Mast Cell Hyperplasia

Whilst the cytokines governing mast cell production have been investigated in great depth, the site of regulation of the mastocytosis remains to be defined. Whether the increase in mast cell numbers is dependent upon resident precursors in the intestine waiting to differentiate following production of cytokines or whether bone-marrow-derived precursors migrate into the intestinal tissue and then differentiate within the gut tissue remains to be completely resolved.

Recent data have generated a hypothesis to suggest that migration may be of major importance and operate in a mechanism similar to that utilised by T cells which home into the intraepithelial niche [66]. Immature mast cells from the bone marrow express the homing receptors $\alpha4\beta7$ and L selectin. These recognise the endothelial ligand MAdCAM-1 which allows mast cells into the lamina propria. Under the influence of cytokines such as IL-3 and SCF, $\alpha4\beta7$ is downregulated whilst α_E is upregulated under the influence of TGF-β (which is produced locally in the intestine) allowing formation of the $\alpha_E\beta7$ integrin complex. Activated mast cells will enable interaction of this complex with its ligand E-cadherin on the epithelium.

Mast Cell Function: The Role of Mast Cell Proteases

It is a consistent finding with many acute infection models (e.g. *N. brasiliensis, T. spiralis, S. venezuelensis,* secondary *H. polygyrus* infections, *T. muris* in resistant strains of mouse) that the kinetics of expulsion are closely mirrored by intestinal mastocytosis (as assessed by histological staining). Nevertheless, histological presence of increased numbers of mast cells does not indicate that the mast cells are functionally active.

In order to try and resolve this issue experiments in *N. brasiliensis*- and *T. spiralis*-infected rats and mice demonstrated that the cells were functionally active by detection of the secretion of proteases specific for mucosal mast cells into the gut lumen, tissue and serum. These data showed that rat mast cell protease II (RMCPII) in the rat [67] and MMCP1 in the mouse [68] were produced in highly elevated levels following infection whereas uninfected animals had negligible levels.

Interestingly, in addition to normal expulsion of parasites, FcγR chain KO mice infected with *T. spiralis* also secrete high levels of MMCPI into the serum reflecting functional activity of the elevated numbers of mast cells in the small intestine [unpubl. observations]. The absence of high affinity IgE receptors on mast cells in these animals again suggests that IgE mediated activation of mucosal mast cells is not necessary and raises the possibility that mast cells are activated by other routes during nematode infection, perhaps by cytokines or parasite secretions directly.

The function of the proteases released by activated mast cells in the gastrointestinal tract is the subject of much speculation. Experiments with RMCPII, which is found in abundance in mucosal mast cells of rats have suggested that laminin and collagen type IV components of the basement membrane in the gut may be potential targets [69]. Recent work from the *N. brasiliensis* system has further shown that release of RMCPII is associated with the rapid development of macromolecular permeability through the epithelium of the intestine in the apparent absence of changes in structural integrity of the gut [70]. The target molecule(s) of the protease remain to be identified, however.

Mast Cells and Host Protection

The generation of a leaky gut through the action of mast cell proteases may be a mechanism by which mast cells may contribute to the expulsion of parasites from the intestine. Indeed the non-specific inflammatory response mediated (at least in part) has long been thought to play a role in the expulsion of several gastrointestinal dwelling nematodes. This has been most consistently shown for *T. spiralis* infections in the mouse. Infections of W/W^v mice which are mast cell deficient have a much delayed expulsion of the parasites from the gut when compared to their mast-cell-competent littermates [65].

These latter exeriments have interesting parallels with studies in the *N. brasiliensis* system in mice and rats. Unlike *T. spiralis* infections, *N. brasiliensis* infections are readily expelled from WW^v mice [71], suggesting that mast cells are not important in resistance to this nematode. Such data are in accordance with studies in which in vivo neutralisation of IL-3 and IL-4 during infection severely depresses the intestinal mastocytosis normally observed but has no effect upon worm expulsion [72]. Also, *N. brasiliensis*-infected rats treated with a polyclonal anti-SCF antiserum depressed the intestinal mast cell hyperplasia observed but had no effect on worm expulsion [73]. These latter studies add to the hypothesis that mast cell hyperplasia and mast cell activity are not major mechanisms involved in resistance to *N. brasiliensis*. Also, interestingly, mast cells do not appear to play a protective role during expulsion of *T. muris* and appear more to reflect the generation of a Th2 reponse [Else, pers. commun.].

T. spiralis, however, may not be the only nematode which may be removed from the gut through mast cell action. A number of interesting studies have been carried out in the *H. polygyrus* system which implicate mast cells as a mechanism of resistance. Primary infections of *H. polygyrus* in most mouse strains are long lasting (many months) although some strains do eventually begin to lose their worms [74]. Analysis of antibody isotype responses suggests that the immune reponse to *H. polygyrus* is predominantly controlled by Th2 cells with elevated IgG1 and IgE levels in the serum of infected mice (indeed there is no detectable IgG2a response; Th1 controlled) [75]. A striking feature, however, is the low level of intestinal mastocytosis accompanying a primary infection [76].

The functional significance of the low mast cell response can be demonstrated from co-infection studies in which expulsion of *T. spiralis* is delayed in *H. polygyrus*-infected mice and this was associated with a depressed intestinal mastocytosis when compared to mice infected with *T. spiralis* alone. A closer examination of cytokine production during infection showed that in mice infected with *T. spiralis* alone elevated levels of the mast-cell-promoting cytokines IL-3, IL-4, IL-9 and IL-10 were produced by mesenteric lymph node cells after in vitro stimulation by mitogen. In mice concurrently infected with both parasites, however, lower levels of IL-9 and IL-10 were observed early after infection [77]. These studies suggest that a differential downregulation of some of the Th2-associated cytokines by *H. polygyrus* may be enough to prevent a potentially effective effector mechanism from developing.

Such hypotheses are strengthened by experiments investigating Th cell cytokine responses during *H. polygyrus* infection in mouse strains which eventually do expel *H. polygyrus*. In strains which expel their parasites, a mucosal mast cell response is eventually generated and this is reflected in the ability to maintain high IL-3 and IL-9 production in comparison with strains which do not expel their worms and do not mount a pronounced mast cell response [75].

Taken together, these data suggest that mast cells may indeed play a protective role in resistance to *H. polygyrus* in situations where worm expulsion occurs, i.e. in the challenge model or during a primary infection of 'responder' mouse strains. It also highlights the observation that a long-lasting or chronic infection by gastrointestinal nematodes can occur during what at first glance appears to be a dominant Th2-mediated immune response. Closer examination, however, suggests that in these situations there may be selective downregulation of certain Th2-associated responses which prevent the appropriate effector mechanism from developing. This kind of observation may have particular relevance to some of the chronic intestinal nematode infections of humans where there are certainly data to show that some Th2-controlled responses are stimulated even though the parasites are still present in the intestine [32].

Intestinal Goblet Cells in Host Protection

A number of other studies using a different approach have also demonstrated a dichotomy in expulsive mechanisms operating against different intestinal dwelling nematodes. Nawa et al.[78] have conducted a number of experiments using *N. brasiliensis* and *Strongyloides* sp. Their data suggest that expulsion of *Strongyloides* is mediated by intestinal mast cells whereas *N. brasiliensis* is mediated by mucins released from goblet cells. Elegant co-infection studies with these two species showed that in situations where goblet cell hyperplasia was observed *N. brasiliensis* but not *Strongyloides* was expelled [79].

More recently this group has shown that changes in the terminal sugars of mucins released by goblet cells and the quantity of mucin produced during infection may be under immunological control [80]. Little is known about the cytokine mediated control of goblet cells and mucin production but it is reasonable to suppose that Th2 cytokines may play a role. This can be inferred from studies showing that CsA treatment of *T. spiralis* infected mice caused a reduction in the goblet cell hyperplasia which accompanies infection [6]. Certainly a role for CD4+ T cells has been implicated in the quantity of mucin produced during intestinal nematode infection [81].

Induction of Th2 Cell Responses during Intestinal Nematode Infection

It is thus quite clear that Th cell responses (through the induction of appropriate effector mechanisms) play a major role in the pathophysiology of intestinal nematode infection. It is also becoming quite clear that the Th2 type response appears to be the dominant type of Th cell subset activated following intestinal nematode infection. This raises the question of the mechanism whereby such Th2 cells are activated.

There is intense interest in this area which has resulted in a number of hypotheses all centered around the induction or production of IL-4 by various accessory cells involved in the early activation of T cells. There are a number of studies which show that the antigen-presenting cell type can influence the activation of Th cell subsets. Briefly, presentation of antigen by macrophages is believed to favour induction of Th1 cell responses whereas antigen presentation by B cells induces Th2-type responses [82]. This also appears to hold true when antigen is initially presented by dendritic cells [83].

This kind of analysis was also extended to the influence of particular co-stimulatory molecules expressed by antigen-presenting cells. Most notably there is emerging evidence to suggest that stimulation through the CD28/CTLA4/B7 axis may be of prime importance [84]. Data from models of autoimmunity in mice strongly suggest that signalling through B7-1 preferentially stimulates a Th1-type response whereas stimulation through B7-2 induces a dominant Th2 response [85, 86]. With regard to intestinal helminth infection, there are data to show that treatment of *H. polygyrus*-infected mice with a soluble construct of CTLA4 caused a downregulation in a number of Th2 cytokine genes and IgE production and eosinophilia in vivo [87]. The importance of B7-2 has also been implicated from studies of the *T. muris* system in which in vivo administration of blocking anti-B7-2 monoclonal antibodies to normally resistant mice changed the Th cell response from a dominant Th2 response into one dominated by Th1 cells with the resultant change in response phenotype of the mice to chronic infection [unpubl. observations].

Recent data also provide evidence to show that the binding affinity of antigenic peptides for MHC class II molecules can influence the type of Th response generated with lower class II binding affinity peptides preferentially inducing Th2 type responses [88]. This type of analysis has not been looked at in intestinal helminth infections to date.

Other cell types have been implicated in IL-4 production and thought to be involved in Th cell responses. One that has received considerable attention is the non-B, non-T, FcεRI+ cell [89]. These cells have been shown to produce considerable amounts of IL-4. Furthemore, *N. brasiliensis* infections in mice induce a considerable increase in the numbers of these cells in the spleen in comparison to non-infected animals, and such cells produce increased amounts of IL-4 on a cell per cell basis compared to naive animals [90].

In terms of responses induced in intestinal epithelium there have been interesting new data generated on IL-4 production by a population of NK1.1+ CD4+ αβ+ T cells. These cells are known to rapidly produce IL-4 following stimulation through CD3 and are related to a population of thymic NK1.1+ T cells that also rapidly produce cytokines upon stimulation [91]. Of greater interest is the fact that these cells are stimulated by CD1 molecules [92]. There is a family of CD1 molecules and they are found to be expressed on the cell surface of a number of species. Studies have shown that these molecules bear structural resemblances to MHC class I molecules and have been presumed to have an immunological function [93]. In mice the CD1 molecule is most prominently expressed upon gastrointestinal epithelium [94].

One of the most fascinating features of CD1 molecules is the nature of the antigens presented to NK1.1+ T cells. Although structurally related to MHC class I molecules, CD1 does not appear to present conventional peptides. Indeed, it appears likely that CD1 molecules do not present peptide at all but rather present lipid or glycolipid molecules [95]. The expression of CD1 by gut epithelium places this molecule in an ideal place to present antigen from intestinal dwelling helminths to NK1.1+ T cells and induce rapid IL-4 production. Their role in such infections, however, remains to be defined.

Other cell types are also well placed to play a role in the induction of Th cell response in the gut. These include γδ T cells which are present in high numbers within the intestinal tissue [96]. γδ T cells produce a variety of cytokines including IL-4 and could influence the development of Th cell responses [97]. Moreover, there are data to suggest that at least some γδ T cells can respond to antigen without the need for conventional processing of antigen [98]. Indeed, it is possible that γδ T cells may respond to antigen presented by CD1 [99]. Thus there are several possible cell types which could profoundly influence the development of Th2 responses.

Normal Control of Intestinal Epithelia by Lymphocytes

The gut has been quoted as the largest immune organ of the body and, therefore, it would not be unreasonable to suppose that lymphocytes are likely to play a significant role in the control of epithelial function. Accordingly, there have been a number of studies which have supported a role for T cells in the maintenance of normal mucosal architecture, with the T cell response to intestinal antigen playing a central role. This hypothesis has been given further support from recent studies in which CD45RBhi CD4+ T cells from normal BALB/c mice can induce colitis after transfer into C.B-17 SCID mice, but colitis can be prevented if CD45RBlo CD4+ T cells were co-transferred [100].

More recently, the intraepithelial T cell pool of the intestine has been characterised for a number of species with perhaps the best defined being the mouse. In adult mice, the intraepithelial T cell population is comparable in size to that of the spleen. This population consists of both αβ and γδ T cells with differences being found between the small and the large intestine [101]. The close association between intraepithelial T cells and the basolateral faces of epithelial cells suggests a functional interaction.

New data have suggested that the γδ T cell population plays a critical role in the generation of intestinal crypt cells and their migration onto the villi of the small intestine. Those data were obtained from δ chain TCR KO mice. Such animals had a reduction in crypt cell numbers and this was associated with a reduction in crypt cell proliferation. Downregulation of MHC class II molecules was also observed in these mice. These changes were not observed in mice with a targetted disruption of the β chain of the T cell receptor [102].

These data suggest that γδ T cells are posed to play an important role in the control of mucosal architecture, presumably through the secretion of cytokines. It is known that there are resident populations of γδ T cells within the gut as well populations that move in from parenteral sites [96]. The contribution of these different populations to epithelial changes under situations such as infection, however, remains to be defined. Nevertheless, it is reasonable to suggest that this population of cells is likely to play some role in the changes which are associated with intestinal helminth infection.

Lessons in Intestinal Pathology from Gene-Targetted Mice

Recently, a number of studies in gene-targetted mice have further empha-sised roles for the immune system in pathological changes seen in the gut and may have relevance to pathological changes induced by intestinal helminth infection. Mice with disruption of T cell receptor genes (e.g. α mutants, δ mutants, β mutants) or MHC class II mutants [103] show a fairly high interest of pathology similar to that seen in ulcerative colitis. Of perhaps greater incidence are mice with disruptions in the cytokine genes IL-2 [104] or IL-10 [105]. IL-2 deficient mice show a more pronounced pathology than TCR KO mice with a thickening of the bowel, ulcerations, infiltration of B cells into the mucosa, loss of goblet cells and general loss of normal crypt architecture [104]. IL-10 deficient mice differ from IL-2 KO mice in that the abnormalities are not restricted to the large bowel and are characterised by a generalised abnormality of the villus (atrophy) and crypts associated with pseudopolyps [105].

The value of these kinds of approaches is the definition of critical roles for immune cells and particular cytokines in the generation of intestinal pathology. It also raises the possibility that cytokines produced by immune cells in response to infection may have major effects upon the pathology of the intestine inducing effects directly or indirectly upon non-immune cells. In this respect interesting new data from both *N. brasiliensis* and *H. polygyrus* infections in SCID mice sug-gest that IL-4 may influence parasite survival by disturbing the local gut physiolo-gy without involving the classical immune response [106].

Overall, it can be seen from a variety of basic and applied studies that the pathology induced in the intestines of helminth-infected mice have a complex mechanistic basis. The full-blown response to natural infection will involve intes-tinal changes induced directly by parasite invasion through mechanical damage and secretion of tissue damaging enzymes by the parasite and immune-mediated changes generated predominantly through the secretion of cytokines by Th cells. With regard to the latter, it is also becoming increasingly clear that the immune system plays an important role in the 'normal' regulatory process of the intestine through the secretion of cytokines. Disturbance of this normal homeostatic mech-anism through the production of the anti-parasite immune responses undoubted-ly plays a major role in the pathological changes observed in the gut following infection some of which will contribute to host-protective immunity.

Acknowledgements

I would like to thank Michael Meredith for his help in the preparation of the manuscript, David Artis for figure 1, John Huntley for figure 2 and all my colleagues in Manchester for their helpful discussions and permission to quote unpublished data.

References

1   Chan MS, Medley GF, Jaimson P, Bundy DAP: The evaluation of potential global morbidity attributable to intestinal nematode infections. Parasitology 1994;109:373–387.
2   Ferguson A, Jarrett EEE: Hypersensitivity reactions in the small intestine. I. Thymus dependence of experimental 'partial villous atrophy'. Gut 1975;16:114–117.
3   Manson-Smith DF, Bruce RG, Parrott DMV: Villous atrophy and expulsion of intestinal *Trichinella spiralis* are mediated by T cells. Cell Immunol 1979;47:285–292.
4   Ruitenberg EJ, Leenstra F, Elgersma A: Thymus dependence and independence of intestinal pathology in a *Trichinella spiralis* infection: A study in congenially athymic (nude) mice. Br J Exp Pathol 1977;58:311–314.
5   Piguet PF, Grau GE, Allet B, Vassalli P: Tumor necrosis factor/cachectin is an effector of skin and gut lesions of the acute phase of graft vs. host disease. J Exp Med 1987;166:1280–1289.
6   Garside P, Grencis RK, McI Mowat A: T lymphocyte dependent enteropathy in murine *Trichinella spiralis* infection. Parasite Immunol 1992;14:217–225.
7   Pritchard DI: The survival strategies of hookworms. Parasitol Today 1995;11:255–259.
8   Drake L, Korchev Y, Bashford L, Djamgoz M, Wakelin D, Ashall F, Bundy D: The major secreted product of the whipworm Trichuris is a pore-forming protein. Proc R Soc Lond B 1994;257:255–261.
9   Lillywhite JE, Bundy DAP, Didier JM, Cooper ES, Bianco AE: Humoral immune responses in human infection with the whipworm *Trichuris trichiura*. Parasite Imunol 1991;13:491–507.
10   Ogilvie BM, Love RJ: Co-operation between antibodies and cells in immunity to a nematode parasite. Transplant Rev 1974;19:147–168.
11   Nawa Y, Miller HRP: Adoptive transfer of the intestinal mast cell response in rats infected with *Nippostrongylus brasiliensis*. Cell Immunol 1979;42:225–239.
12   Urban JF Jr, Katona IM, Finkelman FD: *Heligmosomoides polygyrus:* CD4+ but not CD8+ T cells regulate the IgE response and protective immunity in mice. Exp Parasitol 1991;75:500–511.
13   Grencis RK, Reidlinger J, Wakelin D: L3T4 positive lymphoblasts are responsible for transfer of immunity to *Trichinella spiralis* in mice. Immunology 1985;56:213–218.
14   Bell RG, Korenaga M, Wang CH: Characterisation of a cell population in thoracic duct lymph which adoptively transfers rejection of adult *Trichinella spiralis* to normal rats. Immunology 1987;61:221–227.
15   Reidlinger J, Grencis RK, Wakelin D: Antigen specific T cell lines transfer immunity against *Trichinella spiralis* in vivo. Immunology 1986;58:57–61.
16   Lee TDG, Grencis RK, Wakelin D: Cellular mechanisms of immunity to the nematode *Trichuris muris*. Int J Parasitol 1983;13:349–353.
17   Koyama K, Tamanchi H, Ito Y: The role of CD4+ and CD8+ T cells in protective immunity to the murine parasite *Trichuris muris*. Parasite Immunol 1995;17:161–165.
18   Bell RG, Issekutz T: Expression of a protective intestinal immune response can be inhibited at 3 distinct sites by treatment with anti-α4 integrin. J Immunol 1993;151:4790–4802.
19   Mosmann TR, Coffman RL: Th1 and Th2 cells: Different patterns of lymphokine secretion lead to different functional properties. Annu Rev Immunol 1989;7:145–173.
20   Scott P, Natovitz P, Coffman RL, Pearce E, Sher A: Immunoregulation of cutaneous leishmaniasis. T cell lines that transfer protective immunity or exacerbation belong to different T helper subsets and respond to distinct parasite antigens. J Exp Med 1988;168:1675–1684.

21 Heinzel FP, Sadick MD, Holaday BJ, Coffman RL, Locksley RM: Reciprocal expression of interferon γ or interleukin 4 during the resolution of progression of murine leishmaniasis. Evidence for expansion of distinct T cell subsets. J Exp Med 1989;169:59–72.

22 Finkelman FD, Urban JF Jr: Cytokines: Making the right choice. Parasitol Today 1992;8:311–314.

23 Pearce EJ, Reiner SL: Induction of Th2 responses in infectious disease. Curr Opin Immunol 1995; 7:497–504.

24 Locksley RM: Th2 cells: Help for helminths. J Exp Med 1994;179:1405–1407.

25 Grencis RK: T cell and cytokine basis of host variability in response to intestinal nematode infections. Parasitology, in press.

26 Ogilvie BM, Jones VE: Passive protection with cells or antiserum against *Nippostrongylus brasiliensis* in the rat. Parasitology 1968;58:939–949.

27 Williams DJ, Behnke JM: Host protective antibodies and serum immunoglobulin isotypes in mice chronically infected or repeatedly immunised with the nematode parasite *Nematospiroides dubius.* Immunology 1983;48:37–47.

28 Selby GR, Wakelin D: Transfer of immunity against *Trichuris muris* in the mouse by serum and cells. Int J Parasitol 1973;3:717–722.

29 Roach TIA, Else KJ, Wakelin D, Mclaren DJ, Grencis RK: *Trichuris muris:* Antigen recognition and transfer of immunity in mice by IgA monoclonal antibodies. Parasite Immunol 1991;13:1–12.

30 Urban JF Jr, Katona IM, Paul WE, Finkelman FD: Interleukin 4 is important in protective immunity to a gastrointestinal nematode infection in mice. Proc Natl Acad Sci USA 1991;88:5513–5517.

31 Else KJ, Finkelman FD, Maliszewski CR, Grencis RK: Cytokine mediated regulation of chronic intestinal helminth infection. J Exp Med 1994;179:347–351.

32 Grencis RK, Cooper ES: Enterobius, Trichuris, Capillaria and Hookworm including *Ancylostoma caninum*. Clin Gastroenterol N Am, in press.

33 Finkelman FD, Madden KB, Cheever AW, Katona IM, Morris SC, Gately MK, Hubbard BR, Gause WC, Urban JF Jr: Effects of interleukin 12 on immune responses and host protection in mice infected with intestinal nematode parasites. J Exp Med 1994;179:1563–1572.

34 Wakelin D: Allergic inflammation as a hypothesis for the expulsion of worms from tissues. Parasitol Today 1993;9:115–116.

35 Katona IM, Urban JF Jr, Finkelman FD: The role of L3T4+ and Ly2+ T cells in the IgE response and immunity to *Nippostrongylus brasiliensis.* J Immunol 1988;140:3206–3211.

36 Kopf M, Le Gros G, Bachmann M, Lamers MC, Bleuthmann H, Kohler G: Disruption of the murine IL-4 gene blocks Th2 cytokine response. Nature 1993;362:245–248.

37 Harari Y, Russell DA, Castro GA: Anaphylaxis mediated Cl⁻ secretion and parasite rejection in rat intestine. J Immunol 1987;138:1250–1255.

38 Appleton JA, Schain LR, McGregor DD: Rapid expulsion of *Trichinella spiralis* in suckling rats: Mediation by monoclonal antibodies. Immunology 1988;65:487–492.

39 Moqbel R, Wakelin D, MacDonald AJ, King SJ, Grencis RK, Kay AB: Release of leukotrienes during rapid expulsion of *Trichinella spiralis* from immune rats. Immunology 1987;60:425–430.

40 Bell RG: *Trichinella spiralis:* Evidence that mice do not express rapid expulsion. Exp Parasitol 1992;74:417–430.

41 Rennick DM, Lee FD, Yokota T, Arai, K, Cantor H, Nabel GJ: A cloned MCGF cDNA encodes a multilineage hemopoietic growth factor: Multiple activities of interleukin 3. J Immunol 1985;134: 910–914.

42 Rennick DM, Young G, Muller-Seiburg C, Smith C, Arai N, Tanabe Y, Gemmell L: Interleukin 4 (B cell stimulatory factor 1) can enhance or antagonise the factor-dependent growth of hemopoietic progenitor cells. Proc Natl Acad Sci USA 1987:84:6889–6893.

43 Hültner L, Druez C, Moeller J, Uyutenhove C, Schmitt E, Rüde E, Dörmer P, Van Snick J: Mast cell growth-enhancing activity (MEA) is structurally related and functionally identical to the novel mouse T cell growth factor P40/TCGF III (interleukin 9). Eur J Immunol 1990;20:1413–1416.

44 Thompson-Snipes LA, Dhar V, Bond MW, Mosmann TR, Moore KW, Rennick DM: Interleukin 10: A novel stimulatory factor for mast cells and their progenitors. J Exp Med 1991;173:507–510.

45   Miller HRP: Mast cells in the gastrointestinal tract; in Foreman: Immunopharmacology of Mast Cells and Basophils. Academic Press, 1993, pp 197–215.

46   Sredni B, Friedman MM, Bland CE, Metcalfe DD: Ultrastructural, biochemical and functional characteristics of histamine-containing cells cloned from bone marrow: Tentative identification as mucosal mast cells. J Immunol 1983;131:915–921.

47   Tsuji K, Zsebo KM, Ogawa M: Murine mast cell colony formation supported by IL-3 and IL-4 and recombinant rat stem cell factor, ligand for c-*kit*. J Cell Physiol 1991;148:362–369.

48   Hültner L, Moeller J, Schmitt E, Jäge G, Reisbach G, Ring J, Dörmer P: Thiol-sensitive mast cell lines derived from mouse bone marrow respond to a mast cell growth enhancing activity different from both IL-3 and IL-4. J Immunol 1989;142:3440–3446.

49   Hültner L, Moeller J: Mast cell growth enhancing activity (MEA) stimulates interleukin 6 production in a mouse bone marrow derived mast cell line and a malignant subline. Exp Hematol 1990;18:873–877.

50   Ghildyal N, McNeil HP, Gurish MF, Austen KF, Stevens RL: Transcriptional regulation of the mucosal mast cell specific protease gene, MMCP-2, by interleukin 10 and interleukin 3. J Biol Chem 1992;12:8473–8477.

51   Ghildyal N, McNeil HP, Stechsschulte S, Austen KF, Silberstein D, Gurish MF, Somerville LL, Stevens RL: IL-10 induces transcription of the gene for mouse mast cell protease 1, a serine protease preferentially expressed in mucosal mast cells of *Trichinella spiralis* infected mice. J Immunol 1992; 149:2123–2129.

52   Newlands GFJ, Lammas DA, Huntley JF, Mackellar A, Wakelin D, Miller HRP: Heterogeneity of murine bone marrow derived mast cells: Analysis of their proteinase content. Immunology 1991;72: 434–439.

53   Gurish MF, Pear WS, Stevens RL, Scott ML, Sokol K, Ghildyal N, Webster MJ, Hu X, Austen KF, Baltimore D, Friend DS: Tissue regulated differentiation and maturation of a v-abl-immortalized mast cell committed progenitor. Immunity 1995;3:175–186.

54   Lantz CS, Huff TF: Differential responsiveness of purified mouse c-*kit*+ mast cells and their progenitors to IL-3 and stem cell factor. J Immunol 1995;155:4024–4029.

55   Gordon JR, Burd PR, Galli SJ: Mast cells as a source of multifunctional cytokines. Immunol Today 1990;11:458–464.

56   Galli SJ, Geissler EN, Zsebo KM: The kit ligand, stem cell factor. Adv Immunol 1994;55:1.

57   Grencis RK, Else KJ, Huntley JF, Nishikawa S: The in vivo role of stem cell factor (c-*kit* ligand) on mastocytosis and host protective immunity to the nematode *Trichinella spiralis* in mice. Parasite Immunol 1993;15:55–61.

58   Donaldson LE, Schmitt E, Huntley JF, Newlands GFJ, Grencis RK: A critical role for stem cell factor and c-*kit* in host protective immunity to an intestinal helminth. Int Immunol 1996;8.

59   Williams DE, Eisenman J, Baird A, Rauch C, Ness KV, Cosman D, Lyman SD: Identification of ligand for c-*kit* proto-oncogene. Cell 1990;63:167–174.

60   Flanagan JG, Leder P: A cell surface molecule altered in steel mutant fibroblasts. Cell 1990;63: 185–191.

61   Zsebo KM, Williams DA, Geissler EN, Broudy VC, Martin FH, Atkins HL, Hsu RY, Birkett NC, Okino KH, Murdock DC, Jacobson FW, Langley KE, Smith KA, Takeishi T, Cattanach BM, Galli DSJ, Suggs SV: Stem cell factor is encoded at the *Sl* locus of the mouse and its ligand for the c-*kit* tyrosine kinase receptor. Cell 1990;63:213–224.

62   Huang E, Nocka K, Beier DR, Chu Ty, Buck J, Lahm HW, Wellner D, Leder P, Besmer P: The hematopoietic growth factor KL is encoded by the *Sl* locus and is the ligand of the the c-*kit* receptor, the gene product of the *W* locus. Cell 1990;63:225–232.

63   Nocka K, Tan JC, Chiu E, Chu TY, Ray P, Traktman P, Besmer P: Molecular bases of dominant negative and loss of function mutations at the murine c-*kit*/white spoting locus:W37, Wv, W41 and W. EMBO J 1990;9:1805–1813.

64   Kitamura Y, Go S, Hatanaka K: Decrease of mast cells in W/Wv mice and their increase by bone marrow transplantation. Blood 1978;52:447–452.

65   Alizadeh H, Wakelin D: The intestinal mast cell response to *T. spiralis* infection in mast cell deficient W/Wv mice. J Parasitol 1984;70:767–771.

66 Smith TJ, Weis JH: Mucosal T cells and mast cells share common adhesion receptors. Immunol Today 1996;17:60–63.

67 Woodbury, RG, Miller, HRP, Huntley, JF, Newlands GFJ, Palliser AC, Wakelin D: Mucosal mast cells are functionally active during the spontaneous expulsion of intestinal nematode infections in the rat. Nature 1984;312:450–452.

68 Tuohy M, Lammas DA, Wakelin D, Huntley JF, Newlands GFJ, Miller HRP: Functional correlations between mucosal mast cell activity and immunity to *Trichinella spiralis* in high and low responder mice. Parasite Immunol 1990;12:675–685.

69 King SJ, Miller HRP: Anaphylactic release of mucosal mast cell protease and its relationship to gut permeability in *Nippostrongylus brasiliensis* primed rats. Immunology 1984;62:621–627.

70 Scudamore CL, Thornton EM, McMillan L, Newlands GFJ, Miller HRP: Release of the mucosal mast cell granule chymase, rat mast cell protease II during anaphylaxis is associated with the rapid development of paracellular permeability to macromolecules in rat jejunum. J Exp Med 1995;182: 1871–1881.

71 Crowle PK, Reed ND: Rejection of the intestinal parasite *Nippostrongylus brasiliensis* by mast cell deficient W/W^v anaemic mice. Infect Immun 1981;33:54–58.

72 Madden KB, Urban JF Jr, Ziltner HJ, Schrader JW, Finkelman FD, Katona IM: Antibodies to IL-3 and IL-4 suppress helminth induced intestinal mastocytosis. J Immunol 1991;147:1387–1394.

73 Newlands GFJ, Miller HRP, MacKellar A, Galli SJ: Stem cell factor contributes to intestinal mucosal mast cell hyperplasia in rats infected with *Nippostrongylus brasiliensis* or *Trichinella spiralis*, but anti-stem cell factor treatment decreases parasite egg production during *N. brasiliensis* infection. Blood 1995;86:1968–1976.

74 Wahid FN, Behnke JM: Immunological relationships during primary infection with with *Heligmosomoides polygyrus*. Regulation of fast response phenotype by H-2 and non-H-2 genes. Parasitology 1993;107:343–350.

75 Wahid FN, Behnke JM, Grencis RK, Else KJ, Ben-Smith AW: Immunological relationships during primary infection with *Heligmosomoides polygyrus:* Th2 cytokines and primary response phenotype. Parasitology 1994;108:461–471.

76 Dehlawi MS, Wakelin D, Behnke JM: Suppression of mucosal mastocytosis by infection with the intestinal nematode *Nematospiroides dubius*. Parasite Immunol 1987;12:561–566.

77 Behnke JM, Wahid FN, Grencis RK, Else KJ, Ben-Smith A, Goyal PK: Immunological relationships during primary infection with *Heligmosomoides polygyrus (Nematospiroides dubius)*: Down regulation of specific cytokine secretion (IL-9 and IL-10) correlates with poor mastocytosis and chronic survival of adult worms. Parasite Immunol 1993;15:415–421.

78 Nawa Y, Ishikawa N, Tsuchiya K, Horii Y, Abe T, Khan AI, Shi B, Itoh H, Ide H, Uchiyama F: Selective mechanisms for the expulsion of intestinal helminths. Parasite Immunol 1994;16:333–338.

79 Horri Y, Khan AI, Nawa Y: Persistent infection with *Strongyloides venezuelensis* and normal expulsion of *Nippostrongylus brasiliensis* in mongolian gerbils, *Meriones unguiculatus*, with reference to the cellular responses in the intestinal mucosa. Parasite Immunol 1993;15:175–179.

80 Ishikawa N, Horii Y, Nawa Y: Immune mediated alteration of the terminal sugars of goblet cell mucins in the small intestine of *Nippostrongylus brasiliensis* infected rats. Immunology 1993;78: 303–307.

81 Khan WI, Abe T, Ishikawa N, Nawa Y, Yoshimura K: Reduced amount of intestinal mucus treatment with anti-CD4 antibody interferes with the spontaneous cure of *Nippostrongylus brasiliensis* infection in mice. Parasite Immunol 1993;17:485–491.

82 Gajewski TF, Pinnas M, Wong T, Fitch FW: Murine Th1 and Th2 clones proliferate optimally in response to distinct antigen presenting cell populations. J Immunol 1991;146:1750–1758.

83 Stockinger B, Zal T, Zal A, Gray D: B cells solicit their own help from T cells. J Exp Med, in press.

84 Linsley PS, Ledbetter JA: The role of CD28 receptor during T cell response to antigen. Annu Rev Immunol 1993;11:191–212.

85 Kuchroo VK, Prabhu Das M, Brown JA, Ranger AM, Zamvil SS, Sobel RA, Weiner HL, Nabavi N, Glimcher LH: B7-1 and B7-2 costimulatory molecules activate differentially the Th1/Th2 developmental pathways: Application to autoimmune disease therapy. Cell 1995:80:707–718.

86 Freeman GJ, Boussiotis VA, Anumanthan A, Bernstein GM, Ke XY, Rennert PD, Gray GS, Gribben JG, Nadler LM: B7-1 and B7-2 do not deliver identical co-stimulatory signals since B7-2 but not B7-1 preferentially costimulates the initial production of IL-4. Immunity 1995;2:523–532.

87 Lu P, Di Hou X, Chen SJ, Moorman M, Morris SC, Finkelman FD, Linsley P, Urban JF, Gause WC: CTLA-4 ligands are required to induce an in vivo interleukin 4 response to a gastrointestinal nematode parasite. J Exp Med 1994;180:693–698.

88 Kumar V, Batsala B, Soares L, Alexander J, Sette A, Sercarz E: Major histocompatibility complex binding affinity of an antigenic determinant is crucial for the differential secretion of interleukin 4/5 or interferon γ by T cells. Proc Natl Acad Sci USA 1995;92:9510–9514.

89 Seder RA, Paul WE: Acquisition of lymphokine-producing phenotype by CD4+ T cells. Annu Rev Immunol 1994;12:635–674.

90 Conrod DH, Ben-Sasson SZ, Le Gros G, Finkelman FD, Paul WE: Injection with anti-IgD antibodies markedly enhances Fc receptor mediated interleukin 4 production by non B, non T cells. J Exp Med 1990;171:1497–1508.

91 Yoshimoto T, Bendalac A, Watson C, Hu-Li J, Paul WE: Role of NK1,1+ T cells in a Th2 response and in immunoglobulin E production. Science 1995;270:1845–1847.

92 Bendelac A, Lantz O, Quimby ME, Yewdell JW, Bennink JR, Brutkiewicz RR: CD1 recognition by mouse NK1+ T lymphocytes. Science 1995;268:863–865.

93 Porcelli SA, Modlin RL: CD1 and the expanding universe of T cell antigens. J Immunol 1995;155:3709–3710.

94 Porcelli S: The CD1 family: A third lineage of antigen presenting molecules. Adv Immunol 1995;59:1–28.

95 Sieling PA, Chaterjee D, Porcelli SA, Prigozy TI, Soriano T, Brenner MB, Kronenberg M, Brennen PJ, Modlin RL: Science 1995;269:227–230.

96 Haas W, Pereira P, Tonegawa S: Gamma/delta cells. Annu Rev Immunol 1993;11:637–686.

97 Doherty PC, Allan W, Eichelberger M, Carding SR: Roles of αβ and γδ T cell subsets in viral immunity. Annu Rev Immunol 1992;10;123–151.

98 Schild H, Mavaddat N, Litzenberger C, Ehrich EW, Davies MM, Bluestone JA, Matis L, Draper RK, Chien Y: The nature of major histocompatibility complex recognition by γδ T cells. Cell 1994;76:29–37.

99 Ferrick DA, Schrenzel MD, Mulvania T, Hseih B, Ferlin WG, Lepper H: Differential production of interferon γ and interleukin 4 in response to Th1 and Th2 stimulating pathogens by γδ T cells in vivo. Nature 1995;373:255–257.

100 Powrie F: T cells in inflammatory bowel disease: Protective and pathogenic roles. Immunity 1995;3:171–174.

101 Boll G, Rudolphi A, Spieß S, Reimann J: Regional specialisation of intraepithelial T cells in the murine small and large intestine. Scand J Immunol 1995;41:103–113.

102 Komano H, Fujiura Y, Kawaguchi M, Matsumoto S, Hashimoto Y, Obana S, Mombaerts P, Tonegawa S, Yamamoto H, Itohara S, Nanno M, Ishikawa H: Homeostatic regulation of intestinal epithelia by intraepithelial γδ T cells. Proc Natl Acad Sci USA 1995;92:6147–6151.

103 Momaerts P, Mizoguchi E, Grusby MJ, Glimcher LH, Bahn AK, Tonegawa S: Spontaneous development of inflammatory bowel disease in T cell receptor mutant mice. Cell 1993;75:275–282.

104 Sadlack B, Merz H, Schorle H, Schimpf A, Feller AC, Hovak I: Ulcerative colitis disease in mice with a disrupted interleukin 2 gene. Cell 1993;75:253–262.

105 Kuhn R, Lohler J, Rennick D, Rajewsky K, Muller W: Interleukin 10 deficient mice develop chronic enteridites. Cell 1993;75:263–274.

106 Urban JF Jr, Maliszewski CR, Madden KB, Katona IM, Finkelman FD: IL-4 treatment can cure established gastrointestinal nematode infection in immunocompetent and immunodeficient mice. J Immunol 1995;154:4675–4680.

R.K. Grencis, School of Biological Sciences, 3.239 Stopford Building, University of Manchester, Oxford Road, Manchester, M13 9PT (UK)

Freedman DO (ed): Immunopathogenetic Aspects of Disease Induced by Helminth Parasites.
Chem Immunol. Basel, Karger, 1997, vol 66, pp 62–98

....

Pathogenesis of Human Hookworm Infection: Insights from a 'New' Zoonosis

Paul Prociv

Department of Parasitology, The University of Queensland, Brisbane, Australia

Introduction and Historical Outline

Hookworms are members of the strongylid nematode family, Ancylostomatidae, which includes 18 genera found in a wide range of mammalian hosts [1]. They tend to be highly host specific. The anthropophilic species, *Ancylostoma duodenale* and *Necator americanus*, are endemic in most warm-temperate regions, and infect perhaps 20% of the global human population [2]. A parasite of dogs and cats in Asia, *Ancylostoma ceylanicum*, also matures in the human intestine and so is included here, although its geographical distribution and public health impact are limited. Human infections with these species have been reviewed comprehensively in recent years [3–7].

A recent fundamental discovery in hookworm biology is larval hypobiosis, with all its ramifications (see below). Also important has been the finding that *Ancylostoma caninum*, the most widespread hookworm species, is a human enteric pathogen. It had been presumed incapable of 'normal' migration in man [8], despite sporadic reports of its occurrence in the human intestine [6, 9]. Its pathogenicity was first mooted in 1988, with the finding of a hookworm in histological sections from a patient with eosinophilic enteritis (EE) in tropical Australia [10]. Shortly afterwards, an intact worm was found in another patient and confirmed to be *A. caninum* [11].

EE involves predominantly the small intestine [10,12,13], is characterised histologically by intense eosinophilic infiltration, and is usually accompanied by raised blood eosinophil counts and IgE levels. The aetiology is uncertain; food allergy is often invoked, but rarely confirmed [11,14]. Speculating that some cases result from allergy to hookworm secretions, our group sought, and found, circulating IgG and IgE antibodies to excretory-secretory antigens of adult *A. caninum* in typical patients [15]. Subsequently, a component of molecular weight 68 kD (Ac68) was identified as the most reliable diagnostic antigen [16]. Solitary, not fully mature, adult hookworms have now been found in 15 patients, including those reported previously [9, 13] from Queensland, and serological and colonoscopic findings suggest that infection, both clinical and subclinical, is very common (see below).

The initial conclusion was simple: canine hookworms provoke excessive responses in unsuitable hosts. The general belief is that anthropophilic species in humans do not cause intense inflammation. However, the detailed review presented here contradicts such popular views. Comparison of the clinical, pathological and immunological features of canine and anthropophilic hookworm infections, from larval invasion through to events in the gut, provides novel insights into their molecular pathogenesis, as well as directions for future research. The focus is on human infection, although occasional reference to experimental animal findings is unavoidable.

Larval Invasion

In all described hookworm life cycles, the host skin seems to provide the major, if not exclusive, invasion portal. *A. duodenale*, but not *N. americanus*, also establishes successfully after oral ingestion of third-stage larvae (L3); pulmonary migration seems obligatory for the latter species [7]. It has been proposed (without evidence) that the peroral route is important for *A. duodenale* [17]. Larval invasion of the skin can be asymptomatic, or manifest as cutaneous larva migrans of two distinct patterns: static, maculopapular lesions (ground itch), or progressive, serpiginous, linear rashes (creeping eruption). Having penetrated the skin, L3 may perish or persist there, or proceed into either blood or lymphatic vessels, ultimately reaching the pulmonary circulation. There, they can either perforate alveoli (en route to the gut, by tracheo-oesophageal migration), or proceed into the systemic circulation, thence somatic migration and tissue hypobiosis.

Cutaneous Manifestations
Canine Hookworms. Cutaneous lesions indicating larval invasion have not yet been reported by any patient with EE. Skin invasion by *A. caninum* typically causes ground itch, which becomes evident only with repeated exposure, when lesions increase in severity and can be exacerbated by bacterial invasion [5]. The number of lesions represents about 10–15% of the applied L3 dose (volunteer studies, see below, '*A. caninum* Eosinophilic Enteritis in Humans'), and they

centre on hair follicles, lasting up to 1 week. Larvae are rarely found in biopsies. After heavy exposure (1,000 L3 or more), lesions can persist or recur for extended periods, sometimes developing into short, discontinuous creeping eruptions [5, 8, 18–21]. Superimposed, rapidly migratory, urticarial wheals may confuse the picture, as can secondary bacterial infection [5, 20]. Discontinuity of burrows has been attributed to L3 penetrating deeper tissues then resurfacing at distant points [8].

Only *Ancylostoma braziliense* produces classical creeping eruption [22, 23]. Biopsies may show tunnels in the epidermis and underlying dermis, and intense cellular infiltration, especially by eosinophils [22, 24]. L3 are found rarely, in the deep epidermis, superficial dermis, hair follicles or sweat ducts. Individual lesions can persist and progress intermittently for months, but total numbers spontaneously decline about 50% with each passing week [25].

Anthropophilic Hookworms. Ground itch, the typical response to all three species, first alerted Looss, in 1898, to the mechanism of skin invasion by *A. duodenale* [7]. Initial penetration by either *N. americanus* or *A. duodenale* is often asymptomatic [8, 9, 26–30]. Local prickling commences as early as 5–10 min after exposure, with itchy macules evident by 30 min [27, 31]. On open skin, lesions involve hair follicles, although under swabs or wet clothes, the papules distribute randomly [27, 32], confirming that L3 need leverage against surface films, clothing, abrasions or hair follicles to invade. Numbers of lesions can vary from 15 to 80% of an applied L3 dose [27, 33, 34]. Severity and duration of lesions increase with repeated exposure, leading, in extreme cases, to severe urticaria and oedema, with vesiculation that appears purulent from numerous eosinophils [2, 35]. This hypersensitivity to L3 can persist for years. Only 25% of soldiers suffering acute abdominal symptoms from *A. duodenale* reported ground itch (although 70% had respiratory symptoms; see below, 'Anthropophilic Hookworms') [36].

A. ceylanicum occasionally causes ground itch [4, 37], intensified by repeated exposure. Short linear lesions can develop, persisting up to 3 weeks [37–39]. However, no patients infected in New Guinea recalled any skin rashes [40].

Pulmonary Manifestations
Zoonotic Hookworms. Respiratory symptoms have not preceded EE attributed to *A. caninum* infection, and only once have cough, chest pain and radiological abnormalities been categorically linked to (very heavy) exposure to this species [5]. However, in 2 volunteers who developed severe cutaneous reactions after exposure to 1,000–1500 L3, swellings and burrows recurred at the inoculation sites over the ensuing months, coinciding with symptoms of 'upper respiratory tract infection' [20]; these might have reflected L3 mobilisation and subsequent pulmonary migration (see below, 'Zoonotic Hookworms').

Pulmonary abnormalities more frequently accompany creeping eruption attributed to *A. braziliense*, even in light infections. In 26 (50%) of 52 patients, patchy, transient, migratory infiltrates appeared in chest X-rays 7 or more days after the rash commenced, and persisted for several weeks (in 1 case, from 59 to 89 days after exposure) [41]. Only 9 had mild cough, but none had abnormal chest signs. Blood eosinophilia developed in most, and lasted 4–6 weeks, with eosinophils in the sputum of some. Other case reports of Loeffler's syndrome with creeping eruption indicate that symptoms start from about 7 days after exposure and can persist for more than 4 months [42, 43]; several authors suspected that transient pulmonary opacities indicated allergy to rather than trauma from migrating larvae.

Heavy exposure to either *A. caninum* nor *A. braziliense* may give rise to atypical cutaneous lesions. In a notable case [44], extensive soil contact was followed by severe itching and a diffuse papular rash, complicated 1 week later by dyspnea, wheezing and productive cough. All sputum examined until the 36th post-exposure day contained hookworm L3 of uncertain species. Respiratory signs and symptoms were most severe over weeks 2–3 after infection, yet repeated chest X-rays were clear. Truncated, tortuous tracks, extending slowly from some papules for less than 2.5 cm before gradually resolving, suggested not true creeping eruptions, but gross *A. caninum* exposure, complicated by urticaria and scratching. An intense blood eosinophilia was detected on day 19. Secondary bacterial infection was not excluded.

Anthropophilic Hookworms. Even light infection with *A. duodenale* or *N. americanus* can provoke respiratory symptoms. Laryngo-pharyngitis commences as early as 4 days, but usually about 1 week, after exposure [5, 27, 31, 32, 36, 45], and persists for another 1 week–3 months or more [27, 35, 36]. Among soldiers with abdominal symptoms of acute *A. duodenale* infection [36], 70% had complained of 'foxhole cough', yet chest radiography was invariably normal [46]. In therapeutic *A. duodenale* infection, afebrile tracheo-laryngo-pharyngitis developed 4–5 days after the percutaneous application of 400 L3 to patients [27]. Retrosternal pain and dry cough lasted up to 3 weeks, without clinical or radiological evidence of lower respiratory tract involvement. It was concluded that Loeffler's syndrome did not complicate *A. duodenale* infection, even when cutaneous reactions were severe; symptoms and pharyngeal congestion were attributed to mucosal re-invasion by L3 coughed up in sputum. Repeated infection caused chest pain rather than recurrence of duodenal pain (see below, 'Anthropophilic Hookworm Infections').

However, lower respiratory involvement has been reported in heavily exposed residents of an *A. duodenale*-endemic area [35]. Severe wheezing, dyspnoea and/or productive cough persisted 3 months on average, although continuing re-exposure and probable bacterial superinfection complicated interpretation. In an autopsy study of debilitated children infected with *A. duodenale* [47], pulmonary disease was found in 14/21, but generally reflected bacterial co-infection; invasive larvae were identified in the haemorrhagic lungs of only 1 child.

In Japan, ingested *A. duodenale* L3 were causally implicated in Wakana disease [48]. Nausea, salivation and vomiting occurred soon after eating leafy vegetables, followed a few days later by throat discomfort, dysphonia, wheezing and cough, which was productive in almost 50% cases and lasted for 3 weeks or more. Hookworm larvae were found in sputum, associated with blood eosinophilia and transient infiltrations in the chest X-rays. In almost every case, patent infection and severe anaemia, if not present initially, developed subsequently. Because the disease occasionally followed ingestion of cooked vegetables, it was attributed to allergy to larval products rather than migratory trauma.

The manifestations of *N. americanus* infection are similar. Cough developed within 6 days of percutaneous exposure to 45 L3 in 21% of 29 subjects, and persisted over 4 weeks in some; sore throats and haemoptysis were reported in the second week [34]. Even symptom-free volunteers had mucosal erythema at bronchoscopy 2–8 days after exposure [49].

With *A. ceylanicum*, one subject developed a sore throat and dry cough at 12 days after exposure [4], although 10 others, including 2 exposed to heavy infection (1,200 clean L3 each), did not experience any respiratory symptoms [37, 50].

Larval Hypobiosis

Zoonotic Hookworms. Sporadic re-activation of hypobiotic larvae probably underlies recurrent EE in patients who avoid further exposure to *A. caninum* [11, 51], and might explain the seasonal variation in incidence of EE in Townsville [52, 53]. In dogs, *A. caninum* L3 undergo developmental arrest, in either the intestine or skeletal muscle, by mechanisms that are obscure [54–56] but related to age resistance. In older dogs, fewer invading larvae develop into adult worms, while the remainder probably migrate somatically. They must be able to recognise molecular configurations in skeletal muscle capillaries, penetrate muscle cells and then shut down metabolically. If acquired immunity is involved, its role is unclear [55, 57].

One human case report, and occasional rodent studies, indicate that larvae within skeletal muscle cells elicit minimal inflammation. However, myositis was diagnosed clinically in a man with weakness, tiredness and painful leg muscle swelling after heavy exposure to larvae, presumably of *A. caninum* [58]. Cutaneous lesions, respiratory symptoms and blood eosinophilia were documented shortly after exposure, and a muscle biopsy 3 months later yielded one L3 in 250 sections. In a similar case, pain in back muscles beneath the affected skin responded rapidly to thiabendazole treatment [21], again suggesting local invasion. It is not known whether larvae penetrate muscles after circulatory dispersal, or, as suspected from experimental rodents, directly through overlying skin [59].

Dormant L3 appear to have an intrinsic 'clock' that is overridden by host factors. Their mobilisation seems unaffected by immunity or the presence of adult worms in the canine gut [55, 56], but fluctuates seasonally. In post-parturient bitches, hormonal changes stimulate larval migration to the mammary glands [57, 60], leading to patent infection in the pups.

Larval hypobiosis in the skin (rather than 'resurfacing' at distant points [8]) might explain the discontinuous lesions that follow heavy exposure to *A. caninum* (see above, 'Anthrophilic Hookworms') and the persistence of multiple L3 in human hair follicles 4 weeks after infection [21]. With the passage of many L3 through one follicle, an accumulation of inhibitory secretions could induce hypobiosis in late comers. Gradual dissipation of suppressor molecules would then allow some L3 to remobilise, provoking new skin lesions but again inhibiting their competitors. Immune mechanisms are unlikely to arrest L3 in hair follicles so early after exposure. Such larval congregation also occurs in canine hair follicles [61]. The confusing findings from numerous skin penetration studies in other laboratory animals [8] may reflect such inter-larval competition in high-dose infections.

Anthropophilic Hookworms. Larval hypobiosis seems to occur with *A. duodenale* in most endemic regions [4, 31, 33, 62, 63]. Respiratory symptoms 1–2 weeks after self-infection confirmed larval migration through the lungs [31], while a rising blood eosinophilia 8 months later, 4 weeks preceding the onset of patency, indicated renewed development of worms in the gut [33]. Relapse of acute abdominal symptoms in another case, 12 months after initial exposure and treatment, flagged the reappearance of fertile worms in the intestine [62]. Severe neonatal infections suggest that maternal transmission, most likely transmammary, also occurs with *A. duodenale* [4, 63, 64], although larvae have never been detected in human milk. Rare case reports of melaena and patent infection in the first few days after birth [63], if reliable, indicate that transplacental transmission also occurs. This would require mobilisation of hypobiotic larvae during pregnancy, or placental invasion by newly acquired larvae. However, it could not be demonstrated in bitches exposed to *A. caninum* L3 in mid-gestation and at parturition [65]. Maternal transmission implies a tissue reservoir of hypobiotic larvae. Depot sites have not been identified in humans, but skeletal muscle has been implicated in paratenic hosts [66], consistent with the phylogenetic proximity of *A. duodenale* to *A. caninum* [17].

Intestinal Hookworm Infection

Clinical Features

A. caninum *Infection and Human Eosinophilic Enteritis.* Over the last 10 years, more than 300 cases of *A. caninum*-associated EE have been diagnosed in north-eastern Australia, with two now reported from the USA [67, 68]. Its presentation is variable [9, 10, 13, 51, 69], and most human infection with *A. caninum* probably is subclinical (see below).

The chief complaint is abdominal pain, reported in 75% of biopsy-confirmed cases [13]. It is often colicky, sometimes burning, usually exacerbated by food, generally begins in the epigastrium, moves to the central abdomen or right iliac fossa, and typically becomes chronic or recurs in episodes lasting up to a month. Commonly associated symptoms are anorexia, nausea and diarrhoea. Frank intestinal bleeding occurs rarely, probably arising from small bowel ulcers (see below, 'Human *A. caninum* Enteritis'). Extreme cases are typified by rapidly intensifying colic, suggesting small bowel obstruction or acute appendicitis, accompanied by transient blood neutrophilia that precedes a rising eosinophilia [69]. Severe illness rarely develops in patients who have chronic or recurrent symptoms. The episodes resolve spontaneously (or within 12 h of anthelminthic treatment) but recur in about 50% of cases, usually with diminishing intensity.

Serological evidence of hookworm infection was found in 30% of Townsville patients with undiagnosed abdominal pain and normal blood counts [51], and ELISA readings in people with enteric aphthous ulcers and petechial haemorrhages (presumptive hookworm 'bites') found at colonoscopy were generally higher than in the background population [53]. This suggests the infection is often asymptomatic, or causes abdominal pain without blood eosinophilia. A positive immunoblot in only 63% of histologically confirmed cases [13] indicates that *A. caninum* is not the exclusive cause of EE.

The other common canine hookworm, *A. braziliense*, is not a human intestinal pathogen; early suggestive reports were of misidentified *A. ceylanicum* [70].

Anthropophilic Hookworm Infections. Hookworm disease is usually defined as iron-deficiency anaemia, the major complication of persistent infection when host iron intake fails to match losses to an excessive worm burden [3, 6, 7, 17, 71]. Because the symptomatology of acute infection is often understated, Miller [5] advocated replacing the term 'hookworm disease' with specific reference to either primary (direct effects of worms) or secondary (e.g. anaemia and its consequences) manifestations of infection. Here, the primary effects of anthropophilic and *A. caninum* infections will be shown to be comparable, sharing the common basis of intestinal inflammation.

Numerous reports describe significant abdominal symptoms, predominantly in the early stages but also in chronic infection, accompanied by blood eosinophilia. With *A. duodenale*, pain commences usually during the third week after exposure, when any respiratory symptoms begin to settle [5, 27, 32, 36, 72]. Nausea and vomiting are common. The clinical picture can be indistinguishable from the above description, and pain intensity may justify narcotics for relief [5, 27, 32, 36, 46]. Diarrhoea can be incapacitating, even with a small worm burden [27, 36]. The barium meal may be abnormal in 60% of symptomatic cases [46]. Symptoms gradually resolve spontaneously, usually by 6 weeks (but rapidly after anthelminthic treatment) and, with repeated infections, decline in severity [27]. After very heavy acute exposure, especially in children, melaena or severe, life-threatening, intestinal haemorrhage can occur before the infection becomes patent [5, 32, 63, 64]. Similar acute bleeding occurs in experimentally infected chimpanzees, and in dogs with *A. caninum* [5].

Chronic infection is often asymptomatic [27], although pain or indigestion occur in 20–50% of cases, sometimes reflecting ongoing re-exposure [5]. In one outbreak, abdominal pain commenced 3–10 months after intense exposure, and lasted 3–6 months [35]; most subjects were probably already infected beforehand, with reactivation of hypobiotic larvae explaining their delayed and protracted course. The authors attributed the severe symptoms to high worm burdens, and commented that subacute intestinal obstruction had not been previously described in hookworm infection. However, acute peritonism with abdominal distension had been clearly linked to hookworm infection 20 years earlier [73], and was reminiscent of severe EE (although neither the species of hookworm nor the stage of infection were specified).

Symptoms can be variable and have no 'threshold' level of exposure, although they are usually severe and almost universal following intense exposure [35], when frank rectal bleeding and rapid weight loss can occur [32]. Abdominal complaints were prominent in most patients given 400 L3 [27], but not in a volunteer exposed to 100 L3 [33]. Intraduodenal implantation of 50 adult *A. duodenale* in a 3-year old girl did not cause symptoms on two occasions 20 weeks apart, but 500 worms 16 weeks later provoked transient abdominal discomfort [74]. Larval 'presensitisation' may be important to intestinal inflammation (see below, 'Adult Worm Secretory Activity').

The symptoms of *N. americanus* infection are identical but slightly delayed: pain occurs over the 4th to 7th weeks [5, 34, 49, 75], and diarrhoea persists usually until weeks 7–9 [5]. The impression that *A. duodenale* provokes more severe acute symptoms than *N. americanus* [36] is not supported by the evidence, and has been contradicted [27]. Abdominal pain (exacerbated by meals) occurred in 67% of soldiers who developed patent infection (probably *N. americanus* exclusively), with diarrhoea, flatulence/bloating and nausea/vomiting also being very common

[75]. A dose of 250 L3 has provoked severe pain, nausea and intractable diarrhoea that resembled cholera [29], although subsequent reinfections caused symptoms of declining intensity. As few as 50 L3 provoked symptoms in over 50% of volunteers [34, 49], and pain and blood eosinophilia developed even when infection remained non-patent, indicating that scant worms can trigger inflammation [34]. Pain and diarrhoea usually clear within 2 days of taking mebendazole. Chronic infection can resemble peptic ulcer disease [76, 77].

Acute *N. americanus* infection has rarely been incriminated in severe intestinal haemorrhage, although it may have caused fatal bleeding in two infants aged less than 3 months [78]. Without larval hypobiosis, maternal transmission should not occur.

A. ceylanicum infections tend to be low in worm numbers, longevity and fecundity [4, 50, 79], and clinically resemble *A. caninum* EE, presenting with severe abdominal pain [37, 50]. Doses of 50–150 L3 consistently provoke symptoms, commencing at 15–20 days (1–2 weeks before patency) and resolve spontaneously in 2 weeks (unless aborted by anthelminthics) [37]. After exceptionally heavy exposure (1,200 L3), severe symptoms commenced on day 29 and relapsed intermittently but with declining severity for several months [50], perhaps a result of temporary larval arrest in the skin (see above, 'Zoonotic Hookworms'), or gut.

Intestinal Histopathology

Histological (and intestinal function) studies in hookworm-endemic populations are confounded by associated conditions, including other infections and malnutrition [3, 5, 8]. Hospital patients provide an even more biassed sample, and investigations can be impossible to control. Further, constant site-changing by worms means that histological lesions will be focal and in varying stages of evolution, and blind biopsies (by Crosby capsule) will rarely sample a zone of interest. Even endoscopy can access only the mucosa at either extremity of the small intestine, leaving the preferred habitat of hookworms beyond reach. Autopsy findings provide the best view, but are guaranteed to be non-representative.

Extrapolation from animal models to humans is unreliable, because of major differences in physiological and immune responses, the narrow selection of parasite strains that will develop in laboratory hosts, and size: an adult hookworm assumes monstrous proportions in a mouse or hamster, and causes disproportionate intestinal trauma. While inconspicuously submerged in human gut mucus [3, 7], the same worms in hamsters might induce peristaltic drag, gut obstruction and abrasion (perhaps contributing to the patchy villous clubbing observed in this model [8]).

Human A. caninum *Enteritis.* Most worms have been in the distal ileum, even in laparotomy cases, while none has ever been found in the duodenum or jejunum. Two were in the colon, and another possibly in the rectum [N. Sandford, pers. commun.].

Colonoscopy in patients with an *A. caninum* in situ reveals patchy mucosal inflammation and distinctive, aphthous ulceration with pinpoint haemorrhages in the tips of adjacent mucosal villi, both locally and elsewhere in the terminal ileum, caecum and proximal colon. These haemorrhages fit the description of superficial, tentative 'bites' of *A. caninum* in the dog intestine [80], and identical lesions occur in patients who are seropositive but without a worm [52].

The characteristic surgical finding is an inflamed segment of distal ileum, 2–100 cm long. If a hookworm is present, it is usually attached deep in the mucosa of the central zone. Accompanying features often include mucosal ulceration, intense, submucosal oedema (accounting for ileal obstruction), serositis, enlarged draining mesenteric lymph nodes and variable quantities of peritoneal exudate, sometimes turbid with numerous eosinophils.

Histological details are described elsewhere [13]. Variable eosinophilic infiltration involves any and all layers of the gut wall, as well as the contiguous mesentery and nodes. Macrophages may be numerous, and eosinophil abscesses and granulomas can develop. Mast cells have not yet been examined. At worm attachment sites, the mucosa may be lysed and severely eroded, with obliterated crypt architecture. Extensive ulceration over inflammatory zones explains the occasional bleeding.

Infection in Canine Hosts. A. caninum in dogs probably typifies hookworm infections in specific hosts. Adult worms prefer the second and third quarters of the small intestine, aggregating in the central jejunum. They disperse more widely in heavier infections, even into the colon [3, 8, 56, 81]. In experimental infection, histopathology has varied from minimal to severe [8], perhaps reflecting worm burdens. Lymphocytes infiltrate feeding lesions (see below, 'Hookworm Interaction with Host Intestine') within 2 h, and numerous neutrophils with variable eosinophils are present by 4 h [82, 83]. Cellular infiltration is usually focal and resolves soon after worm detachment. In heavy infection, mesenteric and retroperitoneal nodes are invariably enlarged, oedematous, hyperaemic, and infiltrated with eosinophils and plasma cells [5].

A. ceylanicum infections provoke intense neutrophil and eosinophil infiltration at attachment sites, with villous atrophy [84].

EE is well recognised in dogs, with a predilection for certain breeds. As in humans, food allergy has been incriminated, albeit inconclusively, and published case reports grossly underrepresent its true incidence. Adult hookworms have been found in German shepherd dogs with EE [85].

Anthropophilic Hookworm Infections. Both *N. americanus* and *A. duodenale* aggregate in the proximal small intestine, dispersing further in heavier infections. The former species clusters nearer the duodenum [3, 5, 86]. *A. duodenale* has even been found attached in the rectum [87]. Both species prefer to feed along the antimesenteric mucosa [86].

Biopsy studies of chronic infections have produced inconsistent results [3, 5, 77, 88, 89]. However, in otherwise healthy individuals, mucosal changes are minimal, involve only the attachment sites, and closely resemble *A. caninum* infection in dogs (see above, 'Infection in Canine Hosts'): transient, punctiform haemorrhages and focal erosions (1–2 mm in diameter), engorged local capillaries, oedema and submucosal infiltration with lymphocytes, plasma cells and eosinophils [5]. Occasional intense eosinophil invasion of the jejunal submucosa has been detected using Crosby capsules [89]. Aggregates of macrophages containing haemosiderin granules presumably result from bleeding into the mucosa. Villous atrophy and clubbing, reported sporadically (usually with *A. duodenale*), were unrelated to worm burdens, and did not consistently improve after anthelminthic treatment [8]. Intestinal malabsorption does not occur in uncomplicated cases.

Autopsy studies reveal more florid tissue changes, including jejuno-ileitis, extensive ulceration, severe haemorrhages, transmural oedema, suppuration and fibrinopurulent peritonitis [5, 47, 90]. Petechial haemorrhages and bleeding superficial ulcers might represent hookworm feeding lesions. Rarely, adult worms (always *A. duodenale*, even in the presence of *N. americanus*), fertile eggs and rhabditiform larvae have been found within haemorrhagic submucosal abscesses packed with neutrophils and eosinophils [90, 91]. Cellular infiltration and a peculiar oedema most prominent in the submucosa produce leathery thickening of the heavily parasitised jejunum. Intense transmural eosinophilia and oedema can be indistinguishable from severe EE (see above, 'Human *A. caninum* Enteritis'). Mesenteric nodes can be grossly enlarged and packed with eosinophils, which also infiltrate the splenic pulp and bone marrow.

Clearly, the tissue responses in human EE and anthropophilic hookworm infection (particularly with *A. duodenale*) overlap completely, and closely resemble findings in dogs heavily infected with *A. caninum* [5].

Immunological Responses

Immune Stimulation and Protection
Given the complexity of hookworm life cycles, elaborate host immune responses can be expected. Larval penetration of the skin, involving enzyme secretion, sloughing of cuticular sheaths and surface molecules, and secondary bacterial invasion, undoubtedly stimulates antigen-processing cells and, there-

fore, lymphocyte responses. Larval disintegration would release an even greater diversity of immunoreactive molecules. Systemic responses will be reinforced by L3 negotiating the pulmonary vasculature, alveolar-capillary barriers and tracheobronchial mucosae. Arrival of the L4 in the gut provides a quantum boost in immunostimulation. The rapidly growing L4 and L5, with their bulky 'salivary' glands, overshadow the antigenic output of invasive larvae, and also act in a distinct milieu and chronology that should have major qualitative effects. The intestinal stages are biphasic, simultaneously provoking mucosal and systemic immune responses. The adult worm is bathed in digesting food, host enzymes, biliary secretions, secretory IgA and other antibodies, mucin and associated luminal molecules, while its buccal extremity (and perhaps alimentary tract) encounters effector cells, cytokines, circulating antibodies, complement, clotting factors, host hormones and other reactive molecules. It also frequently changes position, keeping a step ahead of focal reactions, and releases potent lytic and other molecules that affect host responses.

Larval hookworms share many somatic and secretory antigens with adults, even though some ES molecules (see below, 'Adult Worm Secretory Activity') might be stage-specific. Undoubtedly, the worms chemically modulate their own behaviour and development, perhaps synergistically with host molecules, but this has not been investigated in any parasitic nematodes, let alone hookworms. They harbour a bacterial microflora [5] that might have independent as well as adjuvant immunological effects, potentiating responses to hookworm products. Again, this remains unexplored.

Despite significant attrition of larvae at each critical stage in their tissue migration, there is no evidence that immunity is protective in humans, by destroying larval or adult hookworms [92]. This reflects the constraints of human experimentation, and of laboratory models. Studies in rodents invariably utilise massive exposure, which facilitates tracking of larvae, but distorts the outcome. *A. caninum*, *A. braziliense* and *A. ceylanicum* have short life-spans in their natural hosts, generally well below a year, compared with the longevity of anthropophilic species in humans [92]. This characteristic is probably genetic. However, dogs subjected to repeated heavy *A. caninum* infections spontaneously expel numerous immature worms [93]. This phenomenon currently defies explanation, but would involve 'age resistance', mucosal inflammation, larval hypobiosis and possibly mutual inhibition within large worm populations.

Animal experimentation does indicate partial protection after immunization or repeated exposure. Vaccination against *A. caninum* in dogs stimulates immunity that reduces adult worm numbers and blood loss, and can be transferred by lymphocytes from mesenteric nodes [5, 94, 95]. However, it remains unknown whether invading L3 perish in resistant dogs, or simply divert into hypobiotic reservoirs. Similarities in population biology and histopathology between natural

A. caninum and *A. duodenale* infections suggested to Miller [5] that protective immunity also develops in humans, but would be difficult to demonstrate in epidemiological studies. However, his 'minimal threshold to trigger an effective immune response' was an experimental larval dose greatly exceeding what would be encountered under natural conditions; most human infections probably derive from repeated, low-level exposure.

A. caninum *Eosinophilic Enteritis in Humans*

Patients with EE often have circulating antibodies to somatic and excretory-secretory antigens of adult *A. caninum* [15, 16], the latter proving more suitable in immunodiagnosis. In Townsville, 71% of patients with EE and 67% with abdominal pain and blood eosinophilia reacted positively by indirect IgG ELISA [51]. However, of 8 patients with an adult worm, only 4 were positive, by both IgG and IgE ELISA [9]. Specificity and sensitivity were enhanced in IgG and IgE immunoblots (positive being a reaction with Ac68), although a woman with severe EE remained seronegative [9], while an intensely reactive serum (in all tests) was from an asymptomatic man (although clinical disease may have been averted by the serendipitous colonoscopic removal of the worm; his blood eosinophil count was rising). Sera from 11 individuals with patent hookworm infections were all positive by both tests; most had *A. duodenale* [16], but at least 3 had *N. americanus* [unpubl. observations]. Blots detecting IgG4 subclass antibodies to Ac68 may further improve the diagnosis, but will not distinguish anthropophilic infection [96]. In schistosomiasis, specific IgE antibodies have been linked to protective immunity, whereas IgG4 antibodies may retard the development of host resistance [97, 98]; this may pertain to hookworm infections, in relation to tolerance (see below, 'Tolerance').

Clearly, *A. caninum* shares major secretory antigens (including Ac68) with other hookworms; the Western blot has a sensitivity and specificity of 80–90%, but cannot distinguish species. The higher ELISA readings in patent (anthropophilic) infections probably reflect intensity and duration of immune stimulation, for at least two adult worms must have survived beyond the pre-patent period, whereas *A. caninum* have always been solitary and immature. Nevertheless, in *A. caninum* infections, serological reactivity does not always correlate with symptoms, suggesting that circulating antibody levels are unreliable indicators of intestinal inflammation.

The larval 'dose' required for seroconversion is unknown, and would vary among individuals. Because L3 share antigens with adult worms, including Ac68 [16], they should stimulate cross-reacting antibodies. In an unpublished study of 'realistic' percutaneous *A. caninum* exposure, a healthy 40-year-old volunteer, who had been infected 13 years previously with *A. duodenale* [62], received 50 L3 and remained seronegative, with a normal blood count. A 23-year-old woman failed to seroconvert after three doses of 50 L3 at weekly intervals. In a 42-year-old man exposed to 100 L3 each month for 18 months, blood counts remained normal, while serum became positive by Western blot at 5 months and by ELISA after 12 months. This indicates that seroconversion requires considerable exposure to L3, although antibody production might have been boosted if L4 and adult worms began feeding in the gut.

Using adult *A. caninum* antigens in serodiagnosis is complicated by the inevitable contamination of ES preparations with canine mucosa and blood [99], as many people have antibodies to canine antigens. Preabsorbing sera with canine tissue extracts does not entirely resolve the problem. Synthetic recombinant antigens should obviate this difficulty and help further investigations.

Anthropophilic Hookworm Infections

Laboratory animals display significant individual and strain variations in immune responsiveness and susceptibility to hookworms that should also apply in human populations [92]. However, immunodiagnostic investigations have been retarded by the simplicity of coprological detection. Skin testing has predominated in human immunological studies, and demonstrates immediate hypersensitivity to extracts of adult worms and L3 that persists for several years after treatment [5, 48, 72]. Sensitivity generally exceeds 80%, but specificity is poor (<80%), with extensive cross-reactivity between *N. americanus, A. duodenale* and *A. caninum* antigens, and reactions give no indication of worm burden. Circulating antibodies to somatic and secretory antigens have been demonstrated by diverse in vitro tests [5, 72, 92], but again with major cross-reactions between the common species, and between larvae and adults [28, 29]. Even individuals unexposed to hookworms tested positively against larval antigens of *N. americanus* and *A. caninum* [28], and *N. americanus* infection serum cross-reacted by ELISA to ES antigens of the feline hookworm, *A. tubaeforme* [29].

Antibodies of all immunoglobulin isotypes, against adult worm excretory-secretory antigens and larval extracts, were found in *N. americanus* infection in Papua New Guinea [100], but their significance is unknown. Immune responses in endemic populations are complicated by repeated exposure and concurrent infections, so that volunteer studies can provide invaluable information. In *A. duodenale, N. americanus* and *A. ceylanicum* infections, specific IgG and IgM are first detected 2–8 weeks after infection, depending partly on the larval dose and individual factors [49, 50, 72, 92]. Single, light exposure may fail to elicit detectable responses. A dose of 1,200 L3 of *A. ceylanicum* stimulated an early rise in IgM antibodies, peaking at 4–6 weeks; IgG reached maximal levels at 4–6 months, and antibodies of both classes stayed up until treatment [50]. Repeated exposure to *N. americanus* L3 leads to progressive, stepwise increments in antibody responses [28, 29, 72], while total serum IgE levels, as well as specific IgE antibodies, follow a similar pattern [29, 49]. Specific antibody levels, including IgE (and total IgE), decline soon after treatment [92].

Abdominal symptoms often begin to ameliorate when detectable serum antibodies appear. However, mounting immune responsiveness to L3 does not reflect resistance to either larval invasion or adult worms, as subsequent fecal egg outputs increase in proportion to the L3 doses [26, 28, 29, 92]. In dogs, vaccination reduces blood loss to *A. caninum* [5], and serum IgA levels rise with increasing exposure to *A. ceylanicum* [101], but the few studies of serum and intestinal secretory IgA in human hookworm infections were inconclusive.

Only two studies have examined human blood lymphocyte responses to hookworms. In 5 volunteers given 50 *N. americanus* L3, lymphocyte transformation to larval antigens was minimal [49]. One of two subjects exposed to 1,200 L3 *A. ceylanicum* [50] reacted to soluble L3 antigens (peaking at 3 weeks), while responses in both to adult antigens peaked at 4–6 weeks, gradually declined to 12 weeks, and returned to normal by week 30 (4 weeks after treatment). The more responsive individual had previously been infected with anthropophilic hookworms. Neither experimental nor epidemiological studies show any correlation between clinical manifestations and serum antibody or lymphocyte responses to hookworm antigens [72].

Peripheral blood eosinophilia is well documented. Counts start rising within a week of exposure to even small doses of L3 of *N. americanus* or *A. duodenale* [28, 29, 33, 34, 92], but increase sharply usually about 2 weeks before eggs appear in the faeces. This occurs even with delayed patency [33]: in a volunteer infected with 100 *A. duodenale* L3, eosinophil counts rose from 500 to 780/mm^3 by day 5, plateaued until week 33, then climbed to a peak of 5,300/mm^3 at 38 weeks, just 2 weeks before eggs appeared. The count was still high (2,850) at week 78. In a child with polycythemia vera treated by 3 intragastric inoculations of live, adult *A. duodenale* removed from experimentally infected dogs [74], blood eosinophilia developed within 2 weeks of each dose, peaking at 23,000/mm^3 10 weeks after the first inoculation of 50 worms. Subsequent peaks occurred earlier and were lower, despite the final dose comprising 500 worms. Circulating eosinophils in acute responses are metabolically active, showing increased superoxide production, prominent vacuolisation and degranulation [102]. Counts decline rapidly after effective anthelminthic therapy [29, 34, 49].

In hookworm infections, blood eosinophilia occurs almost universally, does not correlate with worm burdens, can be provoked by exposure to L3 of zoonotic species (this is more difficult to analyse in anthropophilic infections), synchronises more closely with parasite development in the gut than migration through lungs, often parallels the severity of intestinal symptoms [72] but does not signify resistance to infection [92]. The parasites seem unperturbed by human gut inflammation. Just as peak eosinophil responses decline with repeated infection, so the symptoms become milder. Abdominal pain and blood eosinophilia even in nonpatent *N. americanus* infections suggest that minimal worm numbers can provoke significant inflammation [34].

Intestinal cellular responses to hookworms have been studied only in experimental rodent hosts [92, 101].

Pathogenesis

The mechanisms underlying anaemia in chronic hookworm infection were for many years subject to controversy [3, 5, 7–9], reflecting the complexity of problems affecting nutritionally compromised populations. Now it is generally accepted that blood loss results from direct sucking by hookworms and oozing from traumatised mucosa, anaemia developing when the worm burden is disproportionate to host iron-protein intake. Losses attributable to individual worms vary widely among studies, for *A. duodenale* ranging 0.05–0.3 ml/day, cf. 0.01–0.04 ml for *N. americanus* [5]. *A. ceylanicum* infection rarely precipitates anaemia, except in Western New Guinea [40]. The blood loss per worm could vary with the worm burden, stage of infection, host age and nutrition, concomitant diseases and, perhaps, immunity and other unknown factors. It might even be exacerbated by anaemia itself, for more blood will be needed to satisfy the worm's oxygen or other requirements.

Here, the host-parasite interactions that underlie acute manifestations will be analysed.

Larval Invasion and Development

Both definitive and paratenic hosts can be infected either percutaneously or orally [56], and L3 of most hookworm species seem capable of invading human skin, although their subsequent fates vary.

In volunteer studies (see above, 'A. caninum Eosinophilic Enteritis in Humans'), ground itch did not occur after first exposure to *A. caninum* L3, but could be induced by reinfection after several weeks. This 'refractory' period masks a phase of intense immunological activity that establishes populations of activated lymphocytes and specific IgE-sensitised mast cells in the skin. Applied larvae greatly outnumber the skin lesions provoked, indicating that most either fail to invade, or use common entry points. Accompanying bacteria might exacerbate cutaneous inflammation [5, 50], although intense pruritus without suppuration is not characteristic of bacterial superinfection. Given the continuing tracks of creeping eruption, and that *A. caninum* L3 in inflamed human hair follicles can be unsheathed [21], the early skin lesions represent allergic reactions to larval secretions rather than discarded cuticular sheaths. Delayed-type hypersensitivity is suggested when the papules last for weeks. Intense skin reactions can occur without detectable serum antibody (including IgE) responses (see above, 'A. caninum Eosinophilic Enteritis in Humans'). The L3 of N. americanus (and probably other species) synthesise eicosanoids, including prostaglandins and leukotrienes, from essential fatty acids in the skin [103]; these products may contribute to inflammation or immunomodulation.

The host epidermal basement membrane seems a major barrier to larvae, and A. caninum, A. ceylanicum and A. braziliense differ in their penetration behaviour [61]. However, study findings may have been distorted by massive larval doses (300–2,000) applied to small areas. L3 of both A. caninum and A. duodenale produce a major metalloprotease of 68 kD and, variably, a minor protease of 38 kD, that might be instrumental in ecdysis and histolysis [104]. A. braziliense, A. caninum and A. tubaeforme all secrete a hyaluronidase of about 87 kD, probably to facilitate penetration of skin and deeper tissues. Maximal enzyme activity in A. braziliense [105, 106] suggests a role in cutaneous larva migrans, although L3 involved in creeping eruption are aberrant (perhaps with sensory organs damaged by immune responses); most probably enter the dermis rapidly and migrate beyond (accounting for pulmonary symptoms; see above, 'Zoonotic Hookworms'). While L3 of different species vary in secretory and penetrating abilities [106], it is premature to implicate specific enzyme production.

Subsequent events are even more poorly understood. Occasional studies show ensheathed L3 in deeper tissues, but most lose their sheaths on skin entry. The proposition that sheaths are discarded as an immunological decoy ('smoke-screen') [107] is unfounded; they are more likely to potentiate responses to cuticular antigens. During their brief transit in the circulation, larvae are directly exposed to antibodies, complement, clotting factors and activated effector cells and, in turn, probably release defensive molecules. On reaching the lungs, L3 might provoke capillary haemorrhages and further immune responses, possibly enhanced by companion bacteria [5]. Larvae might perish there, or be expectorated, although they have been found only once in human lungs [47].

Pharyngitis and cough in the second week after exposure to A. duodenale, even when infection remained non-patent for 9 months [31], strongly links migrating larvae to respiratory symptoms. Brumpt [27] attributed upper respiratory tract symptoms in his patients to mucosal re-invasion by migrating A. duodenale larvae. The missing, essential feature of Loeffler's syndrome, abnormal chest radiology, seems to require high larval doses (see above, 'Zoonotic Hookworms' and 'Anthropophilic Hookworms'), of either zoonotic or anthropophilic species. However, because larvae develop during tracheo-oesophageal passage, to reach the gut in the fourth stage, they may be incapable of penetrating the respiratory mucosa. Their simple transit through the lungs, either along vascular channels (en route to tissue depots) or the mucociliary escalator (to the gut), might be sufficient to provoke a local allergic response. Acute respiratory signs were induced in dogs previously infected with hookworms (species not stated) by allowing them to inhale larval extracts or culture fluid [48]. This implies the presence of IgE-sensitised mast cells in the respiratory mucosa.

The hypothesis that, in Wakana disease, ingestion of larval *A. duodenale* antigens triggers an allergic response in the respiratory tract [48] is problematic. The timing of the gastrointestinal and respiratory manifestations is readily explained on the basis of migrating L3 (which had been found in sputum). Those 10% of patients who had eaten cooked vegetables might have been infected coincidentally from other sources. Significantly, *N. americanus* has not been implicated in Wakana disease; its L3 fail to develop after ingestion [17, 106], whereas respiratory symptoms are well documented after percutaneous exposure.

Hookworm Interaction with Host Intestine

Feeding commences within hours of host invasion, triggered in L3 by serum and other factors [106, 108], and then continues throughout subsequent development. After the third moult, the L4 uses its buccal apparatus to feed on the intestinal mucosa. Experimental observations of *A. caninum* in dogs [3, 80, 82] probably apply to other species. To attach for feeding, the adult worm pushes forwards until its buccal capsule buries in the mucosa, usually among deeper folds. Suction generated in the buccal cavity by oesophageal contractions then locks it into position. Sucking is greatly stimulated by the presence of host blood and a solid matrix for the buccal capsule to engage [3]; this may also apply to secretory activity, for adding collagen rafts to the culture medium enhances acetylcholinesterase release by adult *N. americanus* [109].

Mucosal villi are not essential for attachment, as adult *A. duodenale* have been found in the human colon and rectum [87], and can feed on the gingivolabial folds of the mouth [3]. The hold on the mucosal plug drawn into the buccal cavity is secured by 'teeth' (or cutting plates, in the case of *N. americanus*), scraper-like inward projections of the thickened bilateral 'denticular plates' that reinforce the cavity against collapsing. These structures cannot 'bite' or 'chew' like mandibles, but aid maceration of the incoming tissue by funnelling it across deep buccal teeth and spines. Sections of feeding hookworms fail to convey the dynamism of the mucosal 'plug', streaming into the buccal cavity and being pumped out from its depths. *A. caninum* changes position every 4–6 h, leaving small ulcers which heal within 6–24 h [82, 83]. Adult *A. duodenale* rarely penetrate the muscularis mucosae, although in exceptional cirumstances they can perforate the gut wall [47, 90].

The target mucosa is softened by lytic enzymes from amphidial and excretory glands [110–114], then drawn into the buccal cavity to be injected with dorsal oesophageal gland secretions and shredded by the deep teeth. Subventral gland products are added in the oesophageal lumen. Feeding is intermittent, involving rapid, wavelike, oesophageal contractions (up to 4/s) that pump mucosa and blood into the worm's intestine [3, 80, 82], where transit can take as little as 2 min. Presumably, nutrients are digested and absorbed rapidly.

Little is known of the metabolism of hookworms [115], but their constant activity, fecundity and copious secretory output demand substantial nutrition. They are extravagant feeders, taking in far more than seems required. The colour change in blood passing through the parasite suggests considerable oxygen extraction [3, 80]. Despite the anal ejection of intact red cells, a substantial proportion of ingested blood is lysed [3, 5].

Adult Worm Secretory Activity

This ensures the parasite's nutritional well-being, but also provokes and modulates host reactions at a molecular level. Secretory products have diverse but complementary functions, not necessarily mediated by different molecules; several may share a common role, while some enzymes have multiple actions. These are being subjected to intensifying investigation [106, 107, 114, 116, 117].

Anticoagulation. Host blood loss is exacerbated by anticoagulants, secreted ostensibly to prevent thrombotic obstruction of the worm's gut. This was already known in 1904, but 50 years passed before it was linked to the amphidial glands in *A. caninum* [118], then attributed to a protein of molecular weight 20–50 kD [111]. Anticoagulant has been detected at the attachment sites of *A. ceylanicum* in dogs [119]. A 37-kD elastinolytic metalloprotease, found in homogenates of adult *A. caninum* and *A. duodenale* (and secreted by the latter), exhibits fibrinolytic, anticoagulant properties [120]. Soluble extracts of adult *A. caninum* inhibit platelet aggregation, and contain a low-molecular-weight peptide that inhibits clotting factor Xa (a serine protease) and the tissue-factor complex [106, 121]. It is not known whether this peptide is secreted by the worm, or if any of these anticoagulants are immunogenic in human infections.

Proteolysis. Proteases occur in all life forms, and their functions in parasites include host-tissue invasion, nutrient digestion, immune evasion and anticoagulation [122], the last mentioned above. Of particular interest is the diagnostic protein, Ac68, a putative protease of undetermined function [16]. Immunohistochemical studies using monoclonal antibodies localised it in the excretory glands of adult *A. caninum* (and intestinal cells of tissue larvae), although monospecific human sera bound more strongly to amphidial gland cytoplasm [99, 113]. A possible explanation, that Ac68 comprises at least two different molecules, is suggested by other, unpublished findings.

In schistosomes, hemoglobin is digested by cysteine and aspartic proteases [122–124], and a 'hemoglobinase' with characteristics of cysteine proteases has been found in adult *A. caninum* extracts [125]. A secretory 29-kD cysteine protease originates from both amphidial and excretory glands of adult *A. caninum*, and two transcripts encoding this and a closely related enzyme (labelled AcCP-1 and AcCP-2) have been isolated from a cDNA library [114]. On primary amino acid structure, these enzymes show marked similarity to mammalian cathepsin-B cysteine proteinases and, therefore, probably exhibit endo- as well as exo-proteinase activities [126]. Paradoxically, vigorous cysteine protease activity in the tissues and secretions of adult *A. caninum*, and in the tissues of L3, preferentially cleaves the synthetic substrates of cathepsin L rather than cathepsin B [127]. Perhaps transcripts encoding cathepsin-L-like proteinases will also eventually be located, as they have been in schistosomes [128]. Alternatively, given that several differences in key catalytic-pocket amino acids of AcCP-1 and AcCP-2 distinguish these enzymes from their mammalian cathepsin-B homologues [114], the hookworm proteinases may prefer substrates more specific for cathepsin L than cathepsin B. In fact, homology modelling of their active sites suggests that the cathepsin-B-like transcripts encode cathepsin-L-like proteolytic activity [S. Harrop, pers. commun.]. Synthetic-substrate preferences and/or three-dimensional modelling may help to predict the natural substrates and therefore the function of these and other hookworm enzymes.

ES products of larval and adult *N. americanus* include cysteine proteases that may cleave IgG, IgA and IgM molecules [129], and adult worms release a variety of proteolytic activities with widely ranging pH optima [116]. They hydrolyse haemoglobin and fibrinogen, and have been characterized as a mixture of aspartic, cysteine and serine proteases. Some activities were actually enhanced by serine protease inhibition, suggesting major interactions among secretory proteins. A cDNA transcript encoding an aspartic protease has been isolated recently from *A. caninum* [S. Harrop, pers. commun.].

The pH optima of various enzymes have little meaning until their in vivo functions are determined, for potentially they can act in a multitude of interstitial, cellular and even subcellular compartments, including the host gut lumen, viable or necrotic mucosa, exudates, host circulation, inflammatory cell precincts, and parasite structures (surface, buccal cavity, secretory glands, and alimentary or genital tracts). Their metabolites may alter the microecology, including ambient pH, in ways not evident from in vitro studies.

Except for Ac68, it is not known which, if any, of these proteases is immunogenic in natural infections.

Hyaluronidase. Hyaluronidase activity was first detected in crude extracts of adult *A. duodenale* over 40 years ago [130]. A 65-kD hyaluronidase secreted by adult *A. caninum* almost certainly contributes to mucosal maceration and digestion [131]. Its activity was optimal at pH 6, but its source is not known, nor its immunogenicity. Hyaluronidases in many vertebrate and invertebrate venoms function as 'spreading factors' for other toxic molecules; in hookworms, they potentially could greatly enhance the effectiveness of proteases.

Acetylcholinesterase. In L4 and adult *N. americanus*, acetylcholinesterase (AChE) is released from amphidial and oesophageal glands [112, 132]. Its immunogenicity was first demonstrated in a volunteer exposed to four doses of 250 L3 over 13 months [29]; specific antibodies were detected 12 weeks after the second dose, were boosted by subsequent infections, and declined after treatment (which clearly excludes AChE as a vaccine candidate).

Speculation that the enzyme is a 'chemical holdfast' which suppresses local gut motility and/or secretion [115, 117] may be invalid. Its production by *Ancylostoma* species is relatively negligible [107, 132, 133], yet *A. duodenale* and *N. americanus* have comparable effects on host gut motility. Acetylcholine released by mammalian autonomic nerve endings is inactivated in situ by synaptic enzyme, so that exogenous AChE would have minimal effects in the gut, especially in light infections with worms frequently changing positions. Further, the gut has intrinsic motility in the absence of autonomic stimulation. Secreted by oesophageal glands, AChE would be ingested directly by the parasite, and so could function endogenously. It also occurs in significant quantities in a non-parasitic nematode, *Caenorhabditis elegans* [134]; while secretions of this species were not examined, a high concentration of AChE was found in its pharyngeo-intestinal valve, a non-innervated structure. Interestingly, various molecular forms of AChE also occur in human red blood cells and alimentary mucosae (the major nutrients of hookworms), being concentrated in the tips of small intestinal villi [135], but their role is unknown.

N. americanus AChE probably has functions other than hydrolysis of neural acetycholine. As serine hydrolases, AChEs can be proteolytic (having affinities with trypsin and serine carboxypeptidases), and regulate cell growth [136]. Other potential roles include immunomodulation [117]. The hookworm enzyme should be tested more carefully against a wider range of substrates, and compared with AChE from free-living nematodes. A published Western blot shows significant differences between adult male and female *N. americanus* excretory-secretory antigens in their reactions with AChE-immunised rabbit serum [109]. This sex difference in AChE release indicates it might contribute to, or be modified by, genital tract secretions.

Immunomodulation. Some secretory proteases (see above, 'Proteolysis') might inactivate antibodies and other immune mediators that are noxious to the worm. It is doubtful that cleaving IgA would benefit the parasite (except perhaps nutritionally!). Secretory antibodies effectively immobilise small organisms, such as viruses or bacteria, but are hardly likely to damage the cuticle of nematodes in the intestinal lumen. Further, proteolysis will be maximal at the release site, around the buccal extremity deep in the mucosa; antibody inactivation there might be protective, but effects against cuticle-adherent IgA are questionable.

Neutrophil inhibitory factor (NIF), a novel 41-kD glycoprotein that potently inactivates neutrophils in vitro (by binding to the integrin, CD11b/CD18), has been isolated from *A. caninum* and synthesised by gene cloning [137, 138]. Its in vivo actions are unknown, but the same receptor is involved in eosinophil migration [139, 140]. If NIF originates from intestinal cells, as preliminary evidence suggested [M. Moyle, pers. commun.), then its anti-granulocyte activity should not suppress inflammation at the bite site, but might protect the parasite gut from damage by ingested white blood cells. However, if NIF originated from the amphidial and excretory glands, as indicated by immunohistochemical studies [99], it could influence host tissue responses, perhaps dampening focal inflammation. Screening of infected human sera failed to detect antibodies to NIF [A. Loukas, pers. commun.]. Glutathione-S-transferase and superoxide dismutase secreted by *N. americanus* may protect the worm by inactivating toxic oxidants released in acute inflammation [117].

Miscellaneous. Various other substances would be released by adult hookworms, e.g. digestive enzymes, cuticular components [107], genital tract secretions (including eggs), metabolic wastes and bacterial products. Often overlooked are host antigens, which might not contribute to pathogenesis but will certainly affect immunological investigations [99]. A monoclonal antibody to a canine intestinal mucosal antigen (a major component of excretory-secretory antigen preparations) bound to the epicuticle of live adult *A. caninum* removed from dogs [99]. Such adsorption of host protein may protect the parasite by masking it from immune attack.

Immunopathogenesis of Intestinal Disease: A Hypothetical Reconstruction

Individual Susceptibility. Experimental, clinical and epidemiological studies demonstrate major individual variations in susceptibility and responsiveness to hookworm infections, implicating genetic influences. MHC control of responsiveness to parasitic helminths has been found in inbred animals, and no doubt applies to humans, but the data are lacking [141]. Human allergies share fundamental mechanisms with responses to helminths (see below). Their underlying genetic mechanisms are very complex, and interact with environmental influences [142, 143]. The total serum IgE concentration is linked to markers on chromosome 5, including genes for T_H2 response cytokines in band 5q31.1, and the nearby IL-4 gene [143]. Allergen-specific IgE synthesis is controlled partly by HLA-linked genes on chromosome 6, and responsiveness to specific allergens seems to be associated with particular HLA-D types [142]. However, the characteristics of an antigen which render it allergenic remain obscure [141]. The 'end-organ' of allergic expression (skin, lung, gut) seems to be determined by independent genetic factors, as are components of allergic responses, such as mast cell activity, receptors and mediator generation. Therefore, while there are clear familial links in atopy, there is no characteristic haplotype. In view of the extensive range of hookworm antigens, a simple genetic predisposition to infection, or to severe symptoms (including EE), might not be found.

Epidemiologically, *A. caninum* EE has not been linked with atopy [51], and a limited investigation has not discerned any HLA associations [Dr. J. Croese, pers. commun.]. Occasionally, several members of one family have developed EE (but not simultaneously), perhaps reflecting common exposure rather than genetic predisposition. Further, in the early stages of anthropophilic infections, the frequency of abdominal symptoms indicates that inflammatory reactions occur in most cases, albeit of variable intensity (see above, 'Anthropophilic Hookworm Infections'). If the ulcers found in almost 5% of Townsville colonoscopies [53] are in fact *A. caninum* 'bites', then clinical cases represent a minority of total infections. Significant allergy to hookworm secretions would underlie only severe cases, and the allergen might vary among individuals. There may be contributing factors, e.g. in rats, selenium deficiency predisposes to EE [144].

If individuals are not genetically predisposed either to harbouring adult *A. caninum,* or to developing EE, could the parasite be of a unique, geographically isolated strain? First, there is no evidence that it secretes a unique antigen, or provokes inflammatory responses different from those to anthropophilic species (including *A. ceylanicum*). Second, patent infection does not occur; this is not a human-adapted strain that has arisen in north-eastern Australia. Convincing cases have now been diagnosed in the USA [67, 68]. Sharing a common recent ancestry with *A. duodenale, A. caninum* [17, 115] could be expected occasionally to develop in people. It behaves in humans as in dogs, even exhibiting seasonal reactivation of hypobiotic larvae, but the physiology is not quite compatible. Laboratory strains of *A. duodenale* develop in dogs. Further, EE also occurs in dogs, and it would not be surprising if *A. caninum* provoked some cases. Confirmation of this will require very careful studies.

Timing, Worm Burden and Host Responsiveness. Anthropophilic and *A. caninum* infections differ mainly in the numbers and longevity of the parasites. In the former, symptoms commence usually about 2 weeks before the onset of patency, suggesting a response to mucosal feeding by developing worms (perhaps coinciding with the final molt). The severity of symptoms (and, presumably, the underlying inflammation) often seems unrelated to worm numbers. Frequent absence of symptoms, and of obvious mucosal inflammation in endoscopic and autopsy examinations, indicates that worm activity per se causes only punctate ulcers and haemorrhages. Given the mucosal regenerative capacity, these rarely become more extensive or confluent, even in heavy infections. In cases of severe haemorrhage with intense *A. duodenale* infection, both in infants [63, 64] and adults [7], perhaps the mucosa becomes saturated with histolytic enzymes and anticoagulants. However, complicating factors might be involved, including bacterial or viral infection, gross inflammation, and mucosal repair compromised by protein deficiency [47]. With heavy experimental *A. duodenale* infection in chimpanzees, and *A. caninum* in dogs, blood loss commences with the fourth molt about 21 days after exposure [5], synchronous with rapid parasite growth and, perhaps, secretion of new enzymes. On the other hand, in older, well-nourished and lightly infected hosts, inflammation and haemorrhage signify exaggerated tissue responses to worm antigens, mediated by immune mechanisms.

In *A. caninum* infection, immaturity of the parasite (average length 8 mm) [9] indicates recent arrival, e.g. a 10-mm female worm found in the terminal ileum of an asymptomatic patient just 16 days after he had taken 600 mg mebendazole [9]. Blood eosinophilia was borderline ($520/mm^3$), but the ELISA and Western blot were already strongly positive. The alternative explanation, prolonged survival in the gut of a growth-retarded parasite, seems unlikely. Clinical EE clearly represents intense allergic responses to minimal antigenic provocation.

Molecular Mechanisms. The immunopathology of intestinal helminthiases, despite extensive studies in model systems [8, 72, 92, 101, 145], remains poorly understood [146]. Nematodes provoke infiltration by lymphocytes, mast cells and oeosinophils (particularly in the mucosa and submucosa), oedema, mucus hypersecretion, gut hypermotility, and raised levels of circulating eosinophils and specific and nonspecific IgE antibodies [146–148]. With antigens shared by larval and adult hookworms, initial larval invasion may 'prime' the later intestinal response, although interactions between cutaneous and intestinal presentation of antigens remain unclear, and further complicated by the tissue phases of infection, both larval and adult. In outline, hookworm antigens initially activate epidermal dendritic cells, then macrophages in the lungs and gut (including Peyer's patches and associated lymph nodes), to release IL-1. Lymphocytes are stimulated to proliferate and secrete IL-2 (and promote expression of IL-2 receptors), leading to proliferation of helper, suppressor and cytotoxic T cell populations, with feedback stimulation of macrophages, releasing more IL-1 [141, 145, 148]. The cytokines released by activated lymphocytes, macrophages and other cells orchestrate the subsequent inflammatory response and outcome of the infection [149, 150]. In helminthic infections, CD4+ T cells of the T_H2 phenotype predominate and generate IL-3, IL-4, IL-5, IL-6, IL-9, IL-10 and IL-13 [150], which greatly enhance the synthesis of IgE, and proliferation and migration of mast cells and eosinophils, among other effects.

Adult hookworm antigens are presented on the villous surface (perhaps blocked by IgA) and in the submucosa. Mast cells, primed with IgE and recruited to the feeding site, degranulate on exposure to specific antigens, to release pre-formed histamine, various enzymes, cytokines and membrane-derived lipid mediators [151, 152]. The ensuing complex of events, manifesting as acute inflammation, includes vasodilatation and fluid transudation, increased mucin secretion by goblet cells, the recruitment of eosinophils, smooth muscle contraction and stimulation of vagal reflex arcs [140, 147, 151, 152]. Eosinophilic infiltration ushers in a phase of local tissue damage, in severe cases leading to ulceration and bleeding. Blood eosinophil numbers, reflecting their mobilisation from bone marrow to effector sites, parallel the evolution of intestinal symptoms (see above, 'Anthropophilic Hookworm Infections'). However, in surgical cases of EE, the intestinal eosinophilia (and acute symptoms) develops so rapidly, and can be so extensive, that there is a marked delay before mobilisation is sufficient to raise the circulating eosinophil count [69]. Numbers of hypodense eosinophils rise in acute hookworm infection, their state of activation indicated by superoxide production and chemotactic responsiveness [102].

While the host-protective role of eosinophils remains doubtful (see below, 'Neuro-Endocrine Involvement'), their toxic granule contents and newly synthesised inflammatory mediators are prime agents of tissue damage [140, 147, 153]. For example, platelet-activating factor (PAF), alkyl-acetyl-glyceryl-phosphoryl-choline, is a broad-spectrum mediator synthesised by mast cells, eosinophils and other cells. It is a potent eosinophil chemotaxin and intestinal ulcerogen (at least in the rat), and enhances vagal effects in the lung, exacerbating bronchial smooth muscle spasm, mucus secretion, oedema and exudation [147, 153]. Interestingly, the injurious effects of PAF seem to occur only in the presence of bacterial endo-toxins [154]. Given its partial structural similarities with acetylcholine, examination of its suceptibility to *N. americanus* AChE could shed light on the lower blood losses caused by this species. Of course, PAF acts in concert with numerous other toxic molecules, and even cytokines have been incriminated in the pathogenesis of inflammatory bowel diseases [155].

The localised secretion of large quantities of hookworm antigens in the presence of specific antibodies could predispose to intestinal type III hypersensitivity (Arthus) lesions, and the formation of granulomas in EE [13] indicates delayed-type, cellular responses as well.

Neuro-Endocrine Involvement. Inflammation might involve changes in gastroduodenal hormone secretion, such as gastrin, secretin and cholecystokinin, affecting acid secretion and other functions [145]. Motility disorders, manifesting as nausea, vomiting, diarrhoea, pain and increased secretions, may be induced by inflammatory mediators directly or through the autonomic nervous system. Abnormal upper intestinal motility (accompanying mucosal and gut wall thickening) found in barium meal studies of acute ancylostomiasis was attributed to 'disturbed reflex arcs' [46]. Mounting evidence implicates the autonomic nervous system in allergy and inflammation, including intestinal responses to nematodes [145, 156–158]. Parasympathetic activity is potentiated by allergic reactions in sensitised guinea pig airways, and connections between mast cells and nerve endings have been demonstrated in many tissues, including the gastrointestinal tract [159]. Autonomic neural stimulation in immediate hypersensitivity can increase intestinal mucus secretion and muscle excitation through axon reflexes, so that a point stimulus in the mucosa could be transduced and expressed panmucosally, i.e. a few small, localised parasites might provoke inflammation over large tracts of intestine [145]. Exposure of the gut to parasite antigens can sensitise even distal segments not normally in contact with the parasite (e.g. colon), provoking inflammation on subsequent contact.

Parasympathetic reflex arcs, perhaps interacting with autocrine eosinophil and mast cell products, such as PAF and various cytokines, may account for the varying lengths of inflamed segments in severe *A. caninum* enteritis, which can extend 50 cm either side of the attached worm [13]. This cannot be explained by simple dispersal of allergens through luminal diffusion, or along intestinal vascular channels, or by a migrating, 'biting' worm.

Allergy vs. Protection. The paradigm of T_H2-mediated protection against helminths, spontaneous expulsion of trichostrongyles from ruminants and laboratory rodents, is precipitated by exposure to large numbers of larvae, involves mast cell degranulation (but eosinophil mobilisation only occasionally), and expels immature worms from the gut [156, 160, 161]. Responses in hookworm infection appear similar, but do not expel the parasites, except possibly in heavy *A. caninum* infection in dogs [93]. Hookworms might resist expulsion simply because they have effective anchoring mechanisms and, unlike trichostrongyles, can inactivate noxious molecules by externally 'predigesting' host tissues.

Differences between the pathogenesis of acute allergy and helminthic infection remain contentious [92, 145, 148, 156, 157, 161, 162]. There is no dividing line between 'normal' inflammation and hypersensitivity; the distinction lies in balancing response against stimulus (in terms of size, number and virulence of pathogens). In allergy, inappropriate reactions are provoked by innocuous antigens, without obvious benefit; in helminth-induced enteritis, parasite expulsion might be achieved, but at considerable cost (in terms of disease). Nevertheless, the spectrum of atopic reactions is broad, as is the range of responses to hookworm infection.

Intestinal inflammation from any cause might facilitate transmucosal passage of potential allergens to initiate hypersensitivity [163]. Hookworms may provoke allergy by mechanically breaching the mucosal barrier. While severe *A. caninum* EE has the hallmarks of acute hypersensitivity, the specific allergens remain to be identified. Tantalisingly, helminthic secretory proteases, particularly cysteine proteases, are strong promoters of T_H2 lymphocyte differentiation, and a cysteine protease from dust mites is potently allergenic [149].

The circulating levels of IL-5, a specific promoter of eosinophil proliferation and activation, are raised in helminthiases; its experimental inhibition by monoclonal antibodies suppresses inflammatory responses, but not resistance to infection [140], implicating eosinophils in tissue damage but not host protection. Excessive blood levels of IL-5 in a patient with idiopathic EE coincided with clinical relapses [164], and degranulated eosinophils have been found in the mucosa of others [165, 166].

Clinico-Pathological Correlations. The thickening collar of submucosal oedema in patients with *A. caninum* EE obstructs the distal ileum, exacerbating symptoms that precipitate surgical intervention. The reaction parallels the wheal-and-flare of cutaneous anaphylaxis, the gut flare represented by the zone of cellular infiltrate, and the wheal corresponding to the more limited central region of submucosal oedema. In acute *A. duodenale* infection, the inflammatory reaction can be similar but more diffuse, is caused by larger numbers of developing worms and affects the proximal intestine which, being wider, is less prone to obstruction. Surgery is not undertaken, and infection patency allows specific diagnosis and treatment. Nevertheless, partial small bowel obstruction has been reported in *A. duodenale* (and probably *N. americanus*) infection [35, 36, 73].

While the extent of inflammation in *A. caninum* infection is remarkable, given the size of the single worm involved, also intriguing is the rapid response to anthelminthic therapy – symptoms, and presumably underlying inflammation, generally resolve within 12 h of treatment (see above, '*A. caninum* Infection and Human Eosinophilic Enteritis'). As the common anthelminthics are not recognised anti-inflammatory agents, repair mechanisms must be activated as soon as the stimulus is removed.

Tolerance. Even without treatment, acute EE can be expected to resolve. This might indicate expulsion of the offending parasite, for mature *A. caninum* have never been found in patients. However, in anthropophilic infections, acute symptoms generally subside spontaneously, even though the worms mature and can continue producing eggs for several years. Blood eosinophilia also declines, although not to normal levels. A phase of growing immune tolerance seems to ensue; repeated infection (after treatment) provokes abdominal symptoms of declining severity and duration. This contrasts with skin (and pulmonary) reactivity, which is potentiated by repeated exposure to L3, and the persisting high levels of circulating antibodies.

Tolerance might be induced by the increasing volumes of antigens released into the mucosa and/or the circulation by feeding hookworms. The underlying mechanisms may involve stimulation of CD8+ suppressor T cells, and/or the production of 'blocking' antibodies: IgG subclasses could inactivate the allergen, or rising levels of nonspecific IgE might inhibit cross-linking of FcεRI receptors on mast cells.

While it is impossible to quantify the level of a patient's exposure to *A. caninum* L3, in almost all cases of EE, there has been no history of obvious exposure; conversely, EE has yet to be reported from an individual with documented heavy infection. A reciprocity between cutaneous and intestinal inflammatory responses is also suggested by the relative infrequency of cutaneous lesions preceding symptomatic intestinal anthropophilic infections (see above, 'Anthropophilic Hookworms'). However, as clinical cases of EE represent only a minority of people infected, and heavy exposure occurs rarely, the dose of larvae may be immaterial. Given the antigenic similarities between parasite species, people living in anthropophilic hookworm-endemic regions might become tolerized by the conventional infections, and so will not react severely to gut infection with *A. caninum*.

Conclusions

Hookworms, like all other parasite species, are unique, each with idiosyncratic host-parasite relationships. This applies at every stage of the life cycle, so that extrapolations across host and parasite species may be invalid. Invasive larvae of all the common species may elicit ground itch, except for *A. braziliense*, which produces creeping eruption perhaps related to hyaluronidase secretion. Being an efficient skin penetrator, this species also commonly reaches the lungs. Cutaneous and subsequent pulmonary manifestations are influenced by the larval dose, previous exposure and possibly associated bacterial contamination. Respiratory tract symptoms reflect trauma from larvae, with superimposed inflammation probably reflecting allergic responses. Cutaneous exposure, perhaps with subclinical respiratory involvement, can be sufficient to induce peripheral eosinophilia.

Significant abdominal symptoms occur frequently in early anthropophilic hookworm infection, even after light exposure, and correlate with development of adult worms and rising blood eosinophilia. The underlying cause is immune-mediated intestinal inflammation, triggered by major qualitative or quantitative changes in worm secretory output, and executed by mast cell and eosinophil products, as well as cytokines. The reaction can be severe and affects the proximal intestine, which does not obstruct readily. Patency allows diagnosis, and treatment terminates the symptoms. Generally, inflammation and symptoms will subside without treatment, although abdominal pain may recur indefinitely. This, and declining symptoms in repeated infection, indicate the onset of immune tolerance.

The most widespread hookworm species is *A. caninum*, and many people in endemic areas are likely to carry hypobiotic larvae; these are undetectable with present technology, and most will remain asymptomatic. Neither the longevity of dormant larvae is known, nor the stimuli for their migration to the gut, which probably occurs intermittently. Host incompatibility is indicated by the finding of immature worms, in small numbers, in the distal ileum or beyond. Occasionally, an intense allergic reaction produces EE in the distal small bowel, which can obstruct. The factors determining who will develop clinical enteritis are obscure. There is no clear association with an allergic tendency, and genetic linkages have not been investigated, for infections with either anthropophilic or canine species. Spontaneous decline in symptoms might reflect either induction of tolerance by adult worms, or their demise.

Present diagnostic serology for hookworm infection is inadequate for clinical use, but molecular biotechnology promises the development of suitable antigens. However, blood antibody, eosinophil and lymphocyte responses are but crude indicators of events in the intestine. Improved understanding of inflammation associated with hookworm infection will depend on unravelling the complex immunocytochemical events at all stages of hookworm-host interactions, taking into account confounding variables such as bacterial co-colonisation and host nutrition.

The complexity of immune responses, provoked by migrating larvae and intestinal worms, coupled with the failure of natural and repeated infections to stimulate any obvious host protection, dampen the prospects for an effective vaccine against human hookworm infection. The allergenicity of some hookworm products raises the possibility that vaccines may exacerbate immunopathogenesis. Investing in vaccine development hardly seems justified, given the availability of effective chemotherapy, the high host-specificity of the parasites, their clinical insignificance in many cases, their ready control by simple human behavioural modifications, and their decline internationally with economic and social development. Well-coordinated anthelminthic campaigns have eradicated hookworms from disadvantaged communities, even without changes in living conditions [167]. People who cannot now afford anthelminthic treatment are hardly likely to afford repeated vaccination, for a parasitosis which does not rate highly in the morbidity stakes against many of the other endemic infections.

However, continuing research into hookworm host-parasite relationships is justified by the important discoveries in basic science that will arise, giving detailed insights into the pathogenesis of enteric infections, and allergies. Most intestinal helminths, even the ubiquitous pinworm, *Enterobius vermicularis*, secrete antigens that can interact with host tissues, so investigations of the mechanisms underlying hookworm enteritis are certain to have extensive ramifications.

Acknowledgements

I am indebted to many colleagues, all of whom have contributed substantially to our investigations. In particular, the clinical expertise, observations and provocative ideas of John Croese, combined with basic science and technical input from Joan Opdebeeck, Alex Loukas, Nongyao Sawangjaroen, Paul Brindley and Stephen Harrop (who also commented on the manuscript), are very much appreciated. Our work was funded by the National Health and Medical Research Council of Australia, The Wenkart Foundation and The University of Queensland.

References

1   Lichtenfels JR: No.8. Keys to the genera of the superfamilies Ancylostomatoidea and Diaphano-cephaloidea; in Anderson RC, Chabaud AG, Willmott S (eds): CIH Keys to the Nematode Parasites of Vertebrates. London, Farnham Royal, 1980.
2   Stoll NR: This wormy world. J Parasitol 1947;33:1–18.
3   Roche M, Layrisse M: The nature and causes of 'hookworm anaemia'. Am J Trop Med Hyg 1966; 15:1031–1102.
4   Banwell JG, Schad GA: Hookworm. Clin Gastroenterol 1978;7:129–156.
5   Miller TA: Hookworm infection in man. Adv Parasitol 1979;17:315–384.
6   Beaver PC, Jung RC, Cupp EW: The Strongylida: Hookworms and other bursate nematodes; in Clinical Parasitology. Philadelphia, Lea & Febiger, 1984, pp 269–301.
7   Grove DI: *Ancylostoma duodenale, Necator americanus* and hookworm disease; in A History of Human Helminthology. Oxford, CAB International, 1990, pp 499–541.
8   Behnke JM: Pathology; in Gilles HM, Ball PAG (eds): Human Parasitic Diseases, vol 4: Hookworm Infections. Amsterdam, Elsevier, 1991, pp 51–91.
9   Croese J, Loukas A, Opdebeeck J, Fairley S, Prociv P: Human enteric infection with canine hookworms: An emerging problem in developed communities. Ann Intern Med 1994;120:369–374.
10   Croese TJ: Eosinophilic enteritis – A recent North Queensland experience. Aust NZ J Med 1988;18: 848–853.
11   Prociv P, Croese J: Human eosinophilic enteritis caused by *Ancylostoma caninum*, a common dog hookworm. Lancet 1990;355:1299–1302.
12   Talley NJ, Shorter RG, Phillips SF, Zinsmeister AR: Eosinophilic gastroenteritis: A clinicopathological study of patients with disease of the mucosa, muscle layer and subserosal tissues. Gut 1990; 31:54–58.

13 Walker N, Croese J, Clouston A, Parry M, Loukas A, Prociv P: Eosinophilic enteritis in north-eastern Australia: Pathology, association with *Ancylostoma caninum* and implications. Am J Surg Pathol 1995;19:328–337.

14 Talley NJ: Eosinophilic gastroenteritis; in Sleisenger MH, Fordtran JS (eds): Gastrointestinal Disease: Pathophysiology, Diagnosis, Management, ed 5. Philadelphia, Saunders, 1993, pp 1224–1232.

15 Loukas A, Croese J, Opdebeeck J, Prociv P: Detection of antibodies to secretions of *Ancylostoma caninum* in human eosinophilic enteritis. Trans R Soc Trop Med Hyg 1992;86:650–653.

16 Loukas A, Croese J, Opdebeeck J, Prociv P: Immunologic incrimination of *Ancylostoma caninum* as a human enteric pathogen. Am J Trop Med Hyg 1994;50:69–77.

17 Nelson GS: Hookworms in perspective, in Schad GA, Warren KS (eds): Hookworm Disease: Current Status and New Directions. London, Taylor & Francis, 1990, pp 417–430.

18 Shelmire B: Experimental creeping eruption from a cat and dog hookworm *(Ancylostoma braziliense)*. JAMA 1928;91:938–943.

19 Heydon GM: Creeping eruption or larva migrans in north Queensland and a note on the worm *Gnathostoma spinigerum* (Owen). Med J Aust 1929;i:583–591.

20 Hunter GW, Worth CB: Variations in response to filariform larvae of *Ancylostoma caninum* in the skin of man. J Parasitol 1945;31:366–372.

21 Miller AC, Walker J, Jaworski R, de Launey W, Paver R: Hookworm folliculitis. Arch Dermatol 1991;127:547–549.

22 Kirby-Smith JL, Dove WE, White GF: Creeping eruption. Arch Dermatol Syphilol 1926;13:137–175.

23 White GF, Dove WE: The causation of creeping eruption. JAMA 1928;90:1701–1704.

24 Sandground JH: Creeping eruption in the Netherland East Indies caused by the invasion of the larva of *Ancylostoma braziliense*. Geneeskd Tijdschr Nederland-Indie 1939;72:805–810.

25 Katz R, Ziegler J, Blank H: The natural course of creeping eruption and treatment with thiabendazole. Arch Dermatol 1965;91:420–424.

26 Beaver PC: Immunity to *N. americanus* infection. J Parasitol 1944;31(suppl):18.

27 Brumpt L-C: Déductions cliniques tirées de cinquante cas d'ankylostomose provoquée. Ann Parasitol Hum Comp 1952;27:237–249.

28 Ball PAJ, Bartlett A: Serological reactions to infections with *Necator americanus*. Trans R Soc Trop Med Hyg 1969;63:362–369.

29 Ogilvie BM, Bartlett A, Godfrey FC, Turton JA, Worms MJ, Yeates RA: Antibody in self-infections with *Necator americanus*. Trans R Soc Trop Med Hyg 1978;72:66–71.

30 Turton JA: Studies on primary, secondary, tertiary and quaternary self-infections with *Necator americanus*. Parasitology 1977;75:xxxvi.

31 Schad GA, Chowdhury AB, Dean CG, Kochar VK, Nawalinski TA, Thomas J, Tonascia JA: Arrested development in human hookworm infections: An adaptation to a seasonally unfavorable external environment. Science 1973;180:502–504.

32 Ashford BK, Payne GC, Payne FK: Acute uncinariasis from massive infestation and its implications. JAMA 1933;101:843–847.

33 Nawalinski TA, Schad GA: Arrested development in *A. duodenale:* Course of a self-induced infection in man. Am J Trop Med Hyg 1974;23:895–898.

34 Cline BL, Little MD, Bartholomew RK, Halsey NA: Larvicidal activity of albendazole against *N. americanus* in human volunteers. Am J Trop Med Hyg 1984;33:387–394.

35 Koshy A, Raina V, Sharma MP, Mithal S, Tandon BN: An unusual outbreak of hookworm disease in north India. Am J Trop Med Hyg 1978;27:42–45.

36 Rogers AM, Dammin GJ: Hookworm infection in American troops in Assam and Burma. Am J Med Sci 1946;211:531–538.

37 Wijers DJB, Smit AM: Early symptoms after experimental infection of man with *Ancylostoma braziliense* var. *ceylanicum.* Trop Geogr Med 1966;18:48–52.

38 Maplestone PA: Creeping eruption produced by hookworm larvae. Indian Med Gazette 1933;68:251–256.

39 Bearup AJ: Correspondence: *Ancylostoma braziliense.* Trop Geogr Med 1967;19:161–162.

40 Anten JFG, Zuidema PJ: Hookworm infection in Dutch serviceman returning from West New Guinea. Trop Geogr Med 1964;16:216–224.

41 Wright DO, Gold EM: Löffler's syndrome associated with creeping eruption (cutaneous helminthiasis): Report of twenty-six cases. Arch Intern Med 1946;78:303–312.

42 Kalmon EH: Creeping eruption associated with transient pulmonary infiltration. Radiology 1954; 62:222–226.

43 Guill MA, Odom RB: Larva migrans complicated by Loeffler's syndrome. Arch Dermatol 1978; 114:1525–1526.

44 Muhleisen JP: Demonstration of pulmonary migration of the causative agent of creeping eruption. Ann Intern Med 1953;38:595–600.

45 Smith CA: Uncinariasis in the South, with special reference to mode of infection. JAMA 1904;43: 592–597.

46 Hodes PJ, Keefer GP: Hookworm disease: A small intestinal study. Am J Roentgenol Radium Ther 1945;54:728–742.

47 Zimmerman HM: Fatal hookworm disease in infancy and childhood on Guam. Am J Pathol 1946; 22:1081–1099.

48 Harada Y: Wakana disease and hookworm allergy. Yonago Acta Med 1962;6:109–118.

49 Maxwell C, Hussain R, Nutman TB, Poindexter RW, Little MD, Schad GA, Ottesen EA: The clinical and immunologic responses of normal human volunteers to low dose hookworm (Necator americanus) infection. Am J Trop Med Hyg 1987;37:126–134.

50 Carroll SM, Grove DI: Experimental infection of humans with Ancylostoma ceylanicum: Clinical, parasitological, haematological and immunological findings. Trop Geogr Med 1986;38:38–45.

51 Croese J, Loukas A, Opdebeeck J, Prociv P: Occult enteric infection by Ancylostoma caninum: A previously unrecognised zoonosis. Gastroenterology 1994;106:3–13.

52 Croese J: Seasonal influence on human enteric infection with Ancylostoma caninum. Am J Trop Med Hyg 1995;53:158–161.

53 Croese J, Fairley S, Loukas A, Hack J, Stronach P: Ileal ulceration: An index of cryptic infection by Ancylostoma caninum. J Gastroenterol Hepatol 1996;11:524–531.

54 Schad GA: The role of arrested development in the regulation of nematode populations; in Esch GW (ed): Regulation of Parasite Populations. New York, Academic Press, 1977, pp 111–167.

55 Schad GA, Page MR: Ancylostoma caninum: Adult worm removal, corticosteroid treatment, and resumed development of arrested larvae in dogs. Exp Parasitol 1982;54:303–309.

56 Behnke JM: Laboratory animal models; in Schad GA, Warren KS (eds): Hookworm Disease: Current Status and New Directions. London, Taylor & Francis, 1990, pp 105–128.

57 Gibbs HC: Hypobiosis in parasitic nematodes – an update. Adv Parasitol 1986;25:129–174.

58 Little MD, Halsey NA, Cline BL, Katz SP: Ancylostoma larva in muscle fiber of man following cutaneous larva migrans. Am J Trop Med Hyg 1983;32:1285–1288.

59 Matsusaki G: Studies on the life history of the hookworm. VI. On the development of Ancylostoma caninum in the abnormal host. Yokahama Med Bull 1951;2:154–160.

60 Burke TM, Roberson EL: Prenatal and lactational transmission of Toxocara canis and Ancylostoma caninum: Experimental infection of the bitch before pregnancy. Int J Parasitol 1985;15:71–75.

61 Vetter JCM, Leegwater-v.d. Linden ME: Skin penetration of infective hookworm larvae. III. Comparative studies on the path of migration of the hookworms Ancylostoma braziliense, Ancylostoma ceylanicum, and Ancylostoma caninum. Z Parasitenkd 1977;53:155–158.

62 Prociv P, Luke RL: Evidence for larval hypobiosis in Australian strains of Ancylostoma duodenale. Trans R Soc Trop Med Hyg 1995;89:379.

63 Yu S-H, Jiang Z-X, Xu L-Q: Infantile hookworm disease in China. A review. Acta Trop 1995;59: 265–270.

64 Walker AC, Bellmaine SP: Severe alimentary bleeding associated with hookworm infestation in Aboriginal infants. Med J Aust 1975;1:751–752.

65 Burke TM, Roberson EL: Prenatal and lactational transmission of Toxocara canis and Ancylostoma caninum: Experimental infection of the bitch at midpregnancy and parturition. Int J Parasitol 1985; 15:485–490.

66   Schad GA, Murrell KD, Fayer R, El Naggar HMS, Page MR, Parrish PK, Stewart TD: Paratenesis in *A. duodenale* suggests possible meat-borne human infection. Trans R Soc Trop Med Hyg 1984; 78:203–204.

67   Khoshoo V, Schantz P, Craver R, Stern GM, Loukas A, Prociv P: Dog hookworm: A cause of eosinophilic enterocolitis in humans. J Pediatr Gastroenterol Nutr 1994;19:448–452.

68   Khoshoo V, Craver R, Schantz P, Loukas A, Prociv P: Abdominal pain, pan-gut eosinophilia, and dog hookworm infection. J Pediatr Gastroenterol Nutr 1995;21:481.

69   Croese J, Prociv P, Maguire E, Crawford A: Eosinophilic enteritis presenting as surgical emergencies: A report of six cases. Med J Aust 1990;153:415–417.

70   Yoshida Y: Comparative stages of *Ancylostoma braziliense* and *Ancylostoma ceylanicum.* I. The adult stage. J Parasitol 1971;57:983–989.

71   Migasena S, Gilles HM: Hookworm infection. Clin Trop Med Commun Dis 1987;2:617–627.

72   Ottesen EA: Immune responses in human hookworm infection; in Schad GA, Warren KS (eds): Hookworm Disease: Current Status and New Directions. London, Taylor & Francis, 1990, pp 404–413.

73   Parodi L: Sur les syndromes gastro-duodénaux et péritonéaux de l'ankylostomiase. Méd Trop 1958; 18:937–942.

74   Walterspiel JN, Schad GA, Buchanan GR: Direct transfer of adult hookworms *(A. duodenale)* from dog to child for therapeutic purposes. J Parasitol 1984;70:217–219.

75   Kelley PW, Takafuji ET, Wiener H, Milhous W, Miller R, Thompson NJ, Schantz P, Miller RN: An outbreak of hookworm infection associated with military operations in Grenada. Milit Med 1989; 154:55–59.

76   Gibbes JH: Symptoms suggestive of duodenal ulcer arising from hookworm infection. J SC Med Assoc 1934;30:102–106.

77   Rowland HAK: Dyspepsia, duodenitis and hookworm infection. Trans R Soc Trop Med Hyg 1966; 60:481–485.

78   Pagan MA, Torres de Vega C: Fatal intestinal haemorrhage due to hookworm in infants. Bol Asoc Med Puerto Rico 1963;55:456–462.

79   Chowdhury AB, Schad GA: *Ancylostoma ceylanicum:* A parasite of man in Calcutta and environs. Am J Trop Med Hyg 1972;21:300–301.

80   Wells HS: Observations on the blood sucking activities of the hookworm, *Ancylostoma caninum.* J Parasitol 1931;17:167–182.

81   Krupp, IM: Effects of crowding and of superinfection on habitat selection and egg production in *Ancylostoma caninum.* J Parasitol 1961;47:957–961.

82   Kalkofen UP: Attachment and feeding behaviour of *Ancylostoma caninum.* Z Parasitenkd 1970;33: 339–354.

83   Kalkofen UP: Intestinal trauma resulting from feeding activities of *Ancylostoma caninum.* Am J Trop Med Hyg 1974;23:1046–1053.

84   Carroll SM, Grove DI: Transmission electron microscopical studies of the site of attachment of *Ancylostoma ceylanicum* to the small bowel mucosa of the dog. J Helminthol 1984;58:313–320.

85   Hayden DW, Van Kruiningen: Eosinophilic gastroenteritis in German Shepherd dogs and its relationship to visceral larva migrans. JAVMA 1973;162:379–384.

86   Rep BH: The topographic distribution of *N. americanus* and *A. duodenale* in the human intestine. Trop Geogr Med 1975;27:169–176.

87   Yong T-S, Shin H-J, Im K-I, Kim W-H: An imported case of hookworm infection with worms in the rectum. Korean J Parasitol 1992:30:59–62.

88   Nath K, Sur BK, Samuel KC, Gupta BK, Mital HS, Seth ON, Saxena S: Malabsorption in ankylostomiasis. Indian J Med Res 1971;59:1090–1098.

89   Chaudhuri RN, Saha TK: Jejunal mucosa in hookworm disease. Am J Trop Med Hyg 1964;13: 410–411.

90   Bonne C: Invasion of the wall of the human intestine by ancylostomes. Am J Trop Med Hyg 1942; 22:507–509.

91   Bonne C: Invasion of the submucosa of the human small intestine by *Ancylostoma braziliense.* Am J Trop Med Hyg 1937;17:587–594.

92 Behnke JM: Immunology; in Gilles HM, Ball PAG (eds): Human Parasitic Diseases. Amsterdam, Elsevier, 1991, vol 4: Hookworm Infections, pp 92–155.

93 McCoy OR: Immunity reactions of the dog against hookworm *(A. caninum)* under conditions of repeated infection. Am J Hyg 1931;14:286–303.

94 Miller TA: Vaccination against the canine hookworm diseases. Adv Parasitol 1971;9:153–183.

95 Miller TA: Industrial development and field use of the canine hookworm vaccine. Adv Parasitol 1978;16:333–342.

96 Loukas A, Opdebeeck J, Croese J, Prociv P: IgG subclass antibodies against excretory/secretory antigens of *Ancylostoma caninum* in human enteric infections. Am J Trop Med Hyg 1996;54:672–676.

97 Hagan P, Blumenthal UJ, Dunn D, Simpson AJG, Wilkins HA: Human IgE, IgG4 and resistance to reinfection with *Schistosoma haematobium*. Nature 1991;349:243–245.

98 Demeure CE, Rihet P, Abel L, Outtara M, Bourgeois A, Dessein AJ: Resistance to *Schistosoma mansoni* in humans: Influence of the IgE/IgG4 balance and IgG2 in immunity to reinfection after chemotherapy. J Infect Dis 1993;168:1000–1008.

99 Sawangjaroen N: Studies of excretory-secretory antigens of adult *Ancylostoma caninum*; PhD thesis, The University of Queensland, Brisbane, 1996.

100 Pritchard DI, Walsh EA, Quinell RJ, Raiko A, Edmonds P, Keymer AE: Isotypic variation in antibody responses in a community in Papua New Guinea to larval and adult antigens during infection, and following reinfection, with the hookworm *N. americanus*. Parasite Immunol 1992;14:617–631.

101 Carroll SM: Immunity: Hookworm in animal model systems; in Schad GA, Warren KS (eds): Hookworm Disease: Current Status and New Directions. London, Taylor & Francis, 1990, pp 391–403.

102 White CJ, Maxwell CJ, Gallin JI: Changes in the structural and functional properties of human eosinophils during experimental hookworm infection. J Infect Dis 1986;154:778–783.

103 Salafsky B, Fusco AC, Siddiqui A: *Necator americanus*: Factors influencing skin penetration by larvae; in Schad GA, Warren KS (eds): Hookworm Disease: Current Status and New Directions. London, Taylor & Francis, 1990, pp 329–339.

104 Hotez P, Haggerty J, Hawdon J, Milstone L, Gamble HR, Schad G, Richards F: Metalloproteases of infective *Ancylostoma* hookworm larvae and their possible functions in tissue invasion and ecdysis. Infect Immun 1990;58:3883–3892.

105 Hotez PJ, Narasimhan S, Haggerty J, Milstone L, Bhopale V, Schad GA, Richards FF: Hyaluronidase from infective *Ancylostoma* hookworm larvae and its possible function as a virulence factor in tissue invasion and in cutaneous larva migrans. Infect Immun 1992;60:1018–1023.

106 Hotez P, Hawdon J, Cappello M: Molecular mechanisms of invasion by *Ancylostoma* hookworms; in Boothroyd JC, Komuniecki R (eds): Molecular Approaches to Parasitology. New York, Wiley-Liss, 1995, pp 21–29.

107 Pritchard DI: *Necator americanus:* Antigens and immunological targets; in Schad GA, Warren KS (eds): Hookworm Disease: Current Status and New Directions. London, Taylor & Francis, 1990, pp 340–350.

108 Hawdon JM, Schad GA: Long-term storage of hookworm infective larvae in buffered saline solution maintains larval responsiveness to host signals. J Helm Soc Wash 1991;58:140–142.

109 Pritchard DI, Leggett KV, Rogan MT, McKean PG, Brown A: *N. americanus* secretory acetylcholinesterase and its purification from excretory-secretory products by affinity chromatography. Parasite Immunol 1991;13:187–199.

110 Looss A: The anatomy and life history of *Agchylostoma duodenale* Dub. A monograph. Records of the Egyptian Government School of Medicine. Cairo, National Printing Department, 1905, vol 3.

111 Eiff JA: Nature of an anticoagulant from the cephalic glands of *Ancylostoma caninum*. J Parasitol 1966;52:833–843.

112 McLaren DJ, Burt JS, Ogilvie BM: The anterior glands of adult *Necator americanus* (Nematoda: Strongyloidea). II. Cytochemical and functional studies. Int J Parasitol 1974;4:39–46

113 Sawangjaroen N, Opdebeeck JP, Prociv P: Immunohistochemical localization of excretory/secretory antigens in adult *Ancylostoma caninum* using monoclonal antibodies and infected human sera. Exp Parasitol 1995;17:29–35.

114   Harrop SA, Sawangjaroen N, Prociv P, Brindley PJ: Characterization of cathepsin B proteinase genes expressed by adult *Ancylostoma caninum*. Molec Biochem Parasitol 1995;71:163–171.
115   Schad GA: The parasite; in Gilles HM, Ball PAG (eds): Human Parasitic Diseases. Hookworm Infections. Amsterdam, Elsevier, 1991, vol 4, pp 15–49.
116   Brown A, Burleigh JM, Billett EE, Pritchard DI: An initial characterization of the proteolytic enzymes secreted by the adult stage of the human hookworm, *N. americanus*. Parasitology 1995; 110:555–563.
117   Pritchard DI: The survival strategies of hookworms. Parasitol Today 1995;11:255–259.
118   Thorson RE: The effect of extracts of the amhidial glands, excretory glands, and esophagus of adults of *Ancylostoma caninum* on the coagulation of dog's blood. J Parasitol 1956;42:26–30.
119   Carroll SM, Howse DJ, Grove DI: The anticoagulant effects of the hookworm, *Ancylostoma ceylanicum:* Observations in human and dog blood in vitro and infected dogs in vivo. Thrombosis and Haemostasis 1984;51:222–227.
120   Hotez PJ, Trang NL, McKerrow JH, Cerami A: Isolation and characterization of a proteolytic enzyme from the adult hookworm *Ancylostoma caninum*. J Biol Chem 1985;250:7343–7348.
121   Cappello M, Clyne LP, McPhedran P, Hotez P: *Ancylostoma* factor Xa inhibitor: Partial purification and its identification as a major hookworm anticoagulant in vitro. J Infect Dis 1993;167: 1474–1477.
122   McKerrow JH: Parasite proteases. Exp Parasitol 1989;68:111–115.
123   Dalton JP, Smith AM, Clough KA, Brindley PJ: Digestion of haemoglobin by schistosomes: 35 years on. Parasitol Today 1995;11:299–303.
124   Becker MM, Harrop SA, Dalton JP, Kalinna BH, McManus DP, Brindley PJ: Cloning and characterization of the *Schistosoma japonicum* aspartic proteinase involved in hemoglobin digestion. J Biol Chem 1995;270:24496–24501.
125   Oya Y, Noguchi I: Some properties of hemoglobin protease from *A. caninum* (in Japanese, with English abstract). Jap J Parasitol 1977;26:307–313.
126   Takahashi T, Yonezawa S, Deharani AH, Tang J: Comparative studies of two cathepsin B isozymes from porcine spleen. J Biol Chem 1986;261:9368–9374.
127   Dowd AJ, Dalton JP, Loukas AC, Prociv P, Brindley PJ: Secretion of cysteine proteinase activity by the zoonotic hookworm *Ancylostoma caninum*. Am J Trop Med Hyg 1994;51:341–347.
128   Day SR, Dalton JP, Clough KA, Leonardo L, Tiu WU, Brindley PJ: Characterization and cloning of the cathepsin L proteinases of *Schistosoma japonicum*. Biochem Biophys Res Commun 1995;217: 1–9.
129   Kumar S, Pritchard DI: The partial characterization of proteases present in the excretory/secretory products and exsheathing fluid of the infective (L3) larva of *Necator americanus*. Int J Parasitol 1992;22:563–572.
130   Bruni A, Passalacqua A: Sulla presenza di una mesomucinasi (jaluronidasi) in *Ancylostoma duodenale*. Boll Soc Ital Biol Sper 1954;30:789–791.
131   Hotez P, Cappello M, Hawdon J, Beckers C, Sakanari J: Hyaluronidases of the gastrointestinal invasive nematodes *Ancylostoma caninum* and *Anisakis simplex*: Possible functions in the pathogenesis of human zoonoses. J Infect Dis 1994;170:918–926.
132   McLaren DJ: Sense organs and their secretions; inCroll NA (ed): The Organization of Nematodes. London, Academic Press, 1976, pp 139–161.
133   Wang FL, Ning KB, Wang XZ, Yang GM, Wang JY: Average values of *A. duodenale* and *N. americanus* cholinesterase activity in humans. Chinese Med J 1983;96:60–62.
134   Johnson CD, Russell RL: Multiple molecular forms of acetylcholinesterase in the nematode *Caenorhabditis elegans*. J Neurochem 1983;41:30–46.
135   Sine J-P, Ferrand R, Cloarec D, Lehur P-A, Colas B: Human intestine epithelial cell acetyl- and butyrylcholinesterases. Mol Cell Biochem 1991;108:145–149.
136   Small DH: Acetylcholinesterases: Proteases regulating cell growth and development?; in Massoulie J, Bacou F, Barnard E, Chatonnet A, Doctor BP, Quinn DM (eds): Cholinesterases: Structure, Function, Mechanism, Genetics and Cell Biology. Washington, American Chemical Society Conference Proceedings Series, 1991, pp 374–378.

137   Moyle M, Foster DF, McGrath DE, Brown SM, Laroche Y, De Meutter J, Stanssens P, Bogowitz CA, Fried VA, Ely A, Soule HR, Vlasuk GP: A hookworm glycoprotein that inhibits neutrophil function is a ligand of the integrin CD11b/CD18. J Biol Chem 1994;269:10008–10015.

138   Muchowski PJ, Zhang L, Chang ER, Soule HR, Plow EP, Moyle M: Functional interaction between the integrin antagonist neutrophil inhibitory factor and the I domain of CD11b/CD18. J Biol Chem 1994;269:26419–26423.

139   Wardlaw AJ, Moqbel R: The eosinophil in allergic and helminth-related inflammatory responses; in Moqbel R (ed): Allergy and Immunity to Helminths: Common Mechanisms or Divergent Pathways? London, Taylor & Francis, 1992, pp 154–186.

140   Weller P: Eosinophils: Structure and function. Curr Opin Immunol 1994;6:85–90.

141   Kennedy MW: Genetic control of the antibody response to parasite allergens; in Moqbel R (ed): Allergy and Immunity to Helminths: Common Mechanisms or Divergent Pathways? London, Taylor & Francis, 1992, pp 63–80.

142   Marsh DG, Zwollo P, Huang SK, Ansari AA: Molecular genetics of human immune responsiveness to allergens; in Chadwick D, Evered D, Whelan J (eds): IgE, Mast Cells and the Allergic Response. Ciba Foundation Symposium 147. Chichester, Wiley, 1989, pp 171–187.

143   Marsh DG, Neely JD, Breazeale DR, Ghosh B, Freidhoff LR, Schou C, Beaty TH: Genetic basis of IgE responsiveness; relevance to atopic diseases. Int Arch Allergy Immunol 1995;107:25–28.

144   Hong CB, Chow CK: Induction of eosinophilic enteritis and eosinophilia in rats by vitamin E and selenium deficiency. Exp Mol Pathol 1988;48:182–192.

145   Castro GA: Intestinal pathology; in Behnke JM (ed): Parasites: Immunity and Pathology. London, Taylor & Francis, 1990, pp 283–316.

146   MacDonald TT: Mucosal immunity in human chronic helminthic disease and gut inflammation; in Moqbel R (ed): Allergy and Immunity to Helminths: Common Mechanisms or Divergent Pathways? London, Taylor & Francis, 1992, pp 137–153.

147   MacDonald AJ, Cromwell O, Moqbel R: Allergic mediators in immediate-type hypersensitivity and immune reactions against helminths; in Moqbel R (ed): Allergy and Immunity to Helminths: Common Mechanisms or Divergent Pathways? London, Taylor & Francis, 1992, pp 249–263.

148   Nutman TB: T-cell regulation of immediate hypersensitivity: Lessons from helminth parasites and allergic disease; in Moqbel R (ed): Allergy and Immunity to Helminths: Common Mechanisms or Divergent Pathways? London, Taylor & Francis, 1992, pp 187–204.

149   Finkelman FD, Urban JF Jr: Cytokines: Making the right choice. Parasitol Today 1992;8:311–314.

150   Heinzel FP: Th1 and Th2 cells in the cure and pathogenesis of infectious diseases. Current Opinion in Infectious Dis 1995;8:151–155.

151   Miller HRP: Mast cells: Their function and heterogeneity; in Moqbel R (ed): Allergy and Immunity to Helminths: Common Mechanisms or Divergent Pathways? London, Taylor & Francis, 1992, pp 228–248.

152   Schwartz LB: Mast cells: Function and contents. Curr Opin Immunol 1994;6:91–97.

153   Barnes PJ, Chung KF, Page CP: Platelet-activating factor as a mediator of allergic disease. J Allergy Clin Immunol 1988;81:919–934.

154   Sun X-M, MacKendrick W, Tien J, Huang W, Caplan MS, Hsueh W: Endogenous bacterial toxins are required for the injurious action of platelet-activating factor in rats. Gastroenterology 1995;109:83–88.

155   Sartor RB: Cytokines in intestinal inflammation: Pathophysiological and clinical considerations. Gastroenterology 1994;106:533–539.

156   Rothwell TLW: Immune expulsion of parasitic nematodes from the alimentary tract. Int J Parasitol 1989;19:139–168.

157   Capron A, Dessaint JP, Capron M: Allergy and immune defence: Common IgE-dependent mechanisms or divergent pathways; in Moqbel R (ed): Allergy and Immunity to Helminths: Common Mechanisms or Divergent Pathways? London, Taylor & Francis, 1992, pp 1–16.

158   Crowe SE, Perdue MH: Gastrointestinal tract hypersensitivity: Basic mechanisms of pathophysiology. Gastroenterology 1992;103:1075–1095.

159   Undem BJ, Riccio MM, Weinreich D, Ellis JL, Myers AC: Neurophysiology of mast cell-nerve interactions in the airways. Int Arch Allergy Immunol 1995;107:199–201.

Hookworm Infections   97

160 Miller HRP: The protective mucosal response against gastrointestinal nematodes in ruminants and laboratory animals.Vet Immunol Immunopathol 1984;6:167–259.
161 Wakelin D: Allergic inflammation as a hypothesis for the expulsion of worms from tissues. Parasitol Today 1993;9:115–116.
162 Moqbel R, MacDonald AJ: Immunological and inflammatory responses in the small intestine associated with helminthic infections; in Behnke JM (ed): Parasites: Immunity and Pathology. London, Taylor & Francis, 1990, pp 249–282.
163 Fargeas M-J, Theodorou V, More J, Wal J-M, Fioramonti J, Bueno L: Boosted systemic immune and local responsiveness after intestinal inflammation in orally sensitized guinea pigs. Gastroenterology 1995;109:53–62.
164 Takahashi T, Nakamura K, Nishikawa S, Tsuyuoka R, Suzuki A, Murakami M, Amenomori M, Okuno Y, Imura H: Interleukin-5 in eosinophilic gastroenteritis. Am J Haematol 1992;40:295–298.
165 Torpier G, Colombel JF, Mathieu-Chandelier C, Capron M, Dessaint JP, Cortot A, Paris JC, Capron A: Eosinophilic gastroenteritis: Ultrastructural evidence for a selective release of eosinophilic major basic protein. Clin Exp Immunol 1988;74:404–408.
166 Talley NJ, Kephart GM, McGovern TW, Carpenter HA, Gleich GJ: Deposition of eosinophil granule major basic protein in eosinophilic gastroenteritis and celiac disease. Gastroenterology 1992; 103:137–145.
167 Prociv P, Luke R: Changing patterns of human hookworm infections in Australia. Med J Aust 1995; 162:150–154.

Paul Prociv, Assoc. Prof., Department of Parasitology, University of Queensland, Brisbane, Qld. 4072 (Australia)

Freedman DO (ed): Immunopathogenetic Aspects of Disease Induced by Helminth Parasites.
Chem Immunol. Basel, Karger, 1997, vol 66, pp 99–124

....

Human Toxocariasis and the Visceral Larva Migrans Syndrome: Correlative Immunopathology

Stephen G. Kayes

Department of Structural and Cellular Biology, College of Medicine,
University of South Alabama, Mobile, Ala., USA

As in the case of *Toxocara,* the behavior of larvae in man cannot properly be regarded as reflecting a host-parasite relationship that is in its essential features abnormal.

P.C. Beaver [1]

Introduction

The first recognition that humans could be infected by *Toxocara canis*, the common roundworm of domestic dogs, was made in 1952 by Beaver and his colleagues in New Orleans, La., USA [2]. In this sentinel publication Beaver coined the term visceral larva migrans (VLM) to describe the migration of the second-stage larvae through the visceral organs of the aberrant human host. The term cutaneous larva migrans was reserved for migration exclusively within the skin. In essence, what Beaver and his colleagues reported was the finding in very young children of a syndrome which included high peripheral blood eosinophil counts, hepatomegaly, and hyperglobulinemia. In addition to having dogs in the immediate vicinity of the patients, there was an added risk factor of geophagic pica or the eating of soil contaminated with dog feces containing the eggs of the parasite.

A series of papers published prior to 1952 may have presaged the recognition of *T. canis* as a human pathogen. Common to these reports were the findings of children presenting clinically with chronic, elevated eosinophilia, fever, lethargy, lung and liver involvement. When infection with *Ascaris, Trichuris* or other intestinal helminths could be ascertained, the clinical picture was attributed to them.

However, when no evidence of parasitic infection could be found, diagnoses of Weingarten's disease, Frimodt-Moller's syndrome, familial eosinophilia, eosinophilic pseudoleukemia or eosinophilic leukemoides were made. These more esoteric pronouncements reflected the clinical preoccupation with the exaggerated eosinophilia. The first of the pre-VLM papers was published in 1947 [3] and described eosinophilic granulomata in a liver biopsy of a 2-year old girl in Philadelphia, Pa., USA. Within a short time, several more reports appeared, all describing the symptoms now commonly associated with VLM syndrome [4–6]. In common with each other, all of these papers reported findings of eosinophilic granulomata in liver biopsies done at laparotomy. In 1950, Wilder found nematode larvae in 24 of 46 children's eyes which had been enucleated because of external exudative or hemorrhagic retinitis. The larvae were subsequently identified as *T. canis* by Nichols [7] in 1956. Then in 1951, Beautymann and Woolf [8] found a larva in the left thalamus of an English child whose death was attributed to poliomyelitis. It was against this background, that Beaver and colleagues described their 3 cases which forever changed the way parasitologists, and hopefully physicians and veterinarians, look at the relationship between humans and their canine companions.

VLM syndrome consists of hypereosinophilia, hepatosplenomegaly, hyperglobulinemia and Löffler's pneumonia [2, 9, 10]. VLM syndrome due to infection by the microscopic larvae of the cosmopolitan canine ascarid, *T. canis,* may represent one of the great underrecognized parasitic infections in North America. The consensus of most epidemiological studies based on the use of the *T. canis* excretory-secretory (TEX) antigen enzyme-linked immunosorbent assay (ELISA) to evaluate children of developed countries is that between 7 and 30% are seropositive [11–16]. Because most survey results come primarily from individuals who otherwise were considered healthy, the effects of a *T. canis* infection seem inapparent, and the disease is usually considered self-limiting. However, there is now an expanding body of evidence that tissue-invasive nematodiases, particularly in young children, can and do lead to the development of asthma [17–21] and or promote pulmonary fibrosis. The pathogenetic link in these otherwise unrelated conditions may be the finding [22] that eosinophils, a hallmark of VLM syndrome, express mRNA for transforming growth factor-β and the findings that this factor can stimulate fibroblasts to synthesize collagen in a bleomycin-treated mouse model of pulmonary fibrosis [23] and that eosinophils are intimately associated with collagen fibers in eosinophilic myocarditis [24]. If there is a link between eosinophils and connective tissue injury, especially that involving collagen, then it follows that any condition of chronic pulmonary eosinophilia whether related to asthma, parasites such as *T. canis*, or idiopathic causes could result in damaged or scarred lungs and impaired respiration.

Life Cycle of *Toxocara canis*

To appreciate the insidiousness of the human infection with *T. canis*, it is important to realize the elegance of the relationship between the parasite and its definitive host, the dog. It should be pointed out that during most of this chapter, *T. canis* will be considered the etiological agent of VLM, but other larval parasites including *Baylisascaris procyonis* (from racoons), *Toxocara cati* (from cats) and *Gnathostoma spinigerum* can also infect humans and cause the condition.

Because adult dogs exhibit moderate immunity, toxocariasis can be considered primarily a parasitic disease of young puppies. Adult worms inhabit the small intestine of the dogs and fertile female worms produce prodigious numbers of eggs which pass in the feces and onto the soil. While each female worm has been suggested as being capable of producing upwards of 2×10^5 eggs per day, more recent studies suggest a rate of 25–85 thousand eggs per day per female, but when one considers that a puppy typically harbors 50–100 worms, the number of eggs per infected puppy can easily approach 1–2 million eggs per day [25]. During a period of 3–6 weeks under proper conditions of temperature and humidity, the eggs embryonate and become infective. Each egg contains a single second-stage larva (the term juvenile is technically correct as the older term 'larva' connotes an immature and morphologically distinct stage of insect development; however, the larval nomenclature is used here for consistency). When ingested, the eggs hatch and the larval worms enter the vasculature and a somatic migration ensues which involves the liver and lungs. When the worms reach the lungs, they leave the vasculature, enter the air spaces, molt and ascend the respiratory tree to be swallowed. After descent into the small bowel and a final molt, the young adult worms mate and begin the cycle anew.

In female dogs, not all the worms that begin the somatic migration complete it. In the bitch, some of these worms become dormant and await the onset of pregnancy. When pregnancy occurs, the dormant worms (still in an immature stage) migrate to the uterus and infect the pups in utero. Once within the pups the juvenile worms migrate to the liver and lungs to await parturition. Upon the birth of the pups, they finish their migration as previously described and eggs can appear in the feces as early as 2 weeks after whelping. Puppies can also be infected as they suckle (transmammary transmission) with the milk being contaminated, again, by cohorts of larval worms that were dormant in the bitch. Lastly, the mother dog can become more heavily infected during the act of cleaning the nest. Puppies that are extremely heavily infected can pass more mature larvae in their feces and these worms can be ingested by the mother and become established in her small bowel where they contribute to the heavy contamination of the surrounding environment.

As is typical of all ascarids of land mammals, the eggs of *T. canis* require a period of development on soil before becoming infective. Unlike most ascarids, however, *T. canis* can persist within the tissues of hosts other than the definitive host for extended periods of time. Paratenic host is the term that is used for animals which can become infected with the parasite, maintain the parasite in a viable state for extended periods of time, and move the parasite to a more favorable location from which it can complete the life cycle. This latter phenomenon occurs through the act of predation when the canine definitive host eats the paratenic host. While the paratenic or transport host maintains the parasite through space and time, until it is consumed by the definitive host, it should be pointed out that paratenesis is not an absolute requirement of the parasite to complete its life cycle. Beaver et al. were the first to recognize that toddler-aged children (in actuality any human regardless of age) can serve as a paratenic host of *T. canis*.

Within the paratenic host, the larval worms do not develop or grow but they do migrate through the viscera and thereby give rise to VLM. When these paratenic hosts are consumed by dogs, the second-stage larvae complete their migration and become established in the intestines of the dog. The fact that *T. canis* has so many ways and means to complete its life cycle would seem to suggest that it is an example of an extremely well-adapted host-parasite relationship. The life cycle including the role of paratenic hosts is depicted in figure 1. Because humans typically are not subject to canine predation, they are listed as accidental hosts, but in the grand scheme of things they most certainly qualify as paratenic hosts.

The Clinical Presentation of VLM Syndrome

How VLM presents is dependent on multiple factors including the size of inoculum ingested, genetic factors of the host, and whether or not previous exposure has occurred. Experimental animals are typically infected with a single bolus of infective eggs; however, a 'trickle infection' wherein a few eggs at a time are administered over long periods is more likely the manner in which a natural infection is acquired. Almost all the symptoms are related to the organs through which the larvae are migrating and they tend to be more or less nonspecific, with pulmonary sequelae being the most striking.

The second-stage *T. canis* larva is approximately 350–400 μm long by 20–22 μm in diameter and each egg contains a single worm. After various periods of larval migration, each worm becomes encapsulated in a granulomatous reaction that is surrounded by a collagenous capsule. An exception to this finding is that those worms which invade the central nervous system do not seem to elicit an inflammatory reaction of any kind [26, 27]. However, worms enmeshed in a granulomatous reaction are not permanently imprisoned by this host reaction, as they

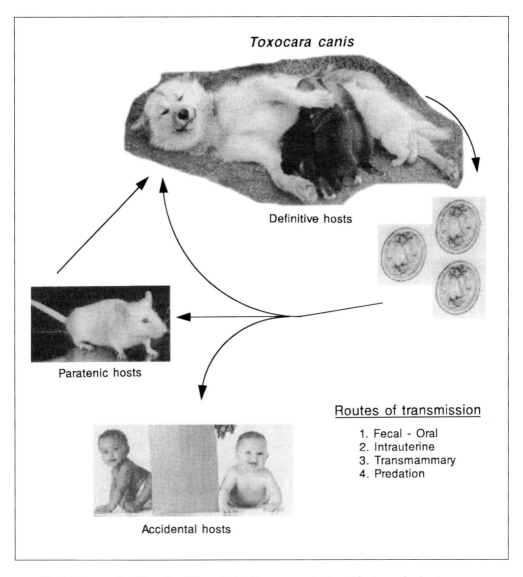

Fig. 1. The complex life cycle of *T. canis.* Adult worms are harbored in the canine hosts and they alone release eggs into the environment. After an appropriate period permitting the ova to embryonate to the infective, second larval stage, other dogs or paratenic hosts, including accidental human hosts can become infected. Intrauterine infection of virtually all puppies born coupled with predation upon paratenic hosts and transmammary infection each contribute to continued parasitism of the definitive canid host.

Table 1. Common signs and symptoms of VLM

Symptoms	Signs
Pica	Hepatomegaly
Fever	Splenomegaly
Cough	Bronchospasm
Wheeze	Lymphadenopathy
Abdominal pain	Eosinophilia
Failure to thrive	
Proximity to dogs (puppies)	

can apparently burrow out of the reaction, migrate elsewhere and elicit the same reaction anew. For this reason, the cellular composition of the granuloma (i.e., acute granulocytic cells such as eosinophils or chronic cells such as multinucleated giant cells or epithelioid macrophages) cannot be used to indicate the length of infection [28].

Most of the nonspecific symptoms of VLM can be attributed to the migration of larvae and the host response to them. As in all paratenic hosts, *T. canis* larvae that are migrating neither molt to the next stage nor increase in size, but they are metabolically active and put out both excretory and secretory materials in addition to shedding epicuticular substances into the extracellular matrices of the host [29, 30]. Thus, the liver's response to these antigenic moieties results in hepatomegaly; pulmonary response leads to pneumonia, bronchitis, and cough; and muscle involvement presents as myalgia associated with eosinophilic polymyositis [28]. Systemically, there is hyperglobulinemia and marked eosinophilia (which will be discussed at length below), but typically the usual constellation of symptoms, listed in table 1, is nonspecific and vague, often resembling 'a case of the flu'.

Of the symptoms that are seen clinically, those associated with the respiratory system are the most common [31]. Typically, parasitic pneumonias such as described by Löffler [10] are associated with cough, wheezing, and transient snowy x-rays which reflect the migration of the larvae through the lungs.

At least three forms of larva migrans have been described reflecting in part both the magnitude of the infection and the overall host response to it. The most common presentation is the classic visceral larva migrans as described by Beaver et al. [2] which consists of the frank eosinophilia, hepatosplenomegaly, and pneumonic problems such as cough, wheeze and eosinophil-rich infiltrates. This is the larva migrans presentation observed in toddler-aged children with a history of pica who ingest substantial numbers of infective eggs. If, on the other hand, the child ingests only a few eggs, the ensuing infection may not be sufficient to reach a threshold of reactivity and there are no symptoms present. This form of the disease has been named clinically inapparent [32] or occult larva migrans and is invoked to explain the results of seroepidemiological studies which identify positive patients who have never sought medical intervention. The eosinophilia and antibody response may be present, but in the absence of noteworthy illness, these signs would go unnoticed. As the child grows older and larger, the worms would become dormant and/or encapsulated in a granulomatous reaction and most likely never be a problem again. In a small number of these cases, however, the worm or worms for some reason becomes reactivated and may begin to migrate again, and if by chance it enters the eye, the third form of larva migrans, namely ocular larva migrans (OLM), is diagnosed. Menarche has been suggested as one stimulus to larva reactivation and it therefore follows that the typical patient with OLM is older than the typical VLM patient (>12.4 years vs. <3 years, respectively) [16, 33]. Thus, because toddler-aged children have oral tendencies and play on the ground or in the dirt or sand boxes frequented by infected dogs, it is easily seen why larva migrans is considered a disease of children. However, recently an outbreak of toxocariasis in adults living in the French Pyrenees has been described [34] and this outbreak has been attributed to the dietary custom of eating undercooked giblets from chickens which had become paratenic hosts of *T. canis* spewed into the environment by the dogs used for hunting. Livers from experimentally infected quail have passed the infection to laboratory mice, suggesting that multiple paratenic hosts are possible within the life cycle [35]. This adult form of the disease presented clinically primarily with lung and abdominal complaints, with elevated IgE being observed more than elevated eosinophilia [36]. The relationship between size of infection and clinical presentation is shown in figure 2.

That the larvae persist in human hosts for extended periods of time and continuously stimulate antibody is suggested by the finding that greater than 7% of 660 healthy blood donors in Canberra Australia were found to be seropositive for *T. canis* [37]. The experimental mouse correlate to these findings is that mice infected a single time with 500 eggs have antigenemias that peak within the first week but never completely disappear over the next half year [38]. A direct relationship between the number of eggs used to infect an animal and the magnitude of the ensuing host responses including antibody titer, eosinophil levels, splenomegaly, in vitro lymphocyte blastogenesis to antigens and mitogens, liver trapping, and the level of circulating antigenemia have been observed by various investigators [38–41].

When laboratory mice are infected with *T. canis* eggs, the larvae disseminate throughout the body and in a relatively short time, with the exception of those larvae in the central nervous system, become encapsulated within an eosinophil-

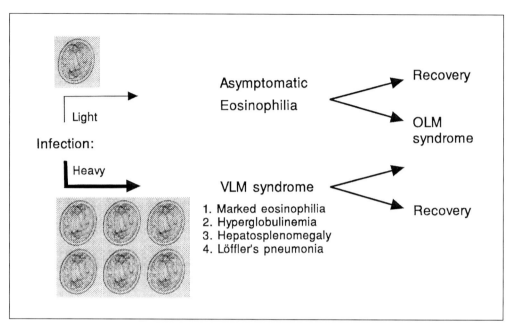

Fig. 2. Schematic diagram depicting relationship between the number of infective *T. canis* ova ingested by human host and clinical presentation. Modified from Schantz [16].

rich granulomatous reaction [26, 28]. Infected mice develop a significant peripheral blood eosinophilia which peaks around day 14 postinfection (PI) and persists at slightly lower levels for months thereafter [42, 43]. Both the granulomatous reaction and the eosinophilia have been shown to be T cell dependent either by abrogating the responses in experimentally infected mice using anti (T) lymphocyte serum [42] or by experimentation in congenitally athymic (T-cell-deficient) nude mice [44, 45]. Concomitant with the cellular reactions (e.g. granuloma formation and eosinophilia), the antibody responses observed in experimental toxocariasis are also CD4+ T cell-dependent [46]. It is this collection of core experiments that suggests that the response to infection with *T. canis* has an immunopathogenic mechanism which underlies the clinical manifestations of the disease.

From the vantage point of the immunologist, experimental *T. canis* infection may be unique among infectious agents. Because the larva neither grows nor molts, it is possible to titrate the exact amount of parasite-specific antigen(s) to which the host is exposed. This is most easily accomplished by varying the number of eggs used to initiate infection and studies using as few as 5 embryonated eggs were able to elicit a small but significant increase in the number of circulating eosinophils [39]. The magnitude of peripheral blood eosinophilia, splenomegaly, lymphocyte proliferation to both mitogens and antigens, and antitoxocara antibody (IgG and IgM, combined) have all been shown to be proportional to the size of the infection over the range of 5–250 eggs [39]. More recently, liver trapping of infective larvae upon subsequent infection and the level of circulating antigenemia have also been found to be proportional to the number of eggs administered. These studies collectively support the belief that ocular larva migrans occurs in patients who ingest so few organisms that little if any immune response is elicited. This allows the worms to migrate until such time as the eye is invaded. It should be noted, however, that OLM can occur in overwhelming infections as well as in minimal infections.

Following a single infection, larval worms are completely, although not evenly, distributed throughout the body of mice within 24–72 h PI [47]. After 1 week PI, worms will tend to avoid the lungs and accumulate in the CNS [27]. Granulomata can be found extensively throughout the anterior musculature (especially the nape of the neck), the liver, kidneys [48], the heart [43, 49, 50] and even on occasion within the eye [28, 51]. The granulomatous reaction begins as an accumulation of eosinophils around the worm and within a week or two, lymphocytes and macrophages replace the early granulocytes. By 6 months PI, the granuloma has contracted in size and the macrophages have become epithelioid in nature, which is suggestive of a response to the secretion of soluble (excretory-secretory) antigens [52, 53] by a viable larva. Many investigators have noted that not every granulomatous reaction examined histologically will contain a viable larva or evidence of dead or dying larvae. It is assumed in these cases that the larva has resumed its migratory ways and moved elsewhere in the body [28, 54].

The Antigens of *Toxocara* and Their Relationship to the Worm's Surface

A major contribution to our understanding of the immunobiology of *T. canis* and to the diagnosis of VLM syndrome was the publication in 1975 by de Savigny [30] of a method to maintain large numbers of L_2 larvae in tissue culture. By collecting the media at weekly intervals, very large quantities of excretory-secretory proteins could be collected (0.5–1.0 mg protein/10^7 worms/week) [41, 54]. With the advent of a TEX-based ELISA, seroepidemiology rapidly revealed the pervasiveness of VLM in populations all over the world [29]. Maizels et al. [55] have recently reviewed the studies characterizing the TEX antigens with the following salient findings: TEX consists of a mixture of at least 5 principal moieties designated TEX or TES-32, -55, -70, -120 and -400 with the numbers reflecting the weight of the individual proteins as visualized on SDS-PAGE gel [56]; all the major proteins are glycosylated [57], the products are extremely antigenic and appear to be released in vivo in amounts consistent with their production in vitro; antibodies raised in different laboratories against TEX react with the carbohydrate residues [58, 59]; and TEX antigens seem to be shared with other *Toxocara* species and even with some other ascarids [60, 61].

A plausible suggestion has been made that TEX contributes to the parasite's adaptation to the host response. There is much circumstantial evidence to support this claim. Smith et al. [62] noted that in order for antiserum to bind to *T. canis,* it was necessary to either chill the organisms to almost freezing or to add protein synthesis inhibitors to disrupt the worm's metabolism. At 37°C, the larval surface rapidly shed fluorescently labeled antibody, which suggested that the metabolic turnover of the surface was, in fact, quite high. These studies were elegantly extended by Badley et al. [63], who incubated L_2 larvae in the presence of immune serum and eosinophils in an attempt to induce antibody-dependent, eosinophil-mediated cytotoxicity. The worms survived. Electron-microscopic examination of larvae before and after the assay revealed the surface of fresh larvae to be covered by a series of uniform annulae but that following the addition of peritoneal exudate cells and immune serum, the surface external to the epicuticle (which was termed diffuse 'electron-dense' granular material) appeared to slough off taking with it the inflammatory cells that had adhered during the experiment. The adherent cells were mostly eosinophils [63]. Preadsorbing the serum used in these experiments with TEX abolished the adherence of peritoneal exudate cells to the larval surface. This was evidence that the diffuse electron-dense granular material was similar, if not identical, to TEX. Finally, Parsons et al. [54] using immunohistochemistry demonstrated anti-TEX-reactive product in serpiginous traces in the liver (of acutely infected mice) and in granulomata or their capsules (in chronically infected mice). This is consistent with the active shedding of the parasite surface during larval migration [41]. Depending on one's point of view, the collective interpretation of these studies is that the deposition of TEX within the parasitized host contributes to the syndrome of VLM by virtue of stimulating antibodies which ultimately lead to immune complex formation and/or deposition; or as viewed from the perspective of the migrating larvae, the shedding of the TEX surface coat serves as a survival mechanism because it cleanses the larval surface of hostile inflammatory cells.

T Cells and Cytokines:
Their Relationships to Eosinophils and Antibody Isotypes

The recognition of the existence of Th1 and Th2 subsets of CD4+ T cells has greatly facilitated the understanding of the immune response of murine [64–69] and human [70–73] hosts to helminthic, protozoan, and bacterial infections. Th1 cells secrete IL-2, interferon-γ (IFN-γ) and mediate delayed-type hypersensitivity reactions and activate macrophages. Th2 cells secrete IL-4, -5 and -10 and regulate humoral immune responses. Based on work with mouse models of leishmaniasis, it has been suggested that Th1 cells mediate immune responses associated with resistance to infection while Th2 cells are thought to mediate susceptibility [74–76] . Additionally, IL-2 can downregulate Th2 cells and IL-10 does likewise to Th1 cells [68]. This cross-regulation would seem to make delayed-type hypersensitivity and antibody responses mutually exclusive. However, the two responses can occur sequentially as reported in *Schistosoma mansoni*-infected mice where the predominant cytokines detected during the prepatent period are those associated with Th1 cells but with the onset of patency, the Th dynamic changes such that Th2 cytokines prevail [66, 74, 77–80].

What determines whether a given parasite will elicit a Th1 or Th2 response is not known with certainty. Toxocariasis exhibits traits of both responses. Granuloma formation is considered a manifestation of delayed-type hypersensitivity (mediated by Th1 cells) and IgE and eosinophilia are thought be hallmarks of Th2 responses. IL-4 is required for the class switch from IgG to IgE and IL-5 is necessary for the production, development, and chemotaxis of eosinophils. Depletion of all Th cells following treatment of mice with anti-CD4 monoclonal antibodies (mAb) abolished *T. canis*-specific IgG1 as well as the IgE response. When mAb against IL-5 was given immediately before infection and then at 7 and 14 days PI, the pulmonary infiltrates in treated mice were devoid of eosinophils, suggesting that *T. canis* did in fact incite a Th2 response [46, p. 106]. Treatment with mAb against IFN-γ (a Th1 cytokine) had no effect on the composition or extent of the pulmonary infiltrate. Using a more direct approach wherein specific cytokine levels were measured, Romagnani [71, 73] has established human T cell clones derived from healthy individuals specific for either *Mycobacterium tuberculosis* or *T. canis*. The mycobacterial-specific clones secreted the Th1 cytokines IL-2 and IFN-γ when exposed to purified protein derivative of *M. tuberculosis*, while the *T. canis*-specific clones elaborated the Th2 cytokines IL-4 and -5 in response to TEX stimulation.

The eosinophil, both in the peripheral blood and in the histological response to larval worm migration, is perhaps the most striking feature of tissue-invasive parasites. There is no consensus as to what role this granulocyte plays in these encounters, although the current dogma suggests that eosinophils with their low-affinity Fc receptors for IgE (i.e., CD23 or FcεRII) are highly efficient antiparasitic killer cells [reviewed in ref. 81, 82]. The mechanism of killing is presumed to involve the attachment of the eosinophil via the IgE Fc receptor to the parasite which has itself become opsonized or coated with parasite-specific IgE. When sufficient numbers of receptors are appropriately occupied and cross-linked, the eosinophil degranulates and exocytoses its toxic granule proteins onto the worm's surface [83–85]. Degranulation leads to a disruption of the parasite surface possibly by inactivation of Na^+-Ca^{2+} exchangers [86], which would then lead to the death of the organism. As discussed below, IgE-dependent eosinophil-mediated helminth toxicity may occur in humans but does not occur in mice [87].

There is now growing evidence from a variety of sources that suggests that eosinophils from different species may not all contain the same repertoire of immunological skills and furthermore, there is reasonably solid evidence that eosinophils may not kill larval parasites at all, and especially not *T. canis*. Capron and his group [88–91] have identified the Fc receptor for IgE on the surface of human eosinophils, while Conrad [92] and our lab have been unable to identify this receptor on mouse eosinophils [87]. Another immunological marker found on human but not on mouse eosinophils is the CD4 molecule (the functional marker for T helper cells and also the cognate receptor for human immunodeficiency virus) [93] which is recognized in mice using mAb L3T4 [46].

Even more compelling evidence that eosinophils are not killer cells comes from the work of Badley et al. [63] and Fattah et al. [94], who showed that eosinophils could attach to *T. canis* larvae in in vitro tissue culture settings but that with time, the larval surface was shed and the worms were not affected by this interaction. *T. canis* larvae are not killed by neutrophils either [95] and this imperviousness to antibody-dependent, cell-mediated cytotoxicity is quite consistent with the in vivo observations that *T. canis* larvae survive the paratenic host's inflammatory reaction. However, given the large body of literature reporting the in vitro killing of parasitic larvae by both human and mouse eosinophils [85, 96–104] it is reasonable to ask whether such a reaction occurs in vivo. Herndon and Kayes [105] reasoned that almost all of the in vitro experiments used extremely long incubation periods of 16 h or more and confined very large ratios of effector eosinophils to target larvae in small volumes and that such conditions most likely did not occur when larval worms were actively migrating within their hosts. This hypothesis was tested in a mouse model of trichinosis by treating mice with mAb against IL-5 to deplete the bone marrow, peripheral blood and connective tissues of eosinophils and then showing that adult worm burdens in the gastrointestinal tract and larval worms in the muscle were unaffected by this treatment as compared to worm recoveries from mice injected with an isotype control mAb or left untreated. Further, the responses of these mice to secondary infection in this well-characterized model of host resistance was also unaffected by depletion of eosinophils.

The Immunopathology of the Cardiopulmonary System

Using a model of artificial granuloma formation, wherein *T. canis* excretory-secretory antigen or TEX are covalently attached to inert particles (Sepharose 4B beads), it has been shown that granulomatous hypersensitivity is a manifestation of cell-mediated immunity. Antigen-specificity was shown when TEX-coated beads were embolized into the lungs of lightly infected mice (25 eggs) and large eosinophil-rich granulomata formed around the beads 6 days after embolic challenge. In contrast to the results observed when embolizing antigen-coated beads into the lungs of infected mice, only minimal foreign body reactions were seen when the same beads were embolized into the lungs of uninfected, normal mice. Adoptive transfer of bronchoalveolar lavage cells derived from acutely infected mice into the lungs of naive mice conferred granulomatous hypersensitivity upon subsequent antigen-coated bead challenge. Interestingly, spleen cells from immune mice were unable to adoptively transfer immunity to naive mice even though these cells would undergo antigen-specific lymphocyte blastogenesis in response to TEX [106, 107]. Subsequently, it has been shown that beads coated with an irrelevant protein (methylated bovine serum albumin) and embolized into the lungs of lightly infected mice or even uninfected mice elicited a foreign body reaction 6 days later. In marked contrast, these same beads elicited large, florid, eosinophil-rich granulomata when embolized into the lungs of mice infected with 100 infective eggs. Such granulomata resembled histologically, the cellular reaction that normally formed around viable L_2 *T. canis* larvae [108]. These results would seem to indicate that mice infected with *T. canis* were hyperreactive and could react stereotypically not only to antigen-specific stimuli but to nonspecific stimuli as well.

These kinds of experiments suggested that the lung might hold the key to understanding many of the immune mechanisms underlying the host immune response to *T. canis*. Following infection of mice with 250 eggs or less, there is a persistent pneumonitis seen in histological sections that begins around 48 h PI and consists of red blood cells and neutrophils [Kayes, unpubl.]. This is the truly acute inflammatory response. By day 6–7, the first eosinophils are observed and this lag is assumed to represent the time necessary for the immune system to produce the requisite cytokines to stimulate the bone marrow and to attract eosinophils into the lung. Macrophages filled with ingested RBCs are seen next, suggesting that these phagocytes are attempting to resolve the pulmonary infiltrates. By 2 weeks PI, the eosinophils are as numerous or more so than the neutrophils seen earlier, and macrophages are now observed engorged not only with RBCs but ghosts of neutrophils and eosinophils. This pneumonitis with a predominance of eosinophils persists for at least 7 weeks PI [106]. The persistence of the pulmonary infiltrate for so long is unexpected because there are few if any migrating worms in the lung after the first week PI [47], but the finding that there are significant levels of circulating antigen in the blood of mice up to 6 months after infection [38] and that these antigens can be visualized within visceral organs [54] suggests that these circulating or soluble antigens may serve as a constant stimulus to the host's immune system.

If, as suggested previously, the eosinophil is not an antihelminth effector cell, then the question becomes what is the significance of its obvious participation in the host response to infection, not just with *T. canis* but with any helminth. There are no known reports of individuals born with a congenital absence of eosinophils possibly because such a condition would be lethal or because the effects of the deficit are negligible. However, hypereosinophilia, defined as greater than 3×10^9 eosinophils per liter, has been associated clinically with endomyocardial fibrosis and myocardial damage [81, 109]. Given that eosinophils are a major hallmark of VLM syndrome, and that there are reports of myocardial involvement in the pediatric literature [49, 50, 110], several studies have looked at the damaging effects of elevated numbers of eosinophils in experimental models of toxocariasis. We have examined the hearts of mice at weekly intervals over an 8-week period of infection for evidence of myocardial damage that might be attributable to eosinophils. Myocardial lesions in the ventricular walls began as focal infiltrates of eosinophils and macrophages, and then progressed into granulomata containing necrotic debris but not infective larvae. Collagen deposition (the encapsulation response) was noted as early as day 21 PI and by 42 day PI, the lesions had contracted greatly due to loss of cellularity and consisted mostly of fibrosis and hemosiderin-laden macrophages. Myocyte damage was characterized by increased eosinophilic staining and necrosis [43]. To determine whether eosinophils had contributed to the development of this myocardial insult, we examined homogenized hearts of mice over a 6-week period for evidence of eosinophil peroxidase (EPO, a specific granule marker indicative of eosinophil degranulation) both biochemically and histochemically. A marked accumulation of EPO was observed in the hearts of infected mice by day 14 PI as compared to uninfected controls, but these elevated levels were resolved by 6 weeks of infection [43]. Whether there is a lasting effect of this eosinophil damage is not known at present. Mice chronically infected with *T. canis* have a shorter life expectancy compared to uninfected litter mates [Kayes, unpubl.].

To pursue further the hypothesis that a causal relationship existed between eosinophils and cardiac damage, we placed hearts from *T. canis*-infected rats on a standard working heart apparatus. This device allows an evaluation of cardiac output, cardiac work, left ventricular pressure and the monitoring of the rate of ventricular contraction and relaxation (+dP/dt and –dP/dt, respectively). Corresponding to an increased number of eosinophils (which, as noted above, is proportional to the size of the infection) in *T. canis*-infected animals as compared to controls, there was a decrease in cardiac performance such that by day 14 PI, cardiac work was down 25%, while −dP/dt (cardiac relaxation) was reduced 10%. Myocardial dysfunction was also observed when hearts from uninfected rats were placed on the working heart apparatus and perfused with buffer in which eosinophils obtained by bronchoalveolar lavage (BAL) from infected rats were degranulated by exposure to the protein kinase C activator, phorbol ester. At the completion of these studies the hearts were removed, and examined histologically for evidence of structural damage. The most striking change was a marked distention of the intermyocyte space accompanied by an increased pericapillary space. Some myocytes demonstrated a focal loss of their striated staining pattern. Control perfused hearts did not show these changes [111]. Unstimulated eosinophils or buffer alone did not alter cardiac structure or function. This suggests that eosinophil degranulation is linked to one or more signal transduction pathways. These data offer further support for the hypothesis that high levels of circulating eosinophils can lead to cardiac damage.

For over 20 years there has been a wide-ranging discussion as to whether nematode infections could be a cause of asthma [112–115]. The common findings of eosinophils in the lungs and elevated levels of IgE in both conditions is the basis for this suggestion. Desowitz et al. [115] reported that 29% of 80 asthmatic children had anti-*T. canis* IgE antibodies as compared to only 6.4% of 96 control children.

Because eosinophils are associated with a variety of lung diseases such as asthma, which have immunological underpinnings, we and others have examined the effects of eosinophils on isolated, perfused rat lungs. Similar to the cardiac studies just described, vascular resistance, capillary filtration coefficient ($K_{f,c}$, a measure of capillary leakiness which can lead to the formation of pulmonary edema) and bronchoconstriction, which in asthma can be fatal, were evaluated. Eosinophils obtained from *T. canis*-infected rat lungs by bronchoalveolar lavage were again activated with phorbol ester and administered to perfused normal rat lungs which were maintained in an isogravimetric state such that the perfusion fluid going into the lung preparation was equal to the fluid coming out. This was measured by a spring balance from which the lung preparation was suspended. Lungs receiving no eosinophils or unactivated eosinophils showed no change in pulmonary hemodynamics or $K_{f,c}$. However, in lungs receiving just 2×10^6 total, activated eosinophils there was a transient 4.8-fold increase in pulmonary vascular resistance that peaked at 30 min, primarily due to the constriction of small arteries and small veins. After the initial pressor response, $K_{f,c}$ was increased to 7.5 times control at 130 min and this resulted in marked interstitial fluid accumulation. Peak airway pressure (P_{aw}) during constant tidal ventilation also increased in lungs receiving activated eosinophils as compared to the control groups (no cells or unactivated cells). These responses were directly correlated to the number

Table 2. Distribution of the CD4 (T helper) and CD8 (cytotoxic T) cell populations in paired spleen (SPL) and BAL of the lungs of mice during infection with *T. canis*

Weeks PI	CD4+ (αL3T4), %		CD8+ (αLYT2), %		CD4/CD8 ratio	
	SPL	BAL	SPL	BAL	SPL	BAL
0	19	ND	12	ND	1.6	–
1	6.7	36.3	3.3	2.3	2.0	15.8
2	10.8	24.8	5.6	2.0	1.9	12.4
4	17.3	45.7	6.7	3.2	2.6	14.3
6	18.4	32.2	9.4	4.4	2.0	7.3

of eosinophils added to the perfusion buffer over the range of $1–4 \times 10^6$ eosinophils added to a 30-ml volume [116]. Buijs et al. [117] also reported that *T. canis*-infected mice were quite similar to infected rats and had increased pulmonary resistance, reduced dynamic compliance, and developed pulmonary edema. Treatment of mice with anti IL-5 producing hybridoma cells abrogated the eosinophilia but not the alterations of pulmonary function. Only the inability of the tracheal smooth muscle to constrict was eosinophil dependent.

BAL of infected laboratory animals has been a useful and productive method to establish the immunological response occurring in the lung and to examine it in the context of the systemic immune responses of the same animal by comparing responses of BAL cells to the responses of spleen cells. BAL cells have been analyzed by flow cytometry to determine the relative percentage of T cell subsets [Kayes, unpubl.]. We have characterized the ratio of helper to cytotoxic or suppressor phenotype of T cells recovered by BAL from infected mice over a 6-week period and compared this ratio to that found in the spleen of the same mice. The results of this study are given in table 2. Several interesting observations are forthcoming from these results.

There was almost a 67% decrease in the total T cell population of the spleen by 8 days PI (CD4+ plus CD8+ combined) which is almost completely reversed by 6 weeks of infection. A similar result is seen for the CD4+ population which is down by 77% after the first week of infection. In contrast to the spleen, the lung had 33% T cells at 1 week and this number rose and declined slightly to the end of the experiment. Even more interesting is the comparison of the ratios of CD4 and CD8 cells in the two compartments. Even though the spleen undergoes extreme enlargement (5-fold increase in mass by day 14 PI [118]), the helper/suppressor ratio is tightly regulated at around 2.0, while in the lung where the inflammatory reaction is occurring, there is a predominance of helper cells. Almost identical T cell distributions were reported by Buijs et al. [119] and this group further reported a sharp increase in the number of IgE+ cells concomitant with increased levels of this isotype in the lavage fluid. Because almost 90% of the cells recovered by BAL are eosinophils, there is ample reason to believe that the CD4+ T cells are of the Th2 subset which secrete IL-4 and IL-5, which would account for the elevated levels of IgE and eosinophils, respectively.

Kusama et al. [44] reported two waves of eosinophilia in *T. canis*-infected mice at 11 and 21 days PI. Only the first wave was seen in T-cell-deficient mice, suggesting that it was T cell independent. Further, anti-IL-5 mAb treatment completely abrogated the accumulation of eosinophils but not other immuno-inflammatory cells in the lung [44, 46, 120]. It should be noted, however, that Th2 cells are not the only cells which can produce IL-5 in the lung. Recently, it has been reported that a population of double negative (i.e., CD4-, CD8-) cells can also produce IL-5 [45, 121].

Buijs et al. [121] and Buijs [36] found that the IgE concentration in bronchoalveolar lavage fluid went up almost 200-fold over normal levels following a 14-day infection with 250 infective *T. canis* ova and up half again as much in mice infected with 1,000 ova. She suggested that based on ratio comparisons between serum and lung lavage IgE concentrations taken at the two times that pulmonary IgE was produced locally. In contrast, IgA levels were also significantly elevated, but there was no indication of local pulmonary IgA production. Jones et al. [87] used flow cytometry to characterize the Fc receptors on BAL eosinophils recovered from *T. canis*-infected mice and compared these cells with lymphocytes from the spleen known to express IgM, IgG, IgA and IgE. Spleen cells expressed Fc receptors capable of binding all the isotypes tested. In stark contrast, eosinophils expressed only the Fc RII for IgG which is recognized by mAb 2.4G2. This receptor binds aggregated IgG which can result from the interaction with specific antigen that leads to immune complex formation. Attempts to induce the low-affinity Fc receptor for IgE (CD23) by culturing BAL eosinophils with optimal concentrations of IL-4 with or without IL-5 failed to induce the expression of CD23. Whether occupying the 2.4G2 recognizable Fc receptor on mouse eosinophils with aggregated IgG leads to signal transduction which then initiates phagocytosis, exocytosis (i.e., degranulation), or some other biologically important process is not known at the present time. It is of historical interest that eosinophils were thought to phagocytose antigen-antibody complexes long before they were shown to kill parasitic larvae [122, 123]. It is disheartening that there is so much evidence linking eosinophils with larvacidal activity. However, in light of the findings of Badley et al. [63] and Fattah et al. [94] that both animal and human eosinophils cannot damage *T. canis* larvae and the studies just described which document the presence of all the components necessary for an antibody-dependent, eosinophil-mediated cytotoxicity reaction together in a single site but then find that eosinophils are incapable of recognizing the antibodies which are present, would suggest that we can no longer ascribe a proactive antiparasitic effector function to the eosinophil in in vivo situations.

The Immunopathology of the Liver

In 1960 Lee [124] published an experimental study of murine larva migrans designed to ask the straightforward question: 'Could a paratenic host develop resistance to *T. canis* infection?' In this study, mice were infected with a bolus of either 1,000 or 2,000 eggs (control groups) or given 2,000 eggs divided among 3–6 doses administered over 6 weeks. Sacrifice was 8 weeks after the initial infection. The study was noteworthy for two things. First there was an apparent resistance induced which resulted in approximately 20% fewer worms recovered by digestion from multiply infected mice than from mice infected only once. The second significant finding was that in mice multiply infected, the worms comprising the subsequent infective doses tended to accumulate in the liver, and many of these larvae were encapsulated in eosinophil-rich granulomatous reactions.

The phenomenon wherein larvae accumulate in the livers of mice previously infected with *T. canis* has been termed 'liver trapping' and has been studied by several laboratories [124–129]. Given this amount of investigative attention to liver trapping, it is not surprising that an immunological basis has been ascribed to it. Sugane and Oshima [130] suggested that liver trapping was a T-cell-dependent reaction because athymic nude mice failed to trap larvae upon a second exposure. Studies by Parsons et al. [126] demonstrated a direct relationship between the magnitude of liver trapping and the size of the initial priming infection in the range of 25–125 eggs. More eggs did not increase the amount of liver trapping significantly [126]. Liver trapping appears to be antigen-specific as mice immunized with TEX in lieu of a priming infection did trap larvae, while mice immunized with the soluble egg antigens derived from *S. mansoni* did not [41]. Because eosinophils are such a prominent participant in the encapsulation response of trapped larvae, Parsons et al. [131] depleted mice of virtually all their eosinophils with mAb against IL-5 and found that eosinophil depletion had no effect on liver trapping. Passive transfer of immune sera from primed mice also failed to confer liver trapping on naive recipients suggesting that antibody was not the effector mechanism either [cited in ref. 41]. Some mouse strains trap larvae better than others, but a strong role for histocompatibility genes is currently lacking [124]. Adoptive transfer of spleen cells conferred moderate liver traping to naive mice, which is consistent with the nude mice studies alluded to above [130] and antibody depletion studies to identify the essential cell type suggested CD4+ cells were required but not CD8+ cells. However, depletion of CD4+ cells did not completely abrogate this host reponse implying that liver trapping is a multi-faceted host response [41].

The Immunopathology of the Eye

The patient presenting with OLM is typically older than the patient with VLM [16, 33]. Duguid [132] described two types of ocular lesions. One was a typical granulomatous encapsulating reaction, usually solitary, located on the temporal pole near the disc and macula. The second type of lesion was a chronic endophthalmitis associated with marked vitreous reaction often accompanied by retinal detachment. Both types of lesions tended to be unilateral, vision disrupt-ing, and frequently diagnosed as retinoblastoma. A third presentation has since been added, that being a peripheral or protean inflammatory mass in an otherwise quiescent eye [133]. In fact, most of the ocular tissues can be or have been invaded by migrating *T. canis* larvae. The inflammation in OLM most likely results from host sensitization to the soluble larval antigens released from dead or dying intraocular second-stage larvae [134]. Wilder [135] examined a series of 46 enu-cleated eyes taken primarily from small children. The cases were chosen based on pathologic findings which included eosinophilic abscesses and granulomatous changes similar to those associated with helminthic infection elsewhere in the body. She identified what she believed to be hookworm larvae, but which were subsequently identified as *T. canis* by Nichols [7]. Thus, the pathological response in the eye is not altogether different from that seen in the liver, lungs, or muscula-ture.

Unlike VLM which can be considered the systemic manifestion of toxocaria-sis, OLM should be considered a compartmentalized form of the infection. The typical patient with OLM is slightly older than 11 years and is assumed to be lightly infected [33]. This is why a serum-based anti-TEX ELISA may be negative as would be the finding of normal levels of circulating eosinophils in peripheral blood. On the other hand, if the infection size was extremely heavy, then the eye can be invaded with systemic complications as well. Clinicians should be alert to both possibilities and in the absence of positive routine laboratory tests consider further testing of the eye before discounting a diagnosis of OLM. An analysis of aqueous and/or vitreous humor in cases of presumptive OLM by TEX ELISA has consistently demonstrated a local IgE production which is often associated with the presence of eosinophils [136]. The intraocular level of IgE is independent of the systemic circulating levels of this isotype (which may reflect an intact blood-eye barrier) and is considered an essential characteristic leading to a diagnosis of

OLM. In contrast, intraocular eosinophilia, while highly suggestive of an intra-ocular infection with *T. canis*, is not specific as it can result from a variety of infectious helminths [137].

Summary

The surface of *T. canis* is now recognized as a dynamic structure which turns over quite rapidly and serves as a renewable source of large quantities of antigen(s). The major host responses to these antigens include a marked eosinophilia and hyperglobulinemia. Both of these responses are apparently ineffective at ridding the body of infective larvae. Both eosin-ophils and IgE antibodies are manifestations of the Th2 subset of T helper cells and the cytokines that they secrete. Further, there is reason to believe that the antigens released from *T. canis* larvae favor the induction of this cellular population. Finally, there is mounting evidence that the chronic production of parasite antigen and its continued stimulation of the host immune system with a concomitant production of eosinophils can lead to a permanent alteration of the normal organization of the cardiopulmonary system. In the absence of any well-documented drugs capable of killing infective larvae, it would seem that immunological intervention may offer the only way to minimize or neutralize this 'gift from man's best friend'.

This chapter was not intended to be an exhaustive review of the literature pertaining to toxocariasis. Several other recent publications will hopefully fulfill the need for more detailed information on the biology of this organism and the clinical spectrum of the disease it produces [16, 138–140]. Finally, a MEDLARS search of the current medical literature should bring anyone up to speed in a very short time.

Acknowledgements

I would like take this opportunity to acknowledge the following individuals for their contribution to my pursuit of understanding the immunopathology of *T. canis*: my friend and teacher, the late Dr. Paul Beaver, who shared with me his fascination with this most incredible organism; to the colleagues who have supported my labors at the bench, Drs. John A. Oaks, Robert B. Grieve, James Parker, Stephen Schaffer, Michael Cookston, Richard E. Jones, Fred J. Herndon, Raymond B. Hester, Witold Ferens, and Fred D. Finkelman, and my technicians Paul Omholt, Martha Stober, and Ed Dimayuga. I wish to extend a very special thank you to Dr. Jannie Buijs, who was kind enough to send me a copy of her docto-ral dissertation just as I was leaving to go on sabbatical. I would also like to acknowledge the National Institutes of Health, American Heart Association, Alabama Affiliate, and the Uni-versity of South Alabama College of Medicine for their financial support of some of the studies cited herein.

References

1   Beaver PC: The nature of visceral larva migrans. J Parasitol 1969;55:3–12.
2   Beaver PC, Snyder CH, Carrera GM, Dent JH, Lafferty JW: Chronic eosinophilia due to visceral larva migrans. Report of 3 cases. J Pediatr 1952;9:7–19.
3   Perlingiero J, György P: Chronic eosinophilia: Report of a case with necrosis of the liver, pulmonary infiltrations, anemia and *Ascaris* infestation. Am J Dis Child 1947;73:34–43.
4   Zeulzer W, Apt L: Disseminated visceral lesions associated with extreme eosinophilia. Am J Dis Child 1949;78:153–181.
5   Mercer R, Lund H, Bloomfield R, Caldwell R: Larval ascariasis as a cause of chronic eosinophilia with visceral manifestations. Am J Dis Child 1950;80:46–58.
6   Behrer M: Hypereosinophilia with eosinophilic granuloma of the liver associated with *Ascaris* infection. J Pediatr 1951;38:635–640.
7   Nichols RL: The etiology of visceral larva migrans. I. Diagnostic morphology of infective second-stage *Toxocara* larvae. J Parasitol 1956;42:349–362.
8   Beautymann W, Woolf A: An ascaris larva in the brain in association with acute anterior poliomyelitis. J Pathol Bacteriol 1951;63:635–647.
9   Beaver PC: Toxocarosis (visceral larva migrans) in relation to tropical eosinophilia. Bull Soc Pathol Exot 1962;55:555–576.
10 Löffler W: Zur Differential-Diagnose der Lungeninfiltrierungen. I. Frühinfiltrate unter besonderer Berücksichtigung der Rückbildungszeiten. II. Über flüchtige succedan-Infiltrate (mit Eosinophilie). Beitr Klin Tuberk spez Tuberk Forsch 1932;79:338–382.
11 Lungström I, van Knapen F: An epidemiological and serological study of *Toxocara* infection in Sweden. Scand J Infect Dis 1989;21:87–93.
12 Gillespie SH: Human toxocariasis. J Appl Bacteriol 1987;63:473–479.
13 Portús M, Riera C, Prats G: A serological survey of toxocariasis in patients and healthy donors in Barcelona (Spain). Eur J Epidemiol 1989;5:224–227.
14 Herrmann N, Glickman LT, Schantz PM, Weston MG, Domanski LM: Seroprevalence of zoonotic toxocariasis in the United States: 1971–1973. Am J Epidemiol 1985;122:890–896.
15 Embil JA, Tanner CE, Pereira LH, Staudt M, Morrison EG, Gualazzi DA: Seroepidemiologic survey of *Toxocara canis* infection in urban and rural children. Public Health 1988;102:129–133.
16 Schantz PM: *Toxocara* larva migrans now. Am J Trop Med Hyg 1989;41:S21–S34.
17 Richards IM, Eady RP, Jackson DM, Orr TSC, Pritchard DI, Vendy K, Wells E: *Ascaris*-induced bronchoconstriction in primates experimentally infected with *Ascaris suum* ova. Clin Exp Immunol 1983;54:461–468.
18 Feldman GJ, Parker HW: Visceral larva migrans associated with the hypereosinophilic syndrome and the onset of severe asthma. Ann Intern Med 1992;116:838–840.
19 Aderle WI, Oduwole O: *Ascaris* and bronchial asthma in children. Afr J Med Sci 1982;11:161–166.
20 Grove DI: What is the relationship between asthma and worms? Allergy 1982;37:139–148.
21 de Sylva DS, Ismail MM, de Silva ID, de Silva P, Gooneratne D, Goonawardana S: Is filariasis a trigger for bronchial asthma? Acta Pediatr Jpn 1990;32:164–168.
22 Wong DTW, Elovic A, Matossian K, Nagura N, McBride J, Gordon JR, Rand TH, Galli SJ, Weller PF: Eosinophils from patients with eosinophilia express transforming growth factor β1. Blood 1991; 78:2702–2707.
23 Phan SH, Kunkel SL: Lung cytokine production in bleomycin-induced pulmonary fibrosis. Exp Lung Res 1992;18:29–43.
24 Kendell KR, Day JD, Hruban RH, Olson JL, Rosenblum WD, Kasper EK, Baughman KL, Hutchins GM: Intimate association of eosinophils to collagen bundles in eosinophilic myocarditis and ranitidine-induced hypersensitivity myocarditis. Arch Pathol Lab Med 1995;119:1154–1160.
25 Lloyd S: *Toxocara canis*: The dog; in Lewis JW, Maizels RM (eds): *Toxocara* and Toxocariasis: Clinical, Epidemiological, and Molecular Perspectives. London, British Parasitological Society with the Institute of Biology, 1993, pp 11–24.
26 Burren CH: Experimental toxocariasis. I. Some observations on the histopathology of the migration of *Toxocara canis*. Z Parasitenkd 1968;30:152–161.

27 Dunsmore JD, Thompson RCA, Bates IA: The accumulation of *Toxocara canis* larvae in the brains of mice. Int J Parasitol 1983;13:517–521.

28 Kayes SG, Oaks JA: Development of the granulomatous response in murine toxocariasis. Initial events. Am J Pathol 1978;93:277–294.

29 de Savigny DH, Voller A, Woodruff AW: Toxocariasis: Serological diagnosis by enzyme immunoassay. J Clin Pathol 1979;32:284–288.

30 de Savigny DH: In vitro maintenance of *Toxocara canis* larvae and a simple method for the production of *Toxocara* ES antigens for use in serodiagnostic tests for visceral larva migrans. J Parasitol 1975;61:781–782.

31 Gillespie SH: The clinical spectrum of human toxocariasis; in Lewis JW, Maizels RM (eds): *Toxocara* and Toxocariasis: Clinical, Epidemiological, and Molecular Perspectives. London, British Parasitological Society with The Institute of Biology, 1993, pp 55–61.

32 Bass JL, Mehta KA, Glickman LT, Eppes BM: Clinically inapparent *Toxocara* infection in children. N Engl J Med 1983;308:723–724.

33 Logar J, Kraut A, Likar M: *Toxocara* antibodies in patients with visceral or ocular disorder in Slovenia. Infection 1993;21:27–29.

34 Glickman LT, Magnaval JF, Domanski LM, Shofer FS, Lauria SS, Gottstein B, Brochier B: Visceral larva migrans in French adults: A new disease syndrome? Am J Epidemiol 1987;125:1019–1034.

35 Maruyama S, Yamamoto K, Katsube Y: Infectivity of *Toxocara canis* larvae from Japanese quails in mice. J Vet Med Sci 1994;56:399–401.

36 Buijs J: *Toxocara* infection and airway function: An experimental and epidemiological study; PhD thesis, Utrecht, 1993.

37 Nicholas WL, Stewart AC, Walker JC: Toxocariasis: A serological survey of blood donors in the Australian Capital Territory together with observations on the risks of infection. Trans R Soc Trop Med Hyg 1986;80:217–221.

38 Bowman DD, Mika-Grieve M, Grieve RB: Circulating excretory-secretory antigen levels and specific IgG and IgM responses in mice infected with *Toxocara canis*. Am J Trop Med Hyg 1987;36: 75–82.

39 Kayes SG, Omholt PE, Grieve RB: Immune responses of CBA/J mice to graded infections with *Toxocara canis*. Infect Immun 1985;48:697–703.

40 Havasiovareiterova K, Tomasovicova O, Dubinsky P: Effect of various doses of infective *Toxocara canis* and *Toxocara cati* eggs on the humoral response and distribution of larvae in mice. Parasitol Res 1995;81:13–17.

41 Grieve RB, Stewart VA, Parsons JC: Immunobiology of larval toxocariasis *(Toxocara canis):* A summary of recent research; in Lewis JW, Maizels RM (eds): *Toxocara* and Toxocariasis: Clinical, Epidemiological, and Molecular Perspectives. London, British Parasitological Society with The Institute of Biology, 1993, pp 117–124.

42 Kayes SG, Oaks JA: *Toxocara canis*: Role of the T lymphoycte in murine visceral larva migrans and its relationship to onset of eosinophilia. Exp Parasitol 1980;79:47–55.

43 Cookston M, Stober M, Kayes SG: Eosinophilic myocarditis in CBA/J mice infected with *Toxocara canis*. Am J Pathol 1990;136:1137–1145.

44 Kusama Y, Takamoto M, Kasahara T, Takatsu K, Nariuchi H, Sugane K: Mechanisms of eosinophilia in Balb/C-nu/+ and congenitally athymic Balb/C-nu/nu mice infected with *Toxocara canis*. Immunology 1995;84:461–468.

45 Takamoto M, Kusama Y, Takatsu K, Nariuchi H, Sugane K: Occurrence of interleukin-5 production by CD4(–) CD8(–) (double-negative) T cells in lungs of both normal and congenitally athymic nude mice infected with *Toxocara canis*. Immunology 1995;85:285–291.

46 Jones RE III: Type 2 CD4+ T lymphocytes mediate the immune response of mice to infections with the parasitic nematode, *Toxocara canis* (Werner, 1782); PhD thesis, University of South Alabama, Mobile, 1992, pp 106–108.

47 Kayes SG, Oaks JA: Effect of inoculum size and length of infection on the distribution of *Toxocara canis* larvae in the mouse. Am J Trop Med Hyg 1976;25:573–580.

48 Hassan AT, el-Manawaty NH: Experimental murine toxocariasis histopathological study of chronic renal infection, transplacental transmission and ultrastructural study of egg shell. J Egypt Soc Parasitol 1994;24:333–339.

49 Friedman S, Hervada AR: Severe myocarditis with recovery in a child with visceral larva migrans. J Pediatr 1960;56:91–96.

50 Vargo TA, Singer DB, Gillette PC, Fernbach DJ: Letters to Editor. Myocarditis due to visceral larva migrans. J Pediatr 1977;90:322–323.

51 Ghafoor SY, Smith HV, Lee WR, Quinn R, Girdwood RW: Experimental ocular toxocariasis: A mouse model. Br J Ophthalmol 1984;68:89–96.

52 Papadimitriou JM, Spector WG: The origin, properties, and fate of epithelioid cells. J Pathol 1971; 105:187–203.

53 Spector WG: The dynamics of granulomas and the significance of epithelioid cells. Pathol Biol (Paris) 1975;23:437–439.

54 Parsons JC, Bowman DD, Grieve RB: Tissue localization of excretory-secretory antigens of larval Toxocara canis in acute and chronic murine toxocariasis. Am J Trop Med Hyg 1986;35:974–981.

55 Maizels RM, Gems DH, Page AP: Synthesis and secretion of TES antigens from Toxocara canis infective larvae; in Lewis JW, Maizels RM (eds): Toxocara and Toxocariasis: Clinical, Epidemio- logical, and Molecular Perspectives. London, British Parasitological Society with The Institute of Biology, 1993, pp 141–150.

56 Maizels RM, de Savigny D, Ogilvie BM: Characterization of the surface and excretory-secretory antigens of Toxocara canis infective larvae. Parasite Immunol 1984;6:23–37.

57 Meghji M, Maizels RM: Biochemical properties of larval excretory-secretory (ES) glycoproteins of the parasitic nematode Toxocara canis. Mol Biochem Parasitol 1986;18:155–170.

58 Bowman DD, Mika-Grieve M, Grieve RB: Toxocara canis: Monoclonal antibodies to larval excre- tory-secretory antigens that bind with genus and species specificity to the cuticular surface of infec- tive larvae. Exp Parasitol 1987;64:458–465.

59 Maizels RM, Kennedy MW, Meghji M, Robertson BD, Smith HV: Shared carbohydrate epitopes on distinct surface and secreted epitopes of the parasitic nematode Toxocara canis. J Immunol 1987;139:207–214.

60 Page AP, Richards DT, Lewis JW, Omar HM, Maizels RM: Comparison of isolates and species of Toxocara and Toxascaris by biosynthetic labelling of somatic and ES proteins from infective larvae. Parasitology 1991;103:451–464.

61 Kennedy MW, Maizels RM, Meghji M, Young L, Qureshi F, Smith HV: Species-specific and com- mon epitopes on the secreted and surface antigens of Toxocara cati and Toxocara canis infective larvae. Parasite Immunol 1987;9:407–420.

62 Smith HV, Quinn R, Kusel JR, Girdwood RWA: The effect of temperature and antimetabolites on antibody binding to the outer surface of second stage Toxocara canis larvae. Mol Biochem Parasitol 1981;4:183–193.

63 Badley JE, Grieve RB, Rockey JH, Glickman LT: Immune-mediated adherence of eosinophils to Toxocara canis infective larvae: The role of excretory-secretory antigens. Parasite Immunol 1987;9: 133–143.

64 Mosmann TR, Coffman RL: Heterogeneity of cytokine secretion patterns and functions of helper T cells. Adv Immunol 1989;46:111–148.

65 Taguchi T, McGhee JR, Coffman RL, Beagley KW, Eldridge JH, Takatsu K, Kiyono H: Analysis of Th1 and Th2 cells in murine gut-associated tissues: Frequencies of CD4+ and CD8+ T cells that secrete IFN-gamma and IL-5. J Immunol 1990;145:68–77.

66 Sher A, Fiorentino D, Caspar P, Pearce E, Mosmann T: Production of IL-10 by CD4+ T lympho- cytes correlates with down-regulation of Th1 cytokine synthesis in helminth infection. J Immunol 1991;147:2713–2716.

67 Mosmann TR, Cherwinski H, Bond MW, Giedlin MA, Coffman RL: Two types of murine helper T cell clones. I. Definition according to profiles of lymphokine activities and screted proteins. J Immunol 1986;136:2348–2353.

68 Street NE, Mosmann TR: Functional diversity of T lymphocytes due to secretion of different cyto- kine patterns. FASEB J 1991;5:171–177.

69 Mosmann TR, Coffman RL: Th1 and Th2 cells: Different paterns of lymphokine secretion lead to different functional properties. Annu Rev Immunol 1989;7:145–173.

70 Romagnani S: Human TH1 and TH2 subsets: 'Eppur si muove!'. Eur Cytokine Netw 1994;5:7– 12.

71   Del Prete GF, De Carli M, Mastromauro C, Biagiotti R, Macchia D, Falagiani P, Ricci M, Romagnani S: Purified protein derivative of *Mycobacterium tuberculosis* and excretory-secretory antigen(s) of *Toxocara canis* expand in vitro human T cells with stable and opposite (type 1 T helper or type 2 T helper) profile of cytokine production. J Clin Invest 1991;88:346–350.

72   Del Prete G, Maggi E, Romagnani S: Human Th1 and Th2 cells: Functional properties, mechanisms of regulation and role in disease. Lab Invest 1994;70:299–306.

73   Romagnani S: Human Th1 and Th2 subsets: Doubt no more. Immunol Today 1991;12:256–257.

74   Scott P, Natovitz P, Coffman RL, Pearce E, Sher A: Immunoregulation of cutaneous leishmaniasis. T cell lines that transfer protective immunity or exacerbation belong to different T helper subsets and respond to distinct parasite antigens. J Exp Med 1988;168:1675–1684.

75   Corry DB, Reiner SL, Linsley PS, Locksley RM: Differential effects of blockade of CD28-B7 on the development of Th1 or Th2 effector cells in experimental leishmaniasis. J Immunol 1994;153: 4142–4148.

76   Schartonkersten T, Afonso LCC, Wysocka M, Trinchieri G, Scott P: IL-12 is required for natural killer cell activation and subsequent T helper 1 cell development in experimental leishmaniasis. J Immunol 1995;154:5320–5330.

77   Sher A, Coffman RL: Regulation of immunity to parasites by T cells and T cell-derived cytokines. Annu Rev Immunol 1992;10:385–409.

78   Grzych JM, Pearce E, Cheever A, Caulada ZA, Caspar P, Heiny S, Lewis F, Sher A: Egg deposition is the major stimulus for the production of Th2 cytokines in murine schistosomiasis mansoni. J Immunol 1991;146:1322–1327.

79   Pearce EJ, Caspar P, Grzych JM, Lewis FA, Sher A: Down regulation of Th1 cytokine production accompanies induction of Th2 responses by the parasitic helminth, *Schistosoma mansoni.* J Exp Med 1991;173:159–166.

80   Pemberton RM, Malaquias LCC, Falcao PL, Silveira AMS, Rabello ALT, Katz N, Amorim M, Mountford AP, Coffman RL, Correa-Oliveira R, Wilson RA: Cell-mediated immunity to schistosomes. Evaluation of mechanisms operating against lung-stage parasites which might be exploited in a vaccine. Trop Geogr Med 1994;46:247–254.

81   Spry CJF: Eosinophils. A Comprehensive Review and Guide to the Scientific and Medical Literature. Oxford, Oxford University Press, 1988.

82   Weller PF: The immunobiology of eosinophils. N Engl J Med 1991;324:1110–1118.

83   Hamann KJ, Barker RL, Ten RM, Gleich GJ: The molecular biology of eosinophil granule proteins. Int Arch Allergy Appl Immunol 1991;94:202–209.

84   Gleich GJ, Loegering DA: Immunobiology of eosinophils. Annu Rev Immunol 1984;2:429–459.

85   Bass DA, Szejda P: Mechanisms of killing of newborn larvae of *Trichinella spiralis* by neutrophils and eosinophils. Killing by generators of hydrogen peroxide in vitro. J Clin Invest 1979;64:1558–1564.

86   Tai P-C, Hayes DJ, Clark JB, Spry CJF: Toxic effects of human eosinophil secretion products on isolated rat heart cells in vitro. Biochem J 1982;204:75–80.

87   Jones RE, Finkelman FD, Hester RB, Kayes SG: *Toxocara canis*: Failure to find IgE receptors (FcεR) on eosinophils from infected mice suggests that murine eosinophils do not kill helminth larvae by an IgE-dependent mechanism. Exp Parasitol 1994;78:64–75.

88   Capron A, Dessaint J-P, Capron M: FcRII and IgE-dependent activation of inflammatory cells. Res Immunol 1990;141:99–105.

89   Prin L, Capron M, Gosset P, Wallaert B, Kusnierz JP, Bletry O, Tonnel AB, Capron A: Eosinophilic lung disease: Immunological studies of blood and alveolar eosinophils. Clin Exp Immunol 1986;63: 249–257.

90   Grangette C, Gruart V, Ouaissi MA, Rizvi F, Delespesse G, Capron A, Capron M: IgE receptor on human eosinophils (FCεRII): Comparison with B cell CD23 and association with an adhesion molecule. J Immunol 1989;143:3580–3588.

91   Capron M, Truong M-J, Aldebert D, Gruart V, Suemura M, Delespesse G, Tourvieille B, Capron A: Eosinophil IgE receptor and CD23. Immunol Res 1992;11:252–259.

92   Conrad DH: FcRII/CD23: The low affinity receptor for IgE. Annu Rev Immunol 1990;8:623–645.

93   Lucey DR, Dorsky DI, Nicholson-Weller A, Weller PF: Human eosinophils express CD4 protein and bind human immunodeficiency virus 1 gp120. J Exp Med 1989;169:327–332.

94 Fattah DI, Maizels RM, McLaren DJ, Spry CJF: *Toxocara canis*: Interaction of human blood eosinophils with the infective larvae. Exp Parasitol 1986;61:421–431.
95 Huwer M, Sanft S, Ahmed JS: Enhancement of neutrophil adherence to *Toxocara canis* larvae by the C3 component of complement and IgG antibodies. Zentralb Bakteriol Mikrobiol Hyg Ser A 1989;270:418–423.
96 Capron M, Bazin H, Joseph M, Capron A: Evidence for IgE-dependent cytotoxicity by rat eosinophils. J Immunol 1981;126:1764–1768.
97 Graziano RF, Looney RJ, Shen L, Fanger MW: Fc(gamma)R-mediated killing by eosinophils. J Immunol 1989;142:230–235.
98 Greene BM, Taylor HR, Aikawa M: Cellular killing of microfilariae of *Onchocerca volvulus*: Eosinophil- and neutrophil-mediated immune serum-dependent destruction. J Immunol 1981;127:1611–1618.
99 Nogueira NM, Klebanoff SJ, Cohn ZA: *Trypanosoma cruzi*: Sensitization to macrophage killing by eosinophil peroxidase. J Immunol 1982;128:1705–1708.
100 Khalife J, Dunne DW, Richardson BA, Mazza G, Thorne KJI, Capron A, Butterworth AE: Functional role of human IgG subclasses in eosinophil-mediated killing of schistosomula of *Schistosoma mansoni*. J Immunol 1989;142:4422–4427.
101 Hamann KJ, Gleich GJ, Checkel JL, Loegering DA, McCall JW, Barker RL: In vitro killing of microfilariae of *Brugia pahangi* and *Brugia malayi* by eosinophil granule proteins. J Immunol 1990;144:3166–3173.
102 Langley JG, Dunne DW: Temporal variation in the carbohydrate and peptide surface epitopes in antibody-dependent, eosinophil-mediated killing of *Schistosoma mansoni* schistosomula. Parasite Immunol 1992;14:185–200.
103 Dunne DW, Richardson BA, Jones FM, Clark M, Thorne KJI, Butterworth AE: The use of mouse/human chimaeric antibodies to investigate the roles of different antibody isotypes, including IgA2, in the killing of *Schistosoma mansoni* schistosomula by eosinophils. Parasite Immunol 1993;15:181–185.
104 Vadas MA, David JR, Butterworth A, Pisani NT, Siongok TA: A new method for purification of human eosinophils and neutrophils, and a comparison of the ability of these cells to damage schistosomula of *Schistosoma mansoni*. J Immunol 1979;122:1228–1236.
105 Herndon FJ, Kayes SG: Depletion of eosinophils by anti-IL-5 monoclonal antibody treatment of mice infected with *Trichinella spiralis* does not alter parasite burden or immunologic resistance to reinfection. J Immunol 1992;149:3642–3647.
106 Kayes SG, Jones RE, Omholt PE: Use of bronchoalveolar lavage (BAL) to compare local pulmonary immunity with the systemic immune response in mice infected with *Toxocara canis*. Infect Immun 1987;55:2132–2136.
107 Kayes SG, Jones RE, Omholt PE: Pulmonary granuloma formation in murine toxocariasis. Transfer of granulomatous hypersensitivity using bronchoalveolar lavage cells. J Parasitol 1988;74:950–956.
108 Kayes SG: Nonspecific allergic granulomatosis in the lungs of mice infected with large but not small inocula of the canine ascarid, *Toxocara canis*. Clin Immunol Immunopathol 1986;41:55–65.
109 Spry CJF: Eosinophils and endomyocardial fibrosis: A review of clinical and experimental studies, 1980–86; in Kawai C, Abelmann WH (eds): Pathogenesis of Myocarditis and Cardiomyopathy. Recent Experimental and Clinical Studies. Tokyo, University of Tokyo Press, 1987, pp 293–310.
110 Dao AH, Virmani R: Visceral larva migrans involving the myocardium: Report of two cases and review of literature. Pediatr Pathol 1986;6:449–456.
111 Schaffer SW, Dimayuga ER, Kayes SG: Development and characterization of a model of eosinophil-mediated cardiomyopathy in rats infected with *Toxocara canis*. Am J Physiol 1992;262:H1428–1434.
112 Tullis DCH: Bronchial asthma associated with intestinal parasites. N Engl J Med 1970;282:370–372.
113 Chacko DD: Intestinal parasites and asthma. N Engl J Med 1970;283:101.
114 Lasch EE: IgE, parasites and allergy. Lancet 1976;ii:255.
115 Desowitz RS, Rudoy R, Barnwell JW: Antibodies to canine helminth parasites in asthmatic and non asthmatic children. Int Arch Allergy Appl Immunol 1981;65:361–366.

116 Fujimoto K, Parker JC, Kayes SG: Activated eosinophils increase vascular permeability and resistance in isolated perfused rat lungs. Am Rev Respir Dis 1990;142:1414–1421.
117 Buijs J, Egbers MWEC, Nijkamp FP: *Toxocara canis*-induced airway eosinophilia and tracheal hyporeactivity in guinea pigs and mice. Eur J Pharmacol 1995;293:207–215.
118 Kayes SG: Spleen cell responses in experimental murine toxocariasis. J Parasitol 1984;70:522–529.
119 Buijs J, Lokhorst WH, Robinson J, Nijkamp FP: *Toxocara canis*-induced murine pulmonary inflammation: Analysis of cells and proteins in lung tissue and bronchoalveolar lavage fluid. Parasite Immunol 1994;16:1–9.
120 Buijs J, Egbers MWEC, Lokhorst WH, Savelkoul HFJ, Nijkamp FP: *Toxocara*-induced eosinophilic inflammation – Airway function and effect of anti-IL-5. Am J Respir Crit Care Med 1995; 151:873–878.
121 Takamoto M, Sugane K: Mechanisms of eosinophilia in *Toxocara canis* infected mice: In vitro production of interleukin 5 by lung cells of both normal and congenitally athymic nude mice. Parasite Immunol 1993;15:493–500.
122 Litt M: Eosinophils and antigen-antibody reactions. Ann NY Acad Sci 1964;116:964–985.
123 Litt M: Studies in experimental eosinophilia. VI. Uptake of immune complexes by eosinophils. J Cell Biol 1964;23:355–361.
124 Lee H-F: Effects of superinfection on the behavior of *Toxocara canis* larvae in mice. J Parasitol 1960;46:583–588.
125 Olson LJ: Organ distribution of *Toxocara canis* larvae in normal mice and mice previously infected with *Toxocara, Ascaris* or *Trichinella*. Tex Rept Biol Med 1962;20:651–657.
126 Parsons JC, Grieve RB: Effect of egg dosage and host genotype on liver trapping in murine larval toxocariasis. J Parasitol 1990;76:53–58.
127 Parsons JC, Grieve RB: Kinetics of liver trapping of infective larvae in murine toxocariasis. J Parasitol 1990;76:529–536.
128 Akao N: Immune response to excretory-secretory products of second stage larvae of *Toxocara canis*: Humoral immune response relating to larval trapping in the livers of reinfected mice. Jpn J Parasitol 1985;34:293–300.
129 Concepcion JE, Barriga OO: Transfer of infection-induced immune protection to *Toxocara canis* in a mouse model. Vet Immunol Immunopathol 1985;9:371–382.
130 Sugane K, Oshima T: Trapping of large numbers of larvae in the livers of *Toxocara canis*-reinfected mice. J Helminthol 1983;57:95–99.
131 Parsons JC, Coffman RL, Grieve RB: Antibody to interleukin 5 prevents blood and tissue eosinophilia but not liver trapping in murine larval toxocariasis. Parasite Immunol 1993;15:501–508.
132 Duguid IM: Chronic endophthalmitis due to *Toxocara*. Br J Ophthalmol 1961;45:705–717.
133 Luxenberg MN: An experimental approach to the study of intraocular *Toxocara canis*. Trans Am Ophthalmol Soc 1979;77:542–602.
134 Byers B, Kimura S: Uveitis after death of a larva in the vitreous cavity. Am J Ophthalmol 1974;77:63–66.
135 Wilder H: Nematode endophthalmitis. Trans Am Acad Ophthalmol 1950;55:99–109.
136 Liotet S, Bloch-Michel E, Petithory JC, Batellier L, Chaumeil C: Biological modifications of the vitreous in intraocular parasitosis: Preliminary study. Int Ophthalmol 1992;16:75–80.
137 Petithory JC, Chaumeil C, Liotet S, Rosseau M, Bisognani AC: Immunological studies on ocular larva migrans; in Lewis JW, Maizels RM (eds): *Toxocara* and Toxocariasis: Clinical, Epidemiological, and Molecular Perspectives. London, British Parasitological Society with the Institute for Biology, 1993, pp 81–89.
138 Glickman LT, Schantz PM: Epidemiology and pathogenesis of zoonotic toxocariasis. Epidemiol Rev 1981;3:230–250.
139 Schantz PM, Glickman LT: Toxocaral visceral larva migrans. N Engl J Med 1978;298:436–439.
140 Lewis JW, Maizels RM: *Toxocara* and Toxocariasis: Clinical, Epidemiological and Molecular Perspectives. London, British Parasitological Society with the Institute of Biology, 1993, pp 169.

Stephen G. Kayes, PhD, Department of Structural and Cellular Biology, 2042 MSB,
University of South Alabama, Mobile, AL 36688-0002 (USA)

Freedman DO (ed): Immunopathogenetic Aspects of Disease Induced by Helminth Parasites.
Chem Immunol. Basel, Karger, 1997, vol 66, pp 125–158

....

Lymphatic Filariasis

T.V. Rajan, A.V. Gundlapalli
Department of Pathology, University of Connecticut Health Center, Farmington,
Conn., USA

Lymphatic filariasis was described in a recent review in *Lancet* as 'the ancient scourge that won't go away' [1]. Towards the end of the last century, the clinical observations of Lewis in India [2] and the epidemiological studies of Manson in China [3] led to the identification of the causative organisms and mode of transmission. Despite nearly 100 years of clinical, epidemiological and, more recently, laboratory work, our understanding of lymphatic filariasis is incomplete. Far from being eradicated or even controlled, the disease appears to be spreading to larger areas of the tropical world, with increasing numbers of cases every year [4]. In this review, we will cover our understanding of the immunopathogenesis of lymphatic filariasis, combining observations in model systems with the clinical/ epidemiological observations on man.

Definition

Lymphatic filariasis is a disease that occurs mainly in tropical countries of the world, from about 41°N to 37°S. It is caused by long, slender worms of the phylum Nematoda, superfamily Filarioidea. Organisms closely related to the human parasites infect most vertebrate species except fish which, because of their aqueous environment, are presumably protected from the bites of mosquitoes. *Wuchereria bancrofti, Brugia malayi* and, much less commonly, *Brugia timori* are the causative agents of human disease. There are an estimated 120 million cases of the disease worldwide, of which more than 90% are caused by *W. bancrofti* [4].

Historical Perspective

Lymphatic filariasis has existed as a recognizable disorder from the beginnings of recorded human history. Both ancient Chinese and Indian writings describe swellings of extremities and the genitalia that are highly reminiscent of filarial lesions. The Indian physician/surgeon Sushruta compiled a textbook of medicine known as the *Sushruta Samhita*; the extant version was probably in its final form by 70 AD [5, 6]. He refers to a disease called *slipada* (*sli* elephant; *pada* leg). The descriptions of this condition appear to include diseases other than lymphatic filariasis; it is nonetheless clear that at least some of the patients exhibiting *slipada* are cases of lymphatic filariasis. Sushruta also correctly noted that the disease is particularly prevalent in individuals who live close to stagnant water. The disease was clearly known to the Arab physicians around the 10th century as well. The famous Persian physician, Rhazes, first described the condition in Arabic; another renowned Persian physician, Avicenna, mentions that the disease was endemic in Alexandria.

One of the earliest Western descriptions of filariasis is by Jean-Nicolas Demarquay [7], a French physician. His sketches of worms he found in the scrotal fluid of a Cuban patient with scrotal 'tumor' leave little doubt but that he saw microfilariae. In 1868, Wucherer [8] described a species of worm in the urine of patients with tropical hematuria in Brazil and clearly distinguished them from *Bilharzia (Schistosoma) haematobium*. Lewis [2], a Welsh physician stationed in India, performed some remarkable studies on lymphatic filariasis, and it is an egregious oversight that no major filarial parasite is eponymously named after him. It is clear, however, that his work had an impact on other workers in the field, since both Manson [3, 9, 10] and Bancroft [11] refer to his work in their own descriptions of lymphatic filariasis. Sir Patrick Manson, a Scottish physician stationed in China during the second half of the 19th century, correctly attributed the profound, deforming swelling of extremities to infestation with filarial parasites. Manson described the periodicity of the microfilariae in peripheral blood [9] and the location of the microfilariae when they are missing from systemic blood [10]. He also demonstrated that mosquitoes transmit the parasite [10]. The demonstration of the adult female worm was left to Joseph Bancroft [11], an English physician stationed in Australia. Bourne [12] later discovered the adult male worm.

In 1927, Lichtenstein [quoted in Turner, 13] reported from the Celebes (now called Sulawesi) that the mosquito vector *Culex fatigans* could not be infected by the locally prevalent microfilarial species, and that elephantiasis of the legs was the main feature of disease in this area, in contrast to the urogenital lesions and chylous manifestations so characteristic of bancroftian filariasis. In 1958, Buckley proposed the genus name *Brugia* for the organism responsible for lymphatic filariasis in this area (formally reported in 1960 [14]).

The Organisms

The etiologic agents responsible for human lymphatic filariasis belong to two genera, *Wuchereria* and *Brugia*. Until recently only one species was recognized in the genus *Wuchereria*. In 1980, a separate species called *Wuchereria kalimantani* was reported to be distinct from *W. bancrofti* [15]. *W. bancrofti* appears to be a strict pathogen for man in nature, even though it can be transmitted to certain other primates under laboratory conditions [16]. *B. malayi*, on the other hand, also occurs as a zoonotic infection in Malaya, Indonesia and other Pacific islands.

Morphology

Adult *W. bancrofti* and *B. malayi* worms are similar in appearance. They are long, slender, tapered, cream-colored round worms. Both male and female *Brugia* worms are somewhat smaller than their *W. bancrofti* counterparts. In both species, the males (up to 4 cm long and 0.1 mm in diameter for *W. bancrofti* and 3.5 cm × 0.1 mm for *B. malayi*) are significantly smaller than the females, which can be as long as 6–10 cm *(W. bancrofti)* or 5–6 cm *(B. malayi)* and 0.2–0.3 mm or 0.1 mm wide, respectively. Aside from their smaller size, the males can be distinguished from the females by a corkscrew-like tail and the presence of two spicules that function as copulatory organs. Male and female adult worms take permanent residence in afferent lymphatics or the cortical sinuses of lymph nodes and generate microscopic live progeny called 'microfilariae'. The microfilariae of *W. bancrofti* and *B. malayi* are approximately the same size, 280 μm by 7 μm. In common with all nematodes studied to date, the development of the filarial parasites involves 4 larval stages (L1–L4). The increasing complexity of the internal organization of these sequential morphogenetic stages is demonstrated in figures 1–4.

Periodicity

Microfilariae migrate up the lymphatic tree and enter the circulation at the left subclavian vein. Their behavior in the vascular circulation is genetically determined and geographically distinct. Thus, if one were to chart the number of microfilariae that appear in the peripheral blood of an infected individual as a function of time of day, one would note distinct patterns. As was first shown by Manson [9], the most prevalent form of *W. bancrofti* shows a distinct nocturnal periodicity, with significantly more microfilariae in peripheral blood during the night than the day. The temporal limitation of appearance in the peripheral circulation correlates with the feeding behavior of the vector responsible for transmitting the parasite in the area. Thus, the predominant vector for *W. bancrofti* is *Culex quinquefasciatus*, a nocturnally feeding mosquito. However, in the eastern

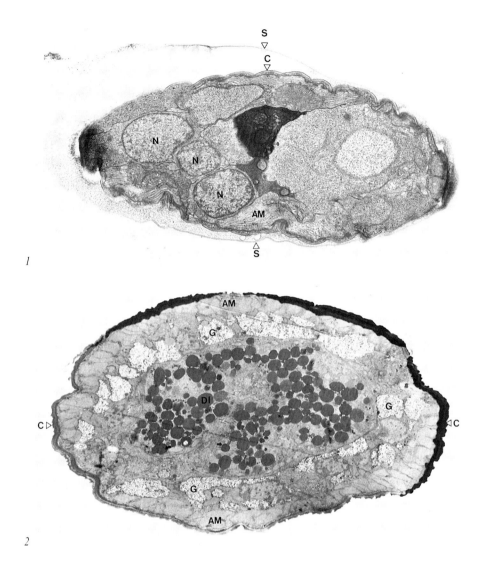

Fig. 1. Cross-section of a microfilarial larva. Note that the sheath (S) is considerably larger than the microfilaria itself; the microfilaria moves freely within the sheath. The space between the sheath and the larval cuticle (C) contains a fluid, as indicated by the electron-dense material. Note the significant diversity of cell structure. Clearly defined muscle cells of the adult type are not developed at this point. However, fibrillar material (AM) suggestive of actomyosin fibers are seen in the areas indicated. N = Nuclei of microfilarial cells.

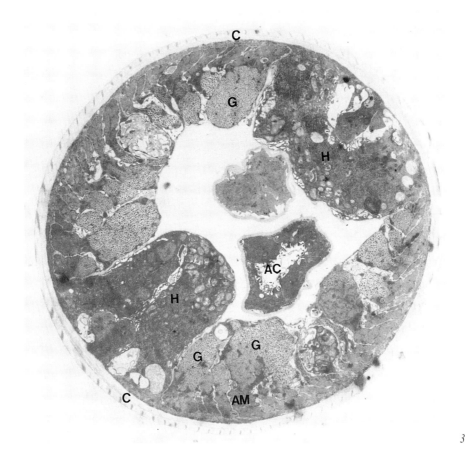

3

Fig. 2. Cross-section of an L3 larva. Unlike the microfilariae, there is no sheath at this stage, and the cuticle (C) is somewhat more prominent. Lying underneath the cuticle are cells that are more clearly recognizable as muscle cells, as indicated by the more peripheral actomyosin fibers (AM) and the more internally located glycogen stores (G). Internal to the glycogen-containing muscle cells are large cells containing dense inclusions (DI). These presumably represent the forerunners of the adult alimentary canal.

Fig. 3. Cross-section of an L4 larva. The lateral hypodermal ridges (H) are more obvious at this stage. Also note the well-developed muscle cells indicated by the peripheral actomyosin fibers (AM) and the internal glycogen stores (G). A well-developed alimentary canal (AC) is noticeable in this stage. Note also the considerably thicker cuticle (C), with the intricate architecture of the outermost layer.

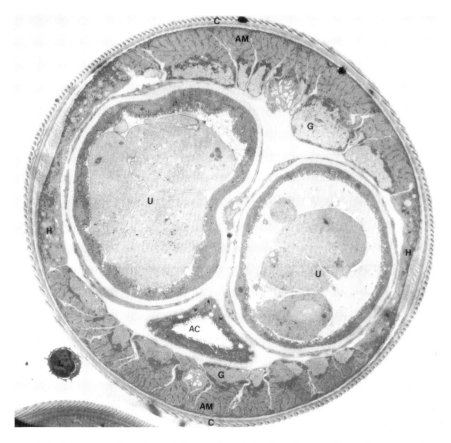

Fig. 4. Cross-section of an adult parasite, with a lymphocyte (L) for size comparison. Note the intricate structure of the outermost layer of the cuticle (C). Lying beneath the cuticle is a layer of the hypodermis (H), most visible in the two lateral aspects. Anteriorly and posteriorly, the muscle cells with characteristic actomyosin fibers (AM) peripherally and glycogen (G) centrally are seen. The two large circular structures (U) represent the gonads in this female adult, and the triangular structure is the alimentary canal (AC), lined by cells that have microvilli on their luminal surface.

Pacific, various species of *Aëdes*, which are daytime feeders, transmit the parasite; in these areas, the parasite appears in peripheral blood essentially throughout the day, with some tendency to an increase during the daylight hours [17].

Manson showed that microfilariae congregate in the deep vessels of the body, particularly in the lung, when they are absent from peripheral blood. The stimuli that induce their appearance in peripheral blood are not clear. Despite the strong correlation with the feeding behavior of the local mosquito population, the vector itself is apparently not the cue. Numerous experiments have documented that reversal of the patient's sleep rhythm causes the microfilariae to reverse their periodicity and become diurnal [17]. These observations strongly imply that periodicity is genetically determined and that the cue to depart from the pulmonary vasculature emanates from signals endogenous to the host. Some studies suggest that the differences in the pCO_2 and pO_2 levels between venous and arterial blood are sensed by the parasite and determine its emergence in the peripheral circulation. Thus, if a patient with microfilariae in the circulation is made to breathe pure oxygen, the microfilariae retreat to the lungs [17].

While fascinating and understandable in a context of epidemiology and evolution, the biological significance of periodicity is obscure. Thus, while the presence of microfilariae in the peripheral circulation is required for entry into the vector, the reasons for their withdrawal elsewhere for the rest of the day are less obvious. There would appear to be no strong selection against such behavior, since eastern Pacific strains of *W. bancrofti* remain in the peripheral circulation for most of the day, with no obvious growth disadvantage. It is likely that the primitive precursor of the parasite was inherently nonperiodic. In any geographic area, variants that exhibit peripheral periodicity consonant with the feeding habits of the local vector would have the highest likelihood of being transmitted and would be subjected to positive selection. This periodicity would then become fixed in that geographic region.

Life Cycle

Man is the only known definitive host in nature for *W. bancrofti*. A number of mammalian species appear to serve as hosts for *B. malayi*, including several species of monkeys and domestic cats. The intermediate host for all lymphatic filarial parasites is the mosquito. *C. quinquefasciatus*, the ubiquitous urban mosquito, is the primary vector for the predominant periodic form of *W. bancrofti*. Various species of *Aëdes* mosquitoes serve as vectors for the aperiodic form found in certain areas of the Pacific. The periodic form of *B. malayi*, which is adapted primarily to humans, is spread by *Anopheline* mosquitoes. *Mansonia* sp. transmit the sub-periodic form.

Microfilariae need to undergo extensive development and metamorphosis to the infective stage in the mosquito in order to continue the natural infection in the mammalian host (fig. 5). The details of the development in the mosquito have been described in numerous excellent reviews [18]. Soon after entry into the mosquito vector, the microfilariae shed their sheath and shorten and thicken to assume the 'sausage' form of the parasite. This development takes from 5 to 105 min. Subsequently, they pierce the midgut of the mosquito to enter the flight muscles where they develop into the L2 larvae. About 2 weeks later, the larvae

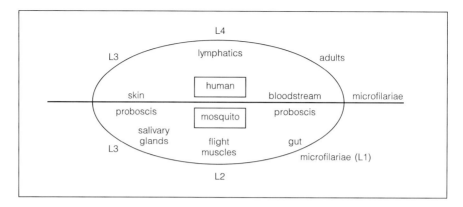

Fig. 5. Life cycle of the filarial worm in the two hosts. Microfilariae in circulation are ingested by mosquitoes, migrate through the midgut into the celomic cavity, and come to rest in the flight muscles. After further maturation, they migrate anteriorly as L3 larvae to the head and exit during a feed. L3 larvae enter the human host, home to the lymphatics and undergo metamorphosis to the L4 and adult forms. Dioecious adults mate, and the female liberates microfilariae which reach the peripheral circulation.

emerge from the mosquito flight muscle as human infective larvae (L3), which migrate anteriorly into the head and the proboscis.

Localization in the Mammalian Host

Perhaps attracted by the host components leaking from the mosquito-generated puncture wound in the skin, the L3 larvae crawl into the subcutaneous tissues at the site of the puncture and migrate towards a lymphatic channel. The mechanisms by which the larvae seek, recognize and colonize the lymphatics are entirely unknown. Human filarial parasites injected into compatible animal hosts likewise home to the lymphatics in these paratenic hosts. This observation suggests that there is a commonality to the signals that denote the lymphatics as such in various mammalian species, and that the cognate receptors in the filarial nematodes are able to recognize these signals. The choice of lymphatic channels for the residence of filarial worms needs explanation. One must suppose that there are unique parasite nutritional needs that are met by the contents of the lymphatics. The identification of these nutritional and/or trophic factors presents an important challenge to workers in filariasis, since they might present us with therapeutic targets.

Molting from the infective L3 stage to the L4 stage takes approximately 2 weeks. By this time, the infective larvae have positioned themselves in the lymphatic channels. Further differentiation and maturation to the adult takes place over the next month in the case of *B. malayi*, and over several months for *W. bancrofti*. The precise life span of adults has not been determined with accuracy. The best estimates are those based on the duration of microfilaremia in individuals removed to a nonendemic area. Based on these data, the longevity of adult worms has been estimated to be between 5 and 8 years [19–21].

Biochemistry

Surprisingly little is known about the biochemistry of the filarial nematodes. The absence of detailed biochemical knowledge becomes particularly obvious when one considers our attempts at rational drug design for the parasites infecting humans. Thus, the spate of acute filariasis in American servicemen in the 1940s prompted an urgent search for chemotherapeutic agents. A group of compounds, the cyanine dyes, were discovered to be important and effective in accomplishing complete cures of cotton rats infected with the model filarial parasite, *Litomosoides carinii*. However, these drugs had no efficacy against the parasites infecting humans. Recent studies have elucidated the reason for this striking disparity. *L. carinii* is aerobic, and since the cyanine dyes interfere with mitochondrial function, they are effective in this organism. In contrast, the human filarial parasites are anaerobic homolactate fermenters, as demonstrated by Wang and Saz [22], and are therefore not susceptible to these agents. This episode highlights the need for further biochemical studies if one were to attempt to design drugs that can target specific metabolic pathways in the parasites. Parenthetically, the near obligate anaerobic metabolism of the adults is surprising, considering that their cells contain cristate mitochondria.

Rew and Saz [23] demonstrated that, unlike adults, microfilariae require oxygen for at least some of their metabolic activities. Thus, microfilariae of a number of filarial species were obtained from appropriate animal models and incubated either aerobically or anaerobically. They found that whereas the parasites remain actively motile under aerobic conditions, they rapidly lose motility under anaerobic conditions. Interestingly, however, if microfilariae were reexposed to oxygen even after a week's incubation in its absence, motility was restored rapidly. These results suggest that microfilariae require aerobic metabolism for motility, but not for survival.

The composition of the nematode cuticle, which represents the interface between the parasite and the host, has been analyzed at the biochemical level. Selkirk et al. [24, 25] and Maizels et al. [26] have shown that the inner aspects of the cuticle are composed of 12–25 collagenous proteins that are heavily cross-linked. The outer cuticle and the epicuticle are not soluble in the aqueous phase even under harsh detergent conditions. However, two presumably nonstructural proteins do partition into the aqueous phase. One has been dubbed the 'ladder protein' because of its tendency to generate a series of bands on SDS-PAGE,

Table 1. Partial list of vaccine candidates evaluated for protection against lymphatic filariasis in animal models

B. malayi antigen	Localization of antigen	Reference
BmA-2, 120 kD	adult, other stages not determined	125
Chitinase, p70 and p75	sheath of microfilariae after maturation in vertebrate host, not found in sheath of uterine microfilariae	32
Aspartyl tRNA synthetase, 62 kD	microfilariae, adult male and female	126
43-kD antigen	not determined ·	33
Paramyosin, 97 kD	L3, adults, microfilariae	30
25-kD antigen	L3, mature adults (internal antigen), microfilariae	127

representing multimers of a unit peptide of molecular weight 17,000. Another, a 29-kD glycoprotein, is highly conserved among the various filarial species. Sequence analyses indicate that it has significant homology to human glutathione peroxidase [27].

Fundamental questions, including the nutritional needs, metabolic pathways that might be unique to the organism, and the mechanisms of nutrient uptake and waste discharge remain completely uncharacterized.

Molecular Biology

Molecular biological analyses of the filarial nematodes have been driven by potential applicability in two areas – the development of DNA probes that could be sensitive and specific for the detection of parasites in the field setting, and the generation of recombinant DNA-based subunit vaccines.

The unique copy DNA sequence complexity of filarial nematodes is about 10^8 base pairs [28]. About 10–12% of the filarial genome is composed of a simple sequence repeat of about 320 base pairs [29]. The very high molar content of this sequence (>30,000 copies per haploid genome) immediately offers the possibility of sequence-specific recognition of the parasite, both in the mosquito vector and in blood films.

In order to define potential candidates that could be used as DNA-based subunit vaccines, investigators have chosen two different approaches. The first is to identify immunogens that are specifically recognized by individuals who are putatively immune to the disease, rather than by individuals that exhibit either the carrier state or disease. Using such a strategy, a number of potential immunogens have been identified (table 1). Most of these candidates have not had significant protective value, with the possible exception of paramyosin. In two different model systems, preimmunization with recombinant filarial paramyosin has resulted in significant host protection. Nanduri and Kazura [30] have shown that preimmunized mice are able to clear a challenge infusion of microfilariae more rapidly than control animals. In a more physiological approach, Li et al. [31] have shown that immunization of jirds with recombinant filarial paramyosin significantly reduces the worm burden following challenge infection with live *B. malayi* L3.

The second approach to the discovery of potential vaccine candidates is to target physiological functions that may be critical to the parasite. Such a function becomes even more attractive if it is unique to the parasite or at least sufficiently different from the host homologue, so that the latter is not affected by the intervention. Invertebrates, in contrast to the vertebrate host, molt in order to escape the constraints of the exoskeleton. This property has been targeted by the work of Fuhrman et al. [32]. A monoclonal antibody, MF-1, was found to significantly reduce circulating microfilaremia in the jird model when administered in vivo. The cDNA encoding the cognate protein has been isolated, and the DNA sequence and inferred amino acid sequence reveal significant homology to bacterial chitinases. Interestingly, a 43-kD antigen has been identified as being closely correlated with protective immunity by Freedman et al. [33] in human populations. Raghavan et al. [34] have cloned the cDNA encoding this protein, which also shares homology with known chitinases, including the MF-1 protein of Fuhrman et al. [32].

A new development that promises to accelerate the rate of acquisition of molecular biological data is the institution of the filarial genome network, sponsored by the WHO [35]. A novel approach to the rapid acquisition of important sequence information has been pioneered by Adams et al. [36] and is referred to as expressed sequence tag (EST) analysis. In this approach, instead of sequencing genomic DNA, investigators generate cDNA libraries representing those genes that are transcribed in multiple tissues and/or stages of the target organism. A feature of nematode nucleic acid biology that facilitates this approach is the spliced-leader RNA [37]. Nilsen [38] has shown that filarial nematodes, in common with all known nematode species, *trans*-splice a short segment of RNA onto many (or all) mRNA molecules. The presence of this tag at the 5′-end of mRNA molecules offers a strategy by which full-length cDNA molecules can be readily obtained. Thus, the first strand can be synthesized using the standard oligo-dT primed reverse-transcriptase reaction. This is followed by PCR using the sense orientation of the spliced-leader sequence as one primer and oligo-dT as the other. Six laboratories have undertaken to produce several hundred ESTs from each of several cDNA libraries. The filariasis research community has chosen *B. malayi* as its model organism because of its ready availability from multiple laboratory animal sources. All data generated in this sequencing effort will be deposited with existing data banks (GenBank and EMBL). Resources can be accessed through the World Wide Web at the FilGenNet Home Page (URL=http://wood-land.bio.ic.ac.uk/fgn). Over 600 ESTs have already been obtained using both traditional and spliced-leader-PCR-generated *B. malayi* L3 cDNA libraries. Scott [pers. commun.] has found that 50% are unique to the *B. malayi* data set in that no significant homology has been discovered with any of the existing sequences in the data banks. Interestingly, the genomes of two bacterial species (*Mycoplasma genitalium* [39] and *Haemophilus influenzae* [40]) have been fully sequenced recently. Here again, nearly 40% of the open reading frames are unique to the organisms.

Epidemiology and Occurrence

One important consideration in any discussion of lymphatic filariasis is that it is restricted to endemic pockets. At this point in time, brugian filariasis is endemic in 8 countries and bancroftian filariasis in about 50. The precise numbers of individuals suffering from lymphatic filariasis is difficult to estimate because of poor reporting and record keeping in many rural areas where the disease is highly prevalent. Recent estimates by the WHO [4], based on a number of assumptions, place the burden of lymphatic filariasis at approximately 120 million, with 90% due to *W. bancrofti*.

Geographic Distribution
Until recently, it was believed that a majority of cases of filarial infection and disease occurred in the Indian subcontinent. Recent reestimates by the WHO suggest that 38% of cases of lymphatic filariasis occur in India and 34% in sub-Saharan Africa [4]. These new data would suggest that the disease is of greater public health concern in sub-Saharan Africa than hitherto believed. Another change from the classical perception of filariasis relates to brugian disease. This was believed to be confined to Indonesia, Malaysia, the Philippines, Vietnam and Korea. More recent studies by the WHO suggest that as many as 32% of all cases of brugian filariasis occur in China and 20% in India. Thus, these two countries bear the majority of the world's burden of brugian filariasis.

Demographics of Disease in Endemic Areas
There are differences in the details of the epidemiological picture of filariasis among endemic areas. This phenomenon is highlighted if one compares human infections in five areas, two with bancroftian and three with brugian filariasis, where the microfilaremia rates vary from 10–20% [41, 42] in the two *W. bancrofti*

endemic areas to 30–50% [13, 43, 44] in the three *B. malayi* endemic areas. These differences have been presumed to be due to differences in the parasite strain indigenous to the area or to regional differences in the host immune responses. Bundy et al. [45] have used mathematical analyses on the available data and suggest that the intensity of transmission alone is sufficient to account for these geographic differences.

Gender Effects on Incidence of Filarial Disease

Gender has an important influence on the prevalence of infection, and the world literature has recently been reviewed by Brabin [46]. According to her survey, the incidence of the chronic sequelae of lymphatic filariasis in males exceeds that in females by a factor of 2. A more recent compilation of data by Pani et al. [47] suggests that the male-female dichotomy may be even greater in India (>12% in males to around 2% in females).

The basis for this gender difference is not clear. It has been speculated that the occupational habits of males bring them in contact with the mosquito vector more frequently [48]. Alternatively, Rosen [49] has suggested that immunity, rather than exposure, is responsible for the observed sexual dimorphism. The basis for this difference in susceptibility is extremely difficult to investigate in humans, and only inferential epidemiological data are available [48–52]. Work in animal models supports the sex differential in susceptibility even when the dose of infective larvae is controlled, suggesting that exposure may not explain the observed differences [53–55]. The data are consistent with a sexual dimorphism in innate immunity, and recent work from Rao et al. [56] suggests that the difference can be abrogated by macrophage blockade. Interestingly, the prevalence of acute lymphatic filariasis is approximately similar in males and females. If there is progression from acute to chronic disease, this would pose a contradiction. One possible explanation is that chronic disease in females is underreported in many areas.

Age Dynamics of Filarial Infection

The prevalence of lymphatic filariasis as a function of age has been determined in a number of geographic locations, and there appears to be an overall concordance of reports. The earliest age when brugian microfilaremia has been detected in an infant is $3^1/_2$ months; for bancroftian filariasis, it is 7–10 months. Day et al. [57] have determined the age dynamics of *W. bancrofti* infection in the East Sepik Province of Papua New Guinea. They collected parasitological data on 126 subjects more than 4 years of age at two time points, 12 months apart, prior to the administration of diethylcarbamazine (DEC). This short-term longitudinal study included analysis of the levels of circulating high-molecular-weight phosphorylcholine-bearing antigen (PC-Ag) as well as microfilaremia. They found that even within this short time interval, there were significant changes in microfilaremia and the concentration of the circulating PC-Ag in subjects who were less than 20 years of age, but not in subjects more than 20 years of age. Similar age-related changes have been noted by Dondero et al. [41] for *W. bancrofti* infection in Howrah, a suburb of Calcutta, India. In a single cross-sectional study, the microfilaremia percentage rose from 0% in the 0–4 age group to 29% in the 20–29 age group, and thereafter remained at the 20–30% level in all subsequent age groups. The numbers of Dennis et al. [43] on age stratification of Timorian microfilaremia are qualitatively similar, though quantitatively higher, with 24% positive in the 0–4 age group, rising to 47% in the 30–39 age group, and thereafter remaining at a plateau for all subsequent age groups [43]. Similar studies of the age-specific rates of acquisition of *W. bancrofti* infection in Pondicherry, Tamilnadu, India [58], once again suggest an age-specific increase in microfilarial rates, from less than 2% under the age of 5 climbing to a maximum of 10% in the 20–30 age group, and declining somewhat in later years. Thus, it would appear that there is an increasing frequency of infection with increasing age, but that all individuals likely to become microfilaremic do so by their third decade of life. An exception to this general formulation may be timorian filariasis; in a village studied by Partono et al. [44], the microfilaremia rates in male residents rose from 0% in the <4-year age group (0 out of 10 subjects) to 100% in residents >50 years of age, while that in the 30–40 age group was lower (about 40%).

Clinical Features of Lymphatic Filariasis

Most textbook discussions of lymphatic filariasis tend to describe clinical features of brugian and bancroftian filariasis together, with relatively little emphasis on the former, since 90% or more of the global incidence of the disease is of the latter variety. However, a careful reading of the literature leads one to the inescapable conclusion that the symptomatology due to brugian parasites (both *B. malayi* and *B. timori*) is significantly different from that due to *W. bancrofti*. Thus, the pathology caused by brugian filariasis is more distinct, dramatic and destructive. One is led to speculate that *W. bancrofti* is better adapted to the human host and is therefore less likely to cause adverse effects. Significant differences between the symptomatology of brugian and bancroftian filariasis will be highlighted where appropriate in the following discussion.

Onset of Clinical Symptoms
In discussing the onset of lymphatic filariasis, it is useful to define two terms, *the incubation period*, which is the time interval between exposure to the parasite and the onset of clinical symptomatology, and *the prepatent period*, which is the

time interval between exposure and appearance of microfilariae in circulation. In an endemic area, where transmission occurs more or less continually, it is difficult to ascertain the precise infective bite. In this regard, therefore, the most informative reports are either experimental infections of man [59, 60] or those instances where individuals have moved from a nonendemic filariasis area to an endemic area [61]. In both instances, the first symptoms of infection occur 4–6 weeks after exposure.

The prepatent period, on the other hand, is the period that ensues between the entry of the L3 larvae into the human host and the appearance of microfilariae in circulation. Individuals exposed for the first time to infection as adults tend, as a rule, not to be productive of microfilariae and therefore do not provide us with this information. The best estimates of the patent period come from parasitological observations on young individuals born in endemic areas. The youngest children seen with *W. bancrofti* microfilaremia are between 7 and 10 months of age, suggesting that this might be a prepatent period for *W. bancrofti*. On the other hand, children as young as $3^1/_2$ months can be microfilaremic for *B. malayi* and *B. timori*. This interval is consistent with the prepatent periods in numerous experimental animals, including jirds, dogs, cats, ferrets and mice.

Spectrum of Clinical Presentation

In many endemic areas, transmission rates are quite high, and the premise is that most individuals are exposed to infective larvae. For instance, Gubler and Bhattacharya [62] conducted a quantitative study of transmission of *W. bancrofti* in Howrah. They estimate that an average resident of a suburb of Calcutta receives over 115,000 bites per year, and of these 1,850 are by infective mosquitoes. They further estimate that each infective bite transmits an average of 3–4 infective larvae, making the total infective larval challenge per individual per year to be approximately 6,000. Other studies have corroborated these numbers suggesting that, in most endemic areas, the average individual is exposed to several hundred to several thousand infective larvae per year. Despite this constant assault, the resultant clinical features are not uniform, and individuals exhibit a spectrum of clinical responses.

One of the fundamental problems of studying lymphatic filariasis is the chronicity of infection and the requirement for long-term longitudinal follow-up in order to determine the course of infection in any given individual. Because of logistical constraints, virtually all studies have been cross-sectional. By their very nature, such studies present a static view, and inferences of the natural history of the disease can be made by following the clinical spectrum in sequential age groups. The premise is that the transitions from one age group to the other represent the evolution of the disease. Bundy et al. [45] have generated mathematical models, based on epidemiological studies, to propose a plausible natural course for the disease. Their models would imply that the natural progression begins with infection, and proceeds through microfilaremia, acute disease, amicrofilaremia and ultimately to the development of chronic symptoms. As with any mathematical models, this scenario must be regarded as tentative. The following discussion is based on the prevailing model of classifying clinical presentations, with no implication that there is an ordered or preferential progression from one clinical manifestation to the other, even though some progression must occur in nature.

Endemic Normals or Asymptomatic Amicrofilaremics. Until recently, it was believed that even in an area which was endemic for lymphatic filariasis and where there was considerable exposure, a large majority of patients exhibited no symptoms of lymphatic filariasis and did not have demonstrable parasite burden. Historically, these individuals, termed 'endemic normals', were believed to represent 60–70% of the population. Freedman et al. [63] and Day [64] have provoked us to reevaluate this picture and have enunciated stringent criteria for the definition of the term 'endemic normal'. These include the absence of any recent or remote history of filarial fever, lymphatic edema or swelling; absence of microfilaremia or reactive discomfort after a provocative dose of DEC; absence of circulating, high-molecular-weight antigen, and the absence of circulating IgG4, an immunoglobulin isotype associated with active infection [65]. If these more stringent criteria are applied to a population, one finds that truly infection-free individuals are rare. In one village in Papua New Guinea, Day [64] found that less than 6% (5 out of 92) were amicrofilaremic and denied any obvious history or symptoms of the disease. When these individuals were tested for circulating 200-kD PC-Ag, widely accepted as an indicator of the presence of adult worm burdens, all were found to be positive. In addition, three out of the five evidenced local and systemic reactions to provocative tests with DEC. Finally, all had detectable levels of filarial-specific IgG4. Thus, if one employs stringent criteria, no individual in this area is an endemic normal. The currently accepted interpretation of available data is that many individuals who are asymptomatic and do not bear obvious signs of parasite burden are nonetheless cryptically infected. Day [64] found that the level of PC-Ag in the microfilaremia-negative individuals is in the same range as that in the microfilaremia-low individuals, suggesting that the two groups may bear similar adult worm burdens. In view of this, this group is perhaps more appropriately designated 'asymptomatic amicrofilaremics'.

It is also worthwhile to remember that this category is probably not a monolithic entity, but may represent diverse responses to the parasite culminating in the same manifest phenotype. Thus, some endemic normals are probably individuals with parasite burdens that are below the levels of detection. Others might be individuals who have had past asymptomatic infections, cleared them without extensive damage to their lymphatic vasculature and have become resistant to reinfection. Other individuals are probably truly immune to the parasite and have never been infected. Even these individuals, however, appear to have been exposed to the parasite at some time in their life, as indicated by the fact that they often display high titers of antifilarial antibodies in their sera and mount vigorous cell-mediated immune responses to filarial antigens.

Asymptomatic Microfilaremics. Many individuals in endemic areas exhibit no symptoms of filarial infection and yet, on routine blood examinations, demonstrate significant parasite load. These individuals would be called carriers in other infectious diseases and are referred to as 'asymptomatic microfilaremics' in the filarial literature. They represent reservoirs of the disease since, being asymptomatic, they would not seek treatment. The parasite burden in such individuals can be dramatically high, exceeding 1,100 microfilariae per milliliter blood. Until recently, these individuals were regarded as being completely free of symptoms or signs of disease. The use of lymphoscintigraphy has revealed that many of these individuals harbor live adult worms in dilated lymphatic vessels, with significant deviations of lymph flow [66–69]. Thus, while they may be free of overt symptomatology, it is clear that some subtle pathological changes are occurring in these patients. In this regard, long-term longitudinal follow-up of this group is critical to our understanding of the evolution of the disease.

Filarial Fever and Adeno-Lymphangitis. Brugian and bancroftiandisease differ in the frequency, intensity and localization of acute symptoms and signs attributable to infection. In brugian filariasis, episodes of fever, adenopathy, lymphangitis, abscesses of affected lymph nodes and local scarring appear to be the rule; many cases of bancroftian filariasis can present with insidious onset of chronic symptoms with no antecedent acute disease.

In brugian filariasis, the classical acute symptoms are enlargement of a single superficial lymph node at a time, most often in the inguinal area [70]. A characteristic retrograde lymphangitis is often associated with this lymphadenitis, with the red, inflamed lymph vessel appearing as a cord-like streak that extends from the lymph node towards the periphery. The lymph node, as well as the associated lymphatic, is often tender and may be painful. In rare instances, the inflammation may spread into the surrounding tissue producing a cellulitis which may involve the entire thigh. The syndrome of recurrent episodes of painful red swellings in the groin area accompanied by fever and malaise is common enough to have earned the colloquial names of 'bowo' in southeast Indonesia and 'mumu' in the Pacific Islands [71]. Many individuals exhibit scars in the groin, conceivably as a result of burst abscesses.

Acute symptoms in bancroftian disease are more often seen in individuals who encounter the parasite for the first time in adulthood, rather than as children. Funiculitis is the most frequent acute manifestation [72, 73].

The role of bacterial infections in acute filarial fever has been a recurring issue in lymphatic filariasis. Manson suggested that the pathological changes in the lymphatics may predispose to bacterial infections, which may be responsible for the acute symptoms [74]. Physicians in endemic areas often report that these episodes respond to broad-spectrum antibiotic treatment that has no known or demonstrable activity on the filarial parasites themselves. This formulation has been greeted with skepticism for the last few decades, but more recently there is increasing acceptance that it may bear some validity. The WHO has recently called for local hygiene as a critical prophylactic against recurrent filarial fever and the development of chronic sequelae [4]. This mode of intervention has been prompted by some recent publications [75, 76] that suggest that bacterial superinfection plays an important role in precipitating febrile episodes, and that recurrent bouts of local inflammation provoke cycles of necrosis and repair, culminating in mechanical blockage of lymphatics.

Conflicting with these data are those of Kar et al. [77] who have examined the humoral immune response against the human filarial parasite in 62 cases of acute disease, presenting with fever and adenolymphangitis in a community with bancroftian filariasis. There was no increase in antibodies to various bacterial antigens, including streptolysin O, but there was an increase in antifilarial titers. Particularly noteworthy was the observation that leukocytosis, a common feature of inflammatory reactions to bacterial infection, did not occur. These data are suggestive of the possibility that filarial fever results from the death of a worm, resulting in local release of filarial antigen and an inflammatory reaction to this antigen.

Part of the problem in investigating the pathogenetic aspects of acute filarial fever is that there is no reproducible model for this disease. However, Denham and Fletcher [78] have pointed out that acute disease is seen clinically in cats as manifested by short-lived lymphadenitis associated with fever at the time of patency, as well as subsequent episodes of sudden increases in the size of a lymph node, with transient lymphedema. Biopsies performed during these episodes document the presence of dead worms in lymphatics, suggesting that sporadic death of worms releases internal antigens resulting in an acute inflammatory reaction.

It is also evident that there is a close correlation between continued residence in an endemic area and the occurrence of acute symptoms. Thus, when a patient with filariasis is transported to a nonendemic area, the episodes of filarial fever gradually subside and disappear with no further treatment [19–21]. It appears reasonable to conclude that continued presence in an area with active transmission is required for eliciting acute symptoms. A model consistent with this observation is that attacks of filarial fever may coincide with the migration of the larvae to the lymphatics and subsequent molting in situ. It is widely believed that fluids released during molting and parturition are highly inflammatory.

In any case, the precise cause of filarial fever is not known. In the case of young children in brugian areas and in the nonendemic bancroftian disease, filarial molting and parturition fluids may be the factors responsible for eliciting inflammatory reactions and fever. On the other hand, acute exacerbations of long-standing chronic disease ('acute on chronic') may be due to secondary, opportunistic bacterial infections of the skin and subcutaneous tissues whose vitality is compromised by long-standing lymph stasis. It is thus conceivable that at least two distinct mechanisms are involved. Consistent with this idea are recent data from Brazil [79]. Individuals with grade I to grade III lymphedema, with none of the cutaneous pathology associated with chronic elephantiasis, exhibited acute adenolymphangitis, without any evidence of bacterial superinfection.

Tropical Pulmonary Eosinophilia. A dramatic manifestation of lymphatic filariasis is tropical pulmonary eosinophilia (TPE). This term was first introduced by Weingarten [80], though there were earlier reports of similar symptoms from India [81]. Individuals present with episodes of acute asthma, and their sputum and pulmonary lavage fluid contain high concentrations of eosinophils. Danaraj [82, 83] has contributed to our understanding of TPE. Following the initial observations of Meyers and Koutenaar, he concluded that the cause of this syndrome is an arsenic-sensitive organism, rather than a reaction to a variety of infectious agents. Subsequently, he confirmed that DEC is effective in curing the condition, suggesting that the cause might be a filarial worm. Immunological studies have indicated that these patients are hyperreactive to filarial antigens and mount a vigorous immune response characterized by high levels of IgE [84]. It is widely believed that in patients with TPE, who are normally not microfilaremic, microfilariae are trapped and lysed in the pulmonary vasculature. This results in antigen-antibody reactions on the surface of mast cells, mediated by cytophilic IgE antibodies. The consequent release of vasoactive amines results in the characteristic symptomatology of TPE.

Chronic Sequelae of Filarial Infection. The most debilitating consequence of lymphatic filariasis is lymphedema. Recent studies from the WHO suggest that the lymphedema follows distinct phases in its evolution and can be classified into three stages. In the first stage, there is pitting edema, which is alleviated by elevating the limb. In stage II, the edema is nonpitting and cannot be reversed by elevation. Finally, in stage III, there is a gross increase in the volume of the limb, with associated changes in the skin and subcutaneous tissues (elephantiasis).

Recent studies in man and in experimental animals reveal that lymphatic dilatation with impairment of lymph flow through the affected region occurs early in infection [66–69]. It is also clear from lymphoscintigraphy studies that there is no mechanical block to lymphatic flow at this early stage. Indeed, it would appear that the adult worms live in lymphatics exhibiting nodular dilatation, swimming freely in a large pool of retained lymph fluid. Studies on immunodeficient animals further document that during this early phase of lymphatic damage, ectasia and stasis do not require a host immune response and appear to be engineered by the parasite through the release of some vasoactive substances. Thus, Vincent et al. [85] and Nelson et al. [86] have clearly demonstrated that soon after the adult worms take residence in the lymphatics of these immunodeficient hosts, there is dilatation, stasis and tortuosity of the lymphatics. Indeed, significant lymphatic dilatation with elephantoid features occurs in C3H/HeJ nude mice in the complete absence of T lymphocytes.

Brugian lymphatic filariasis almost invariably affects the limbs, with elephantiasis of the leg below the knee being the most frequently observed lesion. Less frequently, elephantiasis of the arm below the elbow is seen. The genitalia are seldom, if ever, involved in brugian filariasis, and chyluria has not been reported. In contrast, scrotal disease is the most frequent manifestation of bancroftian filariasis. In many patients, only one scrotal sac is involved and in these cases, it is very often the left. Elephantiasis in bancroftian disease is not limited to the lower leg or arm and tends to involve the entire limb.

According to most textbook descriptions of lymphatic filariasis, individuals with chronic sequelae of lymphatic filariasis are amicrofilaremic. However, there are numerous observations in geographically diverse areas that document continued parasitemia in patients with elephantiasis. Michael et al. [87] have conducted an elegant meta-analysis of available epidemiological data and found that there is no negative correlation between chronic symptoms and microfilaremia.

Histopathology of Lymphatic Filariasis

The histopathology of lymphatic filarial infection has been examined in several species. The most comprehensive description of human pathology is by Wartman [73], who had access to lymph node biopsies from 57 American GIs who had been exposed to lymphatic filariasis in the Pacific Islands at the end of the Second World War. He found that the pathognomonic lesion of acute lymphatic filarial infection was granulomatous inflammation. Lymph vessels showed endothelial hyperplasia, often of a villus nature. There was also marked hyperplasia of the cells of the reticuloendothelial system, tissue eosinophilia and the formation of numerous nodules, which consisted primarily of macrophages with a moderate number of foreign-body-type giant cells. Most of these nodules occurred around adult parasites, but occasionally, microfilariae were seen at the center. Many showed a central area of necrosis, with a border of macrophages arranged in a palisade. In older lesions, where the worms were dead, macrophages and exudative cells were less obvious, and there was a tendency to fibrosis. Recent descriptions from Brazil are consistent with these classical observations [88]. Animal models of filariasis reveal similar histological features [89, 90].

The development of the nude mouse as a model for brugian filariasis has contributed enormously to our understanding of the role of the adaptive immune system in the development of acute histological changes in response to filarial nematodes. Vincent et al. [85] have compared the lymphatic pathology induced by B. pahangi in nude mice and their euthymic littermates. Their descriptions of histological changes in euthymic mice are similar to those of Wartman in human patients. The lesions consist of acute and chronic granulomatous inflammation in and around degenerating worms and cast cuticles. Epithelioid cell granulomas, with significant central liquefaction necrosis and prominent palisading of epithelioid cells around the area of liquefaction are seen, along with an exuberant inflammatory response, including lymphocytes, eosinophils and fibroblasts. In contrast, the histological changes in the nude mice are relatively acellular and progress slowly. Unlike the euthymic mice, nude mice do not develop typical granulomas consisting of epithelioid giant cells. However, certain reactions are seen, including foreign-body reactions to dead worms, perilymphatic inflammation, including polymorphonuclear leukocytes, fibrosis, lymph thrombi and lymphangiectasis. These must be independent of an antigen-specific immune response. Immunological reconstitution of chronically infected nude mice results in progressive fibrosis, obliteration of lymphatics by the formation of thrombi and extensive perilymphangitis associated with necrosis of adult worms and microfilariae.

Immune Responses to the Filarial Parasites

An important advance in our understanding of the vertebrate immune system is the appreciation of the dichotomy of function among CD4+ helper T lymphocytes [91, 92]. With some reservations, CD4+ T cell helper function can be conveniently divided into a Th1-type activity associated with the production of TNF-α and IFN-γ, and a predilection towards cell-mediated immunity. In contrast, Th2 cells have been associated with the production of IL-4 and IL-5, resulting in tissue eosinophilia and the synthesis of IgG4 and IgE. In almost all experimental models that have been analyzed, filarial nematodes evoke a predominantly Th2-type response. Within this overall framework, however, the human immune response to filarial infection is confounded by numerous factors, including the endemic/nonendemic dichotomy and the clinical presentation.

The total serum antibody levels in most individuals living in an endemic zone are more or less equal. There are, however, noticeable differences in the distribution among the various isotypes. Thus, asymptomatic microfilaremic individuals tend to have high levels of IgG4 antibodies directed against filarial antigens, whereas individuals with chronic pathology predominantly display IgG1, IgG2 and IgG3 responses [93]. IgE antibodies are high in TPE, as well as in patients with chronic pathology. The reasons for these observed differences and the mechanisms underlying them are not clear. IgG4 and IgE antibodies recognize the same set of antigens. In contrast to the latter, however, IgG4 antibodies do not trigger mast cells to release effector molecules responsible for acute anaphylactoid reactions. Hussain and Ottesen [94] have speculated that the IgG4 antibodies in patients with high parasite burdens function as 'blocking' antibodies. Thus, because they recognize the same antigens as IgE antibodies, it is conceivable that they bind and neutralize these molecules and prevent them from reacting with mast-cell-bound IgE antibodies. These patterns of isotype distributions seem to establish themselves early in the disease, as indicated by the studies of Hitch et al. [95] in Haiti. They examined the isotype distribution of antifilarial antibodies, in 129 Haitian children 3 months to 15 years of age and found that amicrofilaremic children had predominantly IgG1, IgG2 and IgG3 antibodies, while their microfilaremic counterparts had IgG4 antibodies.

Cell-mediated immune responses to filarial parasites also show similar differences based on clinical presentation. Lymphocytes from patients who are asymptomatic and microfilaremic tend to manifest diminished proliferative responses to filarial antigens, in contrast to those from patients with chronic pathology. The mechanism of the diminished cell-mediated immune response of microfilaremic patients has been examined at the level of T and B cell precursor frequency. King et al. [96] have shown that patients with asymptomatic microfilaremia have a significantly lower frequency of CD3+ T cells than patients with chronic pathology. Similarly, the proportion of lymphocytes producing parasite-specific IgE or IgG was also significantly lower in microfilaremic patients than in patients with chronic pathology. This diminished responsiveness to filarial antigen appears to correlate with an increase in the Th2 response in microfilaremics, in contrast to patients with chronic pathology. Preincubation of peripheral blood mononuclear cells (PBMC) with neutralizing anti-IL-10 or anti-TGF-β antibodies significantly enhances the lymphocyte proliferation response to filarial antigens in the former group. As noted above for humoral responses, these patterns of cellular immunity also appear to establish themselves early. Hitch et al. [97] found that lymphocytes from microfilaremic Haitian children were less reactive to filarial extracts than those from amicrofilaremic counterparts.

For obvious reasons, the kinetics of the immune response to various stages of filarial parasites are better investigated in experimental models, where the longitudinal evolution of the immune response can be more readily studied in individual animals. Numerous investigators have examined murine immune responses to various stages of filarial parasites, including L3 larvae, microfilariae and adult worms [98–101]. Most studies suggest that L3 larvae, as well as implanted adults, evoke a predominantly Th2 response in mice, as judged by IL-4 and IL-5, but not IFN-γ synthesis by local draining lymph node cells, and by splenic T lymphocytes. Surprisingly, however, implantation of microfilariae directly into BALB/c mice evokes high levels of IFN-γ throughout infection, and very little IL-4 at the early stages [98]. Later in infection (28 days after infection), splenocytes from these microfilaria-infected mice reveal some synthesis of IL-4. Pearlman et al. [102] demonstrated that when mice were repeatedly challenged with soluble microfilarial antigens, they were subsequently able to eliminate live microfilariae with accelerated kinetics. This enhanced elimination of microfilariae by immunized mice correlated with the presence of local CD4+ T lymphocytes which secreted predominantly IL-4 and IL-5, but not IFN-γ in response to filarial antigen. In contrast, systemic T lymphocytes (derived from either spleen or lymph node) produced both Th1- and Th2-type cytokines. These data would appear to indicate that the protective immunity against microfilariae may be associated with a local Th2 response. It should, however, be pointed out that this type of immune response is not critical to generating protective immunity against *infective larvae*. Recently, Lawrence et al. [103] have investigated the course of *B. malayi* infection in IL-4 knockout mice which are unable to mount a Th2 response. These mice resist challenge infection with *B. malayi* larvae.

Unresolved Issues in Filariasis

Many fundamental questions about lymphatic filariasis remain unanswered, mostly because of the chronicity of the infection which hampers detailed longitudinal studies, and the lack of optimal animal models. A number of these issues involve the interactions between the parasite and the host immune system.

Immune Deviation in Microfilaremics

By correlating immunological observations with the clinical spectrum, Ottesen [104] has made a persuasive case that the clinical presentation reflects immunological reactivity. As noted above, it is clear that microfilaremic individuals exhibit altered humoral and cellular immune reactivity to filarial, but not unrelated antigens. The mechanism(s) of the deviant immune reactivity towards adult and microfilarial antigens in asymptomatic microfilaremics has been the subject of considerable speculation. Lammie et al. [105], based on studies in Haiti, have generated exciting data that suggest that children born to microfilaremic mothers have a higher propensity to infection. In contrast, there is no correlation between paternal infection and infection in the child. Based on these observations, Lammie et al. [105] have suggested that the transfer of filarial antigen, antibodies or immune complexes to the developing fetus results in neonatal tolerization and a greater tendency to the development of asymptomatic microfilaremia in such children. This suggestion has found support in the studies of Steel et al. [106] in Polynesia. They examined the cellular responses to filarial antigens in 21 children, 17–19 years old, born of microfilaremic or infection-free mothers. They found that the PBMC of the children of microfilaremic mothers showed statistically significant differences from those of uninfected mothers in proliferation and secretion of IL-4, IL-2, IL-5 and GM-CSF in response to filarial antigens. It is interesting that such differences were observed almost 20 years after prenatal exposure to filarial antigens. It is also important to note that the patients used in this study were not currently microfilaremic; therefore, this reduction in specific response to microfilarial antigen is not due to concurrent infection. The reduction in cellular responses appears to be antigen specific, since these individuals respond normally to irrelevant antigens such as streptolysin O and PPD.

Some experiments on animal models have supported the idea of maternal influences on the susceptibility. Schrater et al. [107] examined the effect of maternal infection on the susceptibility of offspring to patent infection in gerbils. They found that female offspring of gerbils were strongly affected by maternal infectious status. Thus, only 4% of female gerbils born to uninfected mothers became microfilaremic following challenge infection; in contrast, 70% of females became infected following challenge infection if they were born of infected mothers. Surprisingly, maternal infection had no effect on the microfilaremia in male gerbils: male gerbils born of both infected and uninfected mothers became microfilaremic at rates exceeding 90%. These data indicate (1) the importance of maternal infection for parasitemia, and (2) significantly higher male susceptibility to parasitemia, even especially in the absence of infection in the parent.

However, other experimental systems do not corroborate the influence of maternal infection on filarial susceptibility in the offspring. Bosshardt et al. [108] and Klei et al. [109] analyzed the outcome of filarial challenge infection in jirds born of microfilaremic or control mothers. They failed to detect an effect of maternal infection on adult worm burdens, though there was a reduction in the severity of histopathological lesions in the offspring of infected mothers. Similarly, Rajan et al. [110] examined the outcome of filarial infection in scid/+ and +/scid heterozygous mice born of microfilaremic or amicrofilaremic homozygous scid mothers. The presence of chronic infection in the mother had no effect on the outcome of filarial challenge in the offspring.

Natural History of Filarial Infection

One of the most puzzling aspects of filariasis is the natural history of the disease in endemic individuals. Is asymptomatic microfilaremia a precursor to acute disease and adenolymphangitis? What determines progression to chronic disease? Since the proportion of asymptomatics is much larger than that of individuals with chronic pathology, what parasitological or host factors predispose to the latter? Since acute exacerbations are not universal in bancroftian filariasis, are there host- or parasite-specific determinants that provoke these severe, debilitating episodes? We do not know the answers to these questions with any certainty, mostly because of the lack of long-term longitudinal studies.

In contrast to the lack of a clear definition of the progression of filarial infection in endemic individuals, we have a better understanding of the natural history in nonendemics. In these instances, the course shows two different outcomes.

As mentioned earlier, several thousand American GIs were stationed in the South Pacific islands towards the end of the Second World War, in an area where filarial transmission was occurring at a significant level [73] . According to some reports, as many as one third of these individuals exhibited acute symptoms of filarial infestation, including funiculitis and scrotal swelling and pain. Many of these individuals were evacuated and brought back to the United States following these episodes. The incidence of filarial fever decreased with time, and no more than 20 of these individuals ever exhibited microfilaremia [111]. Some have been followed for several years and have not exhibited overt elephantiasis of the limbs or scrotum [112]. Thus, it would appear that if the exposure to lymphatic filarial parasites occurs once or a limited number of times in an individual who was not born in an endemic area, the course of infection is acute, with an active inflammatory response, clearance of the parasite and lack of long-term sequelae. The lack of patent infection in these individuals is worthy of note.

A different picture emerges if an individual is brought to an endemic area in postnatal life, but is persistently challenged with infection. In a massive social-engineering effort, a large population in Indonesia was moved from a filariasis-free zone to a filariasis-endemic area [61]. As with the American GIs, many of these individuals responded with acute symptoms of filarial infection. Unlike the situation with the American GIs, however, perhaps as a consequence of repeated exposure to infection, these individuals have demonstrated an accelerated sequence of filarial pathology, with chronic symptoms (lymphedema and elephantiasis) emerging at a much earlier age than is seen in the endemic population [61, 70]. Interestingly, however, most of these individuals have not demonstrated patent infections.

Despite some differences in the progression of disease, it would appear that if a previously nonendemic individual were to be exposed to infection, the response is an immunologically aggressive one, with clearance of the parasite (as demonstrated by the absence of microfilaremia). If the exposure is limited, the infection resolves with no lasting sequelae; if the insult is repetitive, obliterative disease with lymphedema ensues at an accelerated pace.

Concomitant Immunity in Lymphatic Filariasis

The epidemiological studies of Day et al. [57] on the course of filarial infection in Papua New Guinea have suggested that filarial infection frequency increases in the early part of an individual's life and subsequently plateaus with no increase in microfilarial density or antigen concentration in serum through the later years of life. Three influential reviews have suggested that these data are indicative of the development of 'concomitant immunity' as the individual ages [64, 113, 114]. Initially invoked in the field of tumor immunology, the concept of concomitant immunity gained currency in parasitology in the study of schistosomiasis. In this disease, it was observed that after the establishment of a primary infection, subsequent challenge with schistosomulae does not result in an increase in the worm burden. These observations were taken to mean that the presence of the adult worms in the host was 'concomitant' with efficient immune elimination of a different stage of the parasite, namely the schistosomulae. More recent studies have, however, cast doubt upon an immunological explanation for this complex phenomenon. Due to the formation of granulomas and the subsequent development of fibrosis in the liver, portal venous pressure increases, followed by the establishment of portacaval shunts. Challenge schistosomulae, instead of reaching the portal sinusoids, are diverted into the systemic circulation [115–118]. In this nonphysiological site, these organisms are apparently incapable of developing further and perish due to physiological and nutritional reasons.

The role of concomitant immunity in filariasis needs to be examined carefully as well. A fact that needs to be reconciled with this hypothesis is that the life span of adult filariae is about 8 years. This means that the cohort of adult worms that is responsible for microfilaremia in a 20-year-old individual cannot be the same as that which generates microfilaremia in a 50-year-old. The near constant levels of PC-Ag through these three decades of life suggests that the live worm burden remains stable, implying that there is replenishment of adult worms as the individual ages from his/her twenties to the fifties. These data appear to be inconsistent with the hypothesis of concomitant immunity, which would posit that L3 larvae are aborted before maturing into adults. In this scenario, microfilaremia levels would decrease progressively with age and vanish with a mean of 8 years after the establishment of such immunity. These data are, on the other hand, consistent with the hypothesis that in any given individual, the worm burden reaches a certain level beyond which the endogenous population of adults regulates further worm burdens. The death of resident adult worms would permit the replenishment by a fresh cohort, resulting in a steady-state level of worm burden that does not change with the age of the individual. It is well known that nematodes influence their environment by the production of pheromones [119]. Thus, extracts of heavy cultures of *Caenorhabditis elegans*, when added to synchronized, fresh cultures, induce the development of dauer larvae, a resting, dispersal form of this soil-living nematode. Admittedly, the hypothesis of a pheromone-mediated regulation of adult worm numbers is as lacking of factual support as the hypothesis of concomitant immunity.

Host-Protective Immunity in Filarial Infection

Implicit, and sometimes explicit, in much of the recent immunological work in lymphatic filariasis is the premise of adaptive protective immunity in lymphatic filariasis and the possibility of generating recombinant DNA-based subunit vaccines for this disease. In the aforementioned reviews on lymphatic filariasis [64, 113, 114], the issue of concomitant immunity is discussed in a hopeful light, with the implication that the occurrence of concomitant immunity against superinfection implies that it should be possible to generate protective immunity against incoming larvae even in the absence of preacquired worm burden. One observation supporting the feasibility of sterile immunity is the existence of endemic normal individuals. However, as discussed earlier, the very concept of the endemic normal has been challenged [63, 64]. Particularly persuasive are the data from Day [64] that suggest that in an area with high levels of transmission, almost no individual fulfills all the criteria for endemic normalcy. Furthermore, there is little evidence to suggest that if an individual is cured of filarial infection, there is protection against further challenge infection. Overall, data supportive of host-protective, sterilizing immunity are not convincing.

Nonetheless, however, efforts towards the development of prophylactic immunization are important and should persist. Workers seeking to develop such vaccines must also bear in mind the logistics of administering such a vaccine to poor, indigent and largely rural individuals. Furthermore, any vaccine that is generated must be such that its efficacy is boosted by natural infection from mosquitoes, since repeated administration of vaccines, however efficacious, is unrealistic. Finally, in view of the fact that at least the chronic obstructive pathology of lymphatic filariasis is mediated by host immune reaction, the possibility of causing harm by eliciting premature protective immunity must be kept in mind.

The Lethal Hit

The observations of Vincent et al. [120] and Suswillo et al. [121] on nude mice and Nelson et al. [86] on scid mice conclusively demonstrate that antigen-specific (adaptive) immunity plays a critical role in host defense against *B. malayi*. In all these cases, immunodeficient mice were shown to be permissive for *B. malayi* while normal, immunocompetent mice were non-permissive. However, these workers have been unable to decipher the precise mechanism by which lymphocytes mediate antifilarial resistance. The parasite does not express MHC class I antigens, and thus cannot be a target for cytotoxic T lymphocytes. On the other hand, CD4+ helper T cells do not possess a mechanism to lyse or otherwise inactivate pathogens directly. Furthermore, the cuticle is impermeable to antibodies or complement components. This makes it unlikely that antibodies play a major role in host protection.

Thus, while the role of the adaptive (antigen-specific) immune system in antifilarial defense appears to be well documented, the precise component of this system that is the critical effector is unknown. Given the structure of the nematode cuticle, it would appear reasonable to suspect that an effector molecule must be small enough to diffuse through the interstices between the cross-linked collagens of the cuticle and inflict damage on critical cellular functions. Recent literature has highlighted the role of several small reactive molecules generated by mammalian cells in antimicrobial defense [122, 123]. The identification of the molecule(s) that mediate antifilarial defense would be enormously helpful in developing a rational drug design.

Conclusions

Recent advances in immunology, molecular biology and imaging technology have contributed to a deeper understanding of the organisms and immunopathogenesis of lymphatic filariasis. The most significant ideas that have emerged in the recent past have been an appreciation of the mammalian immune response to various stages of the parasite, the realization that clinical presentations form a spectrum that may reflect the immunological status of the host, that early asymptomatic disease is associated with subtle changes in the lymphatics and, somewhat more controversially, that secondary bacterial infection may play a role in the progression of pathological changes. Though much has been learned, there are several unanswered questions about host-parasite interactions in lymphatic filariasis. The International Task Force for Disease Eradication [124] has recently declared lymphatic filariasis to be one of six 'potentially eradicable' diseases. This hopeful pronouncement conflicts with data that suggest that the incidence is rising. The main focus of research should be to understand the host-parasite interactions in greater detail and to amplify available epidemiological data. This knowledge, combined with more complete utilization of the latest diagnostic strategies, mass treatment and vector control strategies, may help realize WHO's goal of controlling this ancient scourge.

Acknowledgements

This work has been supported by grants AI 27773 and AI 30046 from the USPHS. A.V.G. is the recipient of a Graduate Programs Committee Fellowship from the University of Connecticut Health Center.We wish to thank Dr. Art Hand (UCHC) and Ms. Suzie Taylor (Jackson Laboratory, Bar Harbor, Me. USA) for assistance with the electron microscopy; Dr. Eva Peralta for the filarial life cycle figure and the list of vaccine candidates, and Dr. S. Subash Babu for critical reading of the manuscript.

References

1 Anonymous: Lymphatic filariasis – tropical medicine's origin will not go away (editorial). Lancet 1987;1:1409–1410.
2 Lewis TR: On a hematozoan inhabiting human blood, its relation to chyluria and other diseases. Government of India, 1872.
3 Manson P: *Filaria sanguinis hominis*. China Imperial Maritime Customs, 1877.
4 Anonymous: Lymphatic filariasis infection and disease: Control strategies. WHO/CTD/TDR Consultative meeting, Penang. Penang, Malaysia, WHO, 1994, pp i–vi.
5 Routh HB: Elephantiasis. Int J Dermatol 1992;31:845–852.
6 Routh HB, Bhowmik KR: History of elephantiasis. Int J Dermatol 1993;32:913–916.
7 Demarquay J-N: Helminthologie. Gaz Méd Paris 1863;18:665–667.
8 Wucherer OEH: Noticia preliminar sobre vermes de uma especie ainda nao descripta, encontrados na urina de donentes de hematuria intertropical no Brazil. Gaz Med Bahia 1868;3:97–99.
9 Manson P: On filarial periodicity. Br Med J 1899;2:644–646.
10 Manson P: Further observations on *Filaria sanguinis hominis*. China Imperial Maritime Customs, 1877.
11 Bancroft J: Discovery of the adult representative of microscopic filariae. Lancet 1877;ii:70–71.
12 Bourne AG: A note on *Filaria sanguinis hominis* (with a description of a male specimen). Br Med J 1888;1:1050–1051.
13 Turner L: Studies on filariasis in Malaya: The clinical features of filariasis due to *Wuchereria malayi*. Trans R Soc Trop Med Hyg 1959;53:154–169.
14 Buckley JJC: On *Brugia* gen nov for *Wuchereria* spp of the 'malayi' group. Ann Trop Med Parasitol 1960;54:75–77.
15 Palmieri JR, Purnomo, Dennis DT, Marwoto HA: Filarid parasites of South Kalimantan (Borneo) Indonesia. *Wuchereria kalimantani* sp n (Nematoda: Filarioidea) from the silvered leaf monkey, *Presbytis cristatus* Eschscholtz 1921. J Parasitol 1980;66:645–651.
16 Cross JH, Partono F, Hsu MY, Ash LR, Oemijati S: Experimental transmission of *Wuchereria bancrofti* to monkeys. Am J Trop Med Hyg 1979;28:56–66.
17 Hawking F: The 24-hour periodicity of microfilariae: Biological mechanisms responsible for its production and control. Proc R Soc Lond B Biol Sci 1967;169:59–76.
18 Low GC: A recent observation on *Filaria nocturna* in *Culex*: Probable mode of infection of man. Br Med J 1900;i:1456–1457.
19 Jachowski LA, Otto GF, Wharton JD: Filariasis in American Samoa. I. Loss of microfilaria in the absence of reinfection. Proc Helminthol Soc Wash 1951;18:25–28.
20 Bancroft J: New cases of filariasis disease. Lancet 1879;i:698.
21 Leeuwin RS: Microfilaria in Surinamese living in Amsterdam. Trop Geogr Med 1962;14:355–360.
22 Wang EJ, Saz HJ: Comparative biochemical studies of *Litomosoides carinii, Dipetalonema viteae*, and *Brugia pahangi* adults. J Parasitol 1974;60:316–321.
23 Rew R, Saz H: The carbohydrate metabolism of *Brugia pahangi* microfilariae. J Parasitol 1977;63:123–129.

24 Selkirk ME, Blaxter ML: Cuticular proteins of Brugia filarial parasites. Acta Trop 1990;47:373–380.

25 Selkirk ME, Nielsen L, Kelly C, Partono F, Sayers G, Maizels RM: Identification, synthesis and immunogenicity of cuticular collagens from the filarial nematodes *Brugia malayi* and *Brugia pahangi*. Mol Biochem Parasitol 1989;32:229–246.

26 Maizels RM, Gregory WF, Kwan-Lim GE, Selkirk ME: Filarial surface antigens: The major 29 kilodalton glycoprotein and a novel 17–200 kilodalton complex from adult *Brugia malayi* parasites. Mol Biochem Parasitol 1989;32:213–227.

27 Cookson E, Blaxter ML, Selkirk ME: Identification of the major soluble cuticular glycoprotein of lymphatic filarial nematode parasites (gp29) as a secretory homolog of glutathione peroxidase. Proc Natl Acad Sci USA 1992;89:5837–5841.

28 Sim BK, Shah J, Wirth DF, Piessens WF: Characterization of the filarial genome. Ciba Found Symp 1987;127:107–124.

29 McReynolds LA, DeSimone SM, Williams SA: Cloning and comparison of repeated DNA sequences from the human filarial parasite *Brugia malayi* and the animal parasite *Brugia pahangi*. Proc Natl Acad Sci USA 1986;83:797–801.

30 Nanduri J, Kazura JW: Paramyosin-enhanced clearance of *Brugia malayi* microfilaremia in mice. J Immunol 1989;143:3359–3363.

31 Li BW, Chandrashekar R, Alvarez RM, Liftis F, Weil GJ: Identification of paramyosin as a potential protective antigen against *Brugia malayi* infection in jirds. Mol Biochem Parasitol 1991;49:315–323.

32 Fuhrman JA, Lane WS, Smith RF, Piessens WF, Perler FB: Transmission-blocking antibodies recognize microfilarial chitinase in brugian lymphatic filariasis. Proc Natl Acad Sci USA 1992;89:1548–1552.

33 Freedman DO, Nutman TB, Ottesen EA: Protective immunity in bancroftian filariasis. Selective recognition of a 43-kD larval stage antigen by infection-free individuals in an endemic area. J Clin Invest 1989;83:14–22.

34 Raghavan N, Freedman DO, Fitzgerald PC, Unnasch TR, Ottesen EA, Nutman TB: Cloning and characterization of a potentially protective chitinase-like recombinant antigen from *Wuchereria bancrofti*. Infect Immun 1994;62:1901–1908.

35 Blaxter M: The Filarial Genome Network. Parasitol Today 1995;11:441–442.

36 Adams MD, Kerlavage AR, Kelley JM, Gocayne, JD, Fields C, Fraser CM,Venter JC: A model for high-throughput automated DNA sequencing and analysis core facilities. Nature 1994;368:474–475.

37 Van Doren K, Hirsh D: mRNAs that mature through trans-splicing in *Caenorhabditis elegans* have a trimethylguanosine cap at their 5′ termini. Mol Cell Biol 1990;10:1769–1772.

38 Nilsen TW: Trans-splicing in nematodes. Exp Parasitol 1989;69:413–416.

39 Fraser CM: The minimal gene complement of *Mycoplasma genitalium*. Science 1995;270:397–403.

40 Fleischmann RD: Whole genome random sequencing and assembly of *Haemophilus influenzae* Rd. Science 1995;269:496–503.

41 Dondero T, Bhattacharya N, Black H, Chowdrey, AB, Gubler DJ, Inui TS, Mukherjee M: Clinical manifestations of bancroftian filariasis in a suburb of Calcutta, India. Am J Trop Med Hyg 1976;25:64–73.

42 Raccurt CP, Lowrie RC Jr, Katz SP, Duverseau YT: Epidemiology of *Wuchereria bancrofti* in Leogane, Haiti. Trans R Soc Trop Med Hyg 1988;82:721–725.

43 Dennis D, Partono F, Purnomo, Atmosoedjono S, Saroso J: Timor filariasis: Epidemiologic and clinical features in a defined community. Am J Trop Med Hyg 1976;25:797–802.

44 Partono F, Pribadi PW, Soewarta A: Epidemiological and clinical features of *Brugia timori* in a newly established village. Karakuak, West Flores, Indonesia. Am J Trop Med Hyg 1978;27:910–915.

45 Bundy DA, Grenfell BT, Rajagopalan PK: Immunoepidemiology of lymphatic filariasis: The relationship between infection and disease (review). Immunol Today 1991;12:A71–A75.

46 Brabin L: Sex differentials in susceptibility to lymphatic filariasis and implications for maternal child immunity. Epidemiol Infect 1990;105:335–353.

47 Pani SP, Balakrishnan N, Srividya A, Bundy DA, Grenfell BT: Clinical epidemiology of bancroftian filariasis: Effect of age and gender. Trans R Soc Trop Med Hyg 1991;85:260–264.

48 Nelson GS, Heisch RB, Furlong M: Studies in filariasis in East Africa. II. Filarial infections in man, animals and mosquitoes on the Kenya coast. Trans R Soc Trop Med Hyg 1962;56:207–212.

49 Rosen L: Observations on the epidemiology of human filariasis in French Oceania. Am J Hyg 1955; 61:219–248.

50 Jachowski LA, Otto GF: Filariasis in American Samoa. IV. Studies on the factors influencing the epidemiology of infection. Res Rep Naval Med Res Inst 1953;11:869–940.

51 Brabin L: Factors affecting the differential susceptibility of males and females to onchocerciasis. Acta Leiden 1990;59:413–426.

52 Murray WD: Filariasis studies in American Samoa. US Naval Med Bull 1948;48:327–341.

53 Ash L: Preferential susceptibility of male jirds *(Meriones unguiculatus)* to infection with *Brugia pahangi*. J Parasitol 1971;57:777–780.

54 Nakanishi H, Horii Y, Terashima K, Fujita K: Age-related changes of the susceptibility to infection with *Brugia pahangi* in male and female BALB/c mice. J Parasitol 1990;76:283–285.

55 Rajan TV, Nelson FK, Shultz LD, Beamer WG, Yates J, Greiner DL: Influence of gonadal steroids on susceptibility to *Brugia malayi* in scid mice. Acta Trop 1994;56:307–314.

56 Rao UR, Vickery AC, Kwa BH, Nayar JK, Subrahmanyam D: Effect of carrageenan on the resistance of congenitally athymic nude and normal BALB/c mice to infective larvae of *Brugia malayi*. Parasitol Res 1992;78:235–240.

57 Day KP, Grenfell B, Spark R, Kazura JW, Alpers MP: Age-specific patterns of change in the dynamics of *Wuchereria bancrofti* infection in Papua New Guinea. Am J Trop Med Hyg 1991;44:518–527.

58 Vanamail P, Subramanian S, Das PK, Pani SP, Rajagopalan PK, Bundy DA, Grenfell BT: Estimation of age-specific rates of acquisition and loss of *Wuchereria bancrofti* infection. Trans R Soc Trop Med Hyg 1989;83:689–693.

59 Nutman TB: Experimental infection of humans with filariae. Rev Infect Dis 1991;13:1018–1022.

60 Dondero THJ, Mullin SW, Balasinam S: Early clinical manifestations in filariasis due to *Brugia malayi*: Observations on experimental infections in man. Southeast Asian J Trop Med Public Health 1972;3:569–575.

61 Partono F, Purnomo: Clinical features of Timorian filariasis among immigrants to an endemic area in West Flores, Indonesia. Southeast Asian J Trop Med Public Health 1978;9:338–343.

62 Gubler D, Bhattacharya N: A quantitative approach to the study of bancroftian filariasis. Am J Trop Med Hyg 1974;23:1027–1036.

63 Freedman DO, Unnasch TR, Merriweather A, Awadzi K: Truly infection-free persons are rare in areas hyperendemic for African onchocerciasis (letter). J Infect Dis 1994;170:1054–1055.

64 Day K: The endemic normal in lymphatic filariasis: A static concept. Parasitol Today 1991;7:341–343.

65 Kwan LG, Forsyth KP, Maizels RM: Filarial-specific IgG4 response correlates with active *Wuchereria bancrofti* infection. J Immunol 1990;145:4298–4305.

66 Freedman DO, Bui T, De Almeida Filho PJ, Braga C, Maia e Silva MC, Maciel A, Furtado AF: Lymphoscintigraphic assessment of the effect of diethylcarbamazine treatment on lymphatic damage in human bancroftian filariasis. Am J Trop Med Hyg 1995;52:258–261.

67 Freedman DO, de Almeido Filho PJ, Besh S, Maia e Silva MC, Braga C, Maciel A, Furtado AF: Abnormal lymphatic function in presymptomatic bancroftian filariasis. J Infect Dis 1995;171(4): 997–1001.

68 Witte MH, Jamal S, Williams WH, Witte CL, Kumaraswami V, McNeill GC, Can TC, Panicher TM: Lymphatic abnormalities in human filariasis as depicted by lymphangioscintigraphy. Arch Intern Med 1993;153:737–744.

69 Amaral F, Dreyer G, Figueredo-Silva J, Nores J, Cavalcanti A, Samico SC, Santos A, Coutinho A: Live adult worms detected by ultrasonography in human bancroftian filariasis. Am J Trop Med Hyg 1994;50(6):753–757.

70 Partono F: The spectrum of disease in lymphatic filariasis. Ciba Found Symp 1987;127:15–31.

71 Huntington RWJ, Fogel RH, Eichold A, Dickson JG: Filariasis among American troops in a South Pacific island group. Yale J Biol Med 1944;16:529–537.

Lymphatic Filariasis

72 Fogel RH, Huntington RWJ: Genital manifestations of early filariasis. US Navy Med Bull 1944;43: 263–270.

73 Wartman WB: Filariasis in American armed forces in World War II. Medicine 1947;26:333–394.

74 Wilcocks C, Manson-Bahr PEC: Filariasis. Manson's Tropical Diseases, ed 17. London, Bailliere Tindall, 1972.

75 Olzewski WL, Jamal S, Dworozynski A, Swoboda E, Pani SP, Manokaran G, Kumarasurami V, Bryla P: Bacteriological studies of skin, tissue fluid and lymph in filarial lymphedema. Lymphology 1994;27(suppl):345–348.

76 Addiss DG, Eberhard ML, Lammie PJ: 'Filarial' adenolymphangitis without filarial infection (letter). Lancet 1994;343:597.

77 Kar SK, Mania J, Kar PK: Humoral immune response during filarial fever in bancroftian filariasis. Trans R Soc Trop Med Hyg 1993;87:230–233.

78 Denham DA, Fletcher C: The cat infected with *Brugia pahangi* as a model of human filariasis. Ciba Found Symp 1987;127:225–235.

79 Freedman D, Horn T, Silva CE, Braga C, Maciel A: Predominant CD8+ infiltrate in limb biopsies of individuals with filarial lymphedema and elephantiasis. Am J Trop Med Hyg 1995;53:633–638.

80 Weingarten RJ: Tropical eosinophilia. Lancet 1943;i:103–105.

81 Frimodt-Moller C, Barton RM: A pseudo-tuberculous condition associated with eosinophilia. Indian Med Gaz 1940;75:607–613.

82 Danaraj TJ, Schacher JF: Eosinophilic lung (tropical eosinophilia) and its relation to filariasis. Proceedings of the Ninth Pacific Science Congress, 1957, pp 377–385.

83 Danaraj TJ: The treatment of eosinophilic lung (tropical eosinophilia) with diethylcarbamazine. Q J Med 1958;27:243–263.

84 Ottesen EA, Nutman TB: Tropical pulmonary eosinophilia. Annu Rev Med 1992;43:417–424.

85 Vincent A, Vickery A, Lotz M, Desai U: The lymphatic pathology of *Brugia pahangi* in nude (athymic) and thymic mice C3H/HeN. J Parasitol 1984;70:48–56.

86 Nelson FK, Greiner DL, Shultz LD, Rajan TV: The immunodeficient scid mouse as a model for human lymphatic filariasis. J Exp Med 1991;173:659–663.

87 Michael E, Grenfell BT, Bundy DA: The association between microfilaraemia and disease in lymphatic filariasis. Proc R Soc Lond B Biol Sci 1994;256:33–40.

88 Jungmann P, Figueredo-Silva J, Dreyer G: Bancroftian lymphangitis in northeastern Brazil: A histopathological study of 17 cases. J Trop Med Hyg 1992;95:114–118.

89 Schacher J, Sahyoun P: A chronological study of the histopathology of filarial disease in cats and dogs caused by *Brugia pahangi* (Buckley and Edeson, 1956). Trans R Soc Trop Med Hyg 1967;61: 234–243.

90 Hines SA, Crandall RB, Crandall CA, Thompson JP: Lymphatic filariasis. *Brugia malayi* infection in the ferret *(Mustela putorius furo)*. Am J Pathol 1989;134:1373–1376.

91 Mosmann TR: T lymphocyte subsets, cytokines, and effector functions. Ann N Y Acad Sci 1992; 664:89–92.

92 Finkelman FD, Holmes J, Katona IM, Urban JF, Beckman MP, Parte LS, Schooby KA, Coffman RL, Mosmann TR, Paul WE: Lymphokine control of in vivo immunoglobulin isotype selection. Annu Rev Immunol 1990;8:303–333.

93 Maizels RM, Selkirk ME, Sutanto I, Partono F: Antibody responses to human lymphatic filarial parasites. Ciba Found Symp 1987;127:189–202.

94 Hussain R, Ottesen EA: IgE responses in human filariasis. IV. Parallel antigen recognition by IgE and IgG4 subclass antibodies. J Immunol 1986;136:1859–1863.

95 Hitch WL, Hightower AW, Eberhard ML, Lammie PJ: Analysis of isotype-specific antifilarial antibody levels in a Haitian pediatric population. Am J Trop Med Hyg 1991;44:161–167.

96 King CL, Kumaraswami V, Poindexter RW, Kumari S, Jayaraman K, Alling DW, Ottesen EA, Nutman TB: Immunologic tolerance in lymphatic filariasis. Diminished parasite-specific T and B lymphocyte precursor frequency in the microfilaremic state. J Clin Invest 1992;89:1403–1410.

97 Hitch WL, Lammie PJ, Walker EM, Hightower AW, Eberhard ML: Antifilarial cellular responses detected in a Haitian pediatric population by use of a microblastogenesis assay. J Infect Dis 1991; 164:811–813.

Rajan/Gundlapalli

98 Pearlman E, Hazlett FJ, Boom WH, Kazura JW: Induction of murine T-helper-cell responses to the filarial nematode *Brugia malayi*. Infect Immun 1993;61:1105–1112.

99 Lawrence RA, Allen JE, Osborne J, Maizels RM: Adult and microfilarial stages of the filarial parasite *Brugia malayi* stimulate contrasting cytokine and Ig isotype responses in BALB/c mice. J Immunol 1994;153:1216–1224.

100 Bancroft A, Devaney E: The analysis of the humoral response of the BALB/c mouse immunized with radiation attenuated third stage larvae of *Brugia pahangi*. Parasite Immunol 1993;15:153–1462.

101 Bancroft AJ, Grencis RK, Else KJ, Devaney E: Cytokine production in BALB/c mice immunized with radiation attenuated third stage larvae of the filarial nematode, *Brugia pahangi*. J Immunol 1993;150(4):1395–1402.

102 Pearlman E, Kroeze WK, Hazlett FEJ, Chen SS, Mawhorter SD, Boom WH, Kazura JW: *Brugia malayi*: Acquired resistance to microfilariae in BALB/c mice correlates with local Th2 responses. Exp Parasitol 1993;76:200–208.

103 Lawrence RA, Allen JE, Gregory WF, Kopf M, Maizels RM: Infection of IL-4-deficient mice with the parasitic nematode *Brugia malayi* demonstrates that host resistance is not dependent on a T helper 2-dominated immune response. J Immunol 1995;154:5995–6001.

104 Ottesen EA: The Wellcome Trust Lecture. Infection and disease in lymphatic filariasis: An immunological perspective. Parasitology 1992:S71–79.

105 Lammie PJ, Hitch WL, Walker AE, Hightower W, Eberhard ML: Maternal filarial infection as risk factor for infection in children. Lancet 1991;337:1005–1006.

106 Steel C, Guinea A, McCarthy JS, Ottesen EA: Long-term effect of prenatal exposure to maternal microfilaraemia on immune responsiveness to filarial parasite antigens. Lancet 1994;343:890–893.

107 Schrater AF, Spielman A, Piessens WF: Predisposition to *Brugia malayi* microfilaremia in progeny of infected gerbils. Am J Trop Med Hyg 1983;32:1306–1308.

108 Bosshardt SC, McVay CS, Coleman SU, Klei TR: *Brugia pahangi*: Effects of maternal filariasis on the responses of their progeny to homologous infection. Exp Parasitol 1992;74:271–282.

109 Klei TR, Blanchard DP, Coleman SU: Development of *Brugia pahangi* infections and lymphatic lesions in male offspring of female jirds with homologous infections. Trans R Soc Trop Med Hyg 1986;80:214–216.

110 Rajan TV, Bailis JM, Yates JA, Shultz LD, Greiner DL, Nelson FK: Maternal influence on susceptibility of offspring to *Brugia malayi* infection in a murine model of filariasis. Acta Trop 1994;58:283–289.

111 Beaver P: Filariasis without microfilaremia. Am J Trop Med Hyg 1970;19:181–189.

112 Trent S: Reevaluation of World War II veterans with filariasis acquired in the South Pacific. Am J Trop Med Hyg 1963;12:877–887.

113 Maizels RM, Lawrence RA: Immunological tolerance: The key feature in human filariasis? Parasitol Today 1991;7:271–276.

114 Grenfell BT, Michael E, Denham DA: A model for the dynamics of human lymphatic filariasis. Parasitol Today 1991;7:318–323.

115 Mitchell GF: Portal system peculiarities may contribute to resistance against schistosomes in 129/J mice. Parasite Immunology 1989;11:713–717.

116 Mitchell GF: A note on concomitant immunity in host-parasite relationships: A successfully transplanted concept from tumor immunology. Adv Cancer Res 1990;54:319–332.

117 Dean DA, Bukowski MA, Cheever AW: Relationship between acquired resistance, portal hypertension, and lung granulomas in ten strains of mice infected with *Schistosoma mansoni*. Am J Trop Med Hyg 1981;30(4):806–814.

118 Harrison RA, Bickle Q, Doenhoff MJ: Factors affecting the acquisition of resistance against *Schistosoma mansoni* in the mouse. Evidence that the mechanisms which mediate resistance during early patent infections may lack immunological specificity. Parasitology 1982;84:93–110.

119 Thomas JH: Chemosensory regulation of development in *C. elegans*. Bioessays 1993;15:791–797.

120 Vincent AL, Sodeman WA, Winters A: Development of *Brugia pahangi* in nude (athymic) and thymic mice, C3H/HeN. J Parasitol 1980;66:448.

121 Suswillo RR, Owen DG, Denham DA: Infections of *Brugia pahangi* in conventional and nude (athymic) mice. Acta Trop 1980;37:327–335.

122 Hibbs JJ: Synthesis of nitric oxide from *L*-arginine: A recently discovered pathway induced by cytokines with antitumour and antimicrobial activity. Res Immunol 1991;142:565–599.
123 Nathan CF, Hibbs JJ: Role of nitric oxide synthesis in macrophage antimicrobial activity. Curr Opin Immunol 1991;3:65–70.
124 CDC: Morbidity and Mortality Weekly Report 1993;42(No RR-16):1–38.
125 Chenthamarakshan V, Reddy M: Immunoprophylactic potential of a 120 kDa *Brugia malayi* adult antigen fraction, BmA-2, in lymphatic filariasis. Parasite Immunol 1995;17:277–285.
126 Kazura JW, Maroney PA, Pearlman E, Nilsen TW: Protective efficacy of a cloned *Brugia malayi* antigen in a mouse model of microfilaremia. J Immunol 1990;145:2260–2264.
127 Kazura JW, Cicirello H, McCall JW: Induction of protection against *Brugia malayi* infection in jirds by microfilarial antigens. J Immunol 1986;136:1422–1426.

T.V. Rajan, Department of Pathology, University of Connecticut Health Center,
Farmington, CT 06030-3105 (USA)

Freedman DO (ed): Immunopathogenetic Aspects of Disease Induced by Helminth Parasites.
Chem Immunol. Basel, Karger, 1997, vol 66, pp 159–176

....

Immunologic Basis of Disease and Disease Regulation in Schistosomiasis

Allen W. Cheever[a,b]*, George S. Yap*[b]

[a] Biomedical Research Institute, Rockville, Md., and
[b] Immunobiology Section, Laboratory of Parasitic Diseases, National Institute of
Allergy and Infectious Diseases, National Institutes of Health, Bethesda, Md., USA

Schistosomes infect some 200 million people, mainly in South America, Africa and Asia. *Schistosoma mansoni* and *Schistosoma japonicum* live in venules of the intestine and affect mainly the liver and gut, while *Schistosoma haematobium* lives mainly in venules of the urinary tract and damages mainly the bladder and ureters.

Schistosome larvae are shed into fresh water from infected snails and enter humans by penetrating the skin. Over the next month or two, they migrate through the vasculature of the lungs and to the portal veins of the liver, where male and female worms mature, mate and then migrate as generally monogamous pairs to intestinal *(S. mansoni* and *S. japonicum)* and/or urogenital *(S. haematobium)* venules, where they begin to lay eggs. The adult worms cause no direct local reaction, although the large quantities of antigens shed from the worms may cause systemic reactions. Most tissue pathology is related to the host's immune reaction to the eggs. Up to half the eggs pass through the venules into the feces or urine. If they reach fresh water, the embryos hatch and infect new snails. The remainder of the eggs lodge in the tissues in which they are laid or, in the case of those laid by worms in the mesenteric venules, are carried to the liver. They provoke the formation of granulomas in either site.

Most chronically infected individuals have few or no symptoms, but perhaps 5–10% develop serious disease. Acute and chronic schistosomiasis are distinct in the disease they produce, as well as in the populations that they affect. Acute disease occurs in immunologically naive hosts and chronic disease mainly in individuals residing in endemic areas.

Acute Toxemic Schistosomiasis

Acute schistosomiasis develops almost exclusively in previously uninfected individuals and is caused by hyperreactivity to schistosome worm and egg antigens. Acute schistosomiasis is virtually unknown in individuals born in endemic areas and is a disease of tourists, peace corps workers, vacationing relatives from neighboring cities and invading armies. Fever, loss of appetite, abdominal pain and weakness are frequent symptoms, and diarrhea and marked eosinophilia are common signs. Lightly infected individuals may become ill [1], but symptoms are related to the intensity of infection, and both of these are related to the levels of circulating immune complexes [2]. Symptoms are usually intensified at the time the worms begin to lay eggs. The granulomas around schistosome eggs are large and exudative in the acute stage. Proliferation of peripheral blood mononuclear cells (PMBC) to schistosome antigens is vigorous [3–5]. Disease symptoms, granuloma size, immune complexes and proliferation of PMBC are downregulated (modulated) in the next 1–3 months [1].

Experimental schistosome infections in mice, monkeys and other hosts produce acute disease manifested by ruffled fur, diarrhea, eosinophilia and large granulomas. The acute manifestations ameliorate, as in humans, but no rigorous comparison with human infections has been made. Downregulation of cell-mediated hypersensitivity and granuloma size have been extensively studied, as noted below.

Pathology of Chronic Human and Experimental Schistosomiasis

Granulomas around schistosome eggs are the basic unit and most studied feature of the immunopathology of schistosomiasis. Nearly half the cells in granulomas are eosinophils, the remainder being mostly macrophages and lymphocytes. *S. japonicum* granulomas frequently show numerous polymorphonuclear neutrophils as well. Fibrosis is the principal cause of serious disease. Hepatic fibrosis is the most common cause of death in *S. mansoni* and *S. japonicum* infections [6, 7]. Hepatic fibrosis is characteristic in appearance and forms a dense cuff visible to the naked eye around portal vein branches. A proportion of patients with obstructed portal veins shunt numerous eggs from the mesenteric circulation to the lungs and develop granulomatous arteritis which obstructs the pulmonary circulation, causing pulmonary hypertension and hypertrophy of the right heart [6, 7]. Most intestinal symptoms are not associated with fibrosis and are probably caused by the inflammatory reaction to the eggs and by lesions resulting from the passage of eggs through the mucosa into the gut lumen. Glomerulonephritis and the nephrotic syndrome also develop in some patients with portal fibrosis and are probably mediated by immune complexes [8]. The nephrotic syndrome is not seen, however, in the acute stage. Experimentally infected animals may develop glomerulonephritis, but without the nephrotic syndrome [9].

S. haematobium infections often result in mass lesions of the bladder and ureters which may block urine flow and cause damage to the kidneys. Cellular inflammatory lesions regress with time or antischistosomal treatment, but fibrotic obstruction is more persistent [10].

Circumoval granulomas in experimental infections are similar to those in infected persons, although nearly all experimental infections are massive compared to infections in humans [11].

Immunopathogenesis of Circumoval Granulomas

Synchronous granulomas can be produced in naive or infected animals by intravenously injecting schistosome eggs harvested from other infected animals and examining granulomas around eggs lodged in the pulmonary arterioles. Most studies have used this 'pulmonary model' [12] in mice and have employed S. mansoni eggs. The results are not always equivalent to those in infected mice, probably because eggs recovered from the tissues are not as antigenically potent as those laid by the worms [13]. The 'lung model' nonetheless appears to generally reflect the process of granuloma formation in infected animals, and it is amenable to manipulation and sequential analysis of the events governing granuloma formation and immune regulation. Most studies have used granuloma size as the principal indicator of both hypersensitivity and modulation.

Warren et al. [14] demonstrated clearly that S. mansoni egg granulomas were cell-mediated and that immune serum was not important for the formation or modulation of the lesions. Buchanan et al. [15] subsequently demonstrated the importance of T cells. Reactions to S. haematobium eggs have been little studied, but are similar to those for S. mansoni eggs [16].

Role of Cytokines in Granuloma Formation Schistosoma mansoni

CD4+ T helper (Th) lymphocytes have been divided into Th1 and Th2 subsets on the basis of the cytokines secreted by Th clones. Th1 cells secrete primarily IFN-γ and IL-2, while Th2 cells secrete IL-4, which is associated with IgE production, IL-5, which stimulates the production of eosinophils, and IL-10 [17].

Th-mediated reactions can be polarized into Th1-like and Th2-like types, because IFN-γ secreted by Th1 cells inhibits the development of Th2 cells, and IL-10 secreted by Th2 cells inhibits the development of Th1 cells. The direction of the polarization is thus greatly influenced by the initial cytokine response [18]. A predominantly Th2 response is seen in draining lymph nodes 7–10 days after the injection of eggs into the footpad of mice [19], and in *S. mansoni*-infected mice, cytokine mRNA in the liver evolves from a Th0 to a Th2 pattern at 5–6 weeks [20–22], the time at which egg laying begins.

Th2 cytokines are of paramount importance for the development of large granulomas in infected mice and in the lung model using *S. mansoni* eggs [20–22]. In the lung model, mice treated with anti-IL-4 antibodies developed minute granulomas around injected eggs [21–23]. Anti-IL-2 antibodies were equally effective [21, 23], and this treatment was also associated with an inhibition of the Th2 response [21, 23]. Treatment with anti-IFN-γ antibodies enhanced both granuloma size and Th2 responses, measured by cytokine secretion or mRNA for IL-4 and IL-5 [23–25]. However, Th0, Th1 and Th2 clones or cell lines all augmented pulmonary granuloma formation in naive recipient mice [26, 27; Jankovic, D., unpubl. observations]. Treatment of *S. mansoni*-infected mice with antibodies to intercellular adhesion molecule-1, lymphocyte-function-associated antigen-1 or very late antigen-4 inhibited lymphocyte proliferation to soluble egg antigens (SEA) and the production of IL-2 and IL-4 [28], and also diminished the size of granulomas around injected eggs [29].

Anti-IL-5 treatment of *S. mansoni*-infected mice inhibited tissue eosinophilia, but had minimal effect on granuloma size [30]. No effect on hepatic fibrosis was seen. Anti-IL-4 treatment had a moderate to minimal effect on the size of granulomas around *S. mansoni* eggs in infected animals, but treated mice had much lower levels of hepatic fibrosis [23, 31]. Surprisingly, *S. mansoni*-infected IL-4 knockout mice had granulomas and hepatic fibrosis equivalent to wild-type mice, although pulmonary granulomas around injected eggs were smaller [32]. It is possible that compensatory mechanisms exist for IL-4 functions in these knockout mice which would not be present in antibody treated animals.

Anti-IL-2 treatment also had a much more marked effect on hepatic fibrosis than on granuloma size and, as in the lung model, anti-IL-2 diminished Th2 responses [33]. Targeted destruction of cells bearing the high-affinity IL-2 receptor caused dramatic reduction in both granuloma size and hepatic fibrosis in *S. mansoni*-infected mice [34]. Anti-IFN-γ treatment had no significant effect in *S. mansoni*-infected mice [30]. The size of granulomas at 8 weeks of infection was unaffected in mice genetically deficient in IFN-γ [Yap, G. et al., unpubl. observations].

Cytokine treatment of infected mice generally had the effects expected from the anti-cytokine treatments noted above. IFN-γ treatment decreased granuloma size and inhibited hepatic fibrosis [35]. IL-2 and IL-4 administration increased the size of granulomas in mice and reversed the downregulation of granuloma size in chronically infected mice [36, 37]. IL-12 dramatically downregulated the size of granulomas around injected eggs, largely through stimulation of IFN-γ production from natural killer cells [24].

Immunodeficient (nude and scid) mice have minimal reactions to *S. mansoni* eggs. However, scid mice given tumor necrosis factor-α (TNF-α) by Amiri et al. [38] formed granulomas nearly as large as those in intact mice. We have been unable to influence granuloma formation with recombinant TNF-α in CB17 scid mice infected with *S. mansoni* or *S. japonicum* [Cheever, A. et al., unpubl. observations]. Joseph and Boros [39] noted downregulation of granuloma volume in mice treated with anti-TNF-α and upregulation of granuloma size in *S. mansoni*-infected mice treated with TNF-α. One probable mechanism of action of TNF on granuloma formation is the upregulation of intercellular adhesion molecule-1 [28] which is important for cell-cell interactions and for the migration of cells across the endothelium.

Mice repeatedly injected intraperitoneally with large numbers of *S. mansoni* eggs had a diminished response to eggs injected i.v. [40]. Wynn et al. [24] confirmed this finding and, in addition, pushed the reaction toward a Th1 response by immunizing mice with eggs plus IL-12. These mice showed diminished Th2 and augmented Th1 reactions, as assayed by analysis of cytokine mRNA in the tissues and by secretion of cytokines by spleen cells stimulated with *S. mansoni* antigens in vitro, and the reaction to i.v. *S. mansoni* eggs was dramatically reduced. Hepatic granuloma size was significantly reduced in mice repeatedly immunized with *S. mansoni* eggs together with IL-12 and subsequently infected. Hepatic fibrosis was diminished markedly in these mice, which showed augmented Th1 and diminished Th2-like responses [41].

Chemotactic factors derived from the eggs may play a direct role in the recruitment of cells, in addition to the effects of cytokines elicited from host cells [42].

Role of Cytokines in Granuloma Formation Schistosoma japonicum

S. japonicum-egg-induced granulomas are also T cell mediated, [43] and Th2-like cytokine patterns predominate, as in *S. mansoni* infection [44].

Granulomas in anti-IFN-γ and anti-IL-5 treated *S. japonicum*-infected mice were reduced in size, in contrast to the effects of these antibodies in *S. mansoni* infection. However, as in *S. mansoni* infection, there was no effect on fibrosis [45, 46]. A trivial explanation for the difference in the effects of these antibodies on granuloma size may be the substantially greater amount of collagenous matrix associated with *S. mansoni* granulomas, preserving granuloma size with reduced cellularity, while the more cellular *S. japonicum*-induced granulomas may more readily shrink with loss of cells. We have not determined the density of cells in the granulomas to examine this hypothesis. Anti-IL-2 treatment of *S. japonicum*-infected mice, as in *S. mansoni* infection, reduced granuloma size but had a more marked effect on fibrosis, and Th2 responses were reduced [46].

In summary, Th2-type responses seem the predominant driving force in the formation of *S. mansoni*- and *S. japonicum*-egg-induced granulomas, which may be viewed as a type of Th2-delayed hypersensitivity. IFN-γ generally diminishes both granuloma size and hepatic fibrosis.

The cytokine patterns in infected humans are less clear. Zwingenberger et al. [47] found serum IL-4 levels elevated and IFN-γ levels decreased in schistosome-infected patients, and IL-4 levels after in vitro polyclonal stimulation of PMBC correlated with the intensity of schistosome infection, and they correlated negatively with IFN-γ production. Williams et al. [48] also found a trend toward Th2 responses in infected patients. More detailed studies of infected patients are needed, particularly of antigen-specific responses.

Immune Downregulation (Modulation) of the Granulomatous Response during Chronic Schistosoma mansoni Infection

In schistosome-infected mice, the size of newly formed hepatic granulomas peaks at 8 weeks after infection and subsequently diminishes as the infection proceeds into the chronic phase (Fig. 1) [40]. This immune downregulation is accompanied by decreased cutaneous reactions to injected SEA and smaller granulomatous responses to pulmonary challenge with eggs. Furthermore, splenic and lymph node T cells derived from chronically infected mice exhibit decreased proliferative responses and lymphokine production in response to SEA [49–52].

Immune Modulation Results from an Active Suppressor-Cell Mediated Process

The loss or diminution of CD4+ T cell responsiveness to antigens can be explained by mechanisms involving clonal deletion, clonal inactivation/anergy, effector deviation or active suppression or combinations thereof. Two observations are consistent with the idea of active suppression of Th cell responses to SEA. First, adoptive transfer of modulation has been demonstrated [53]. Diminution of hepatic granulomatous responses, assayed at 8 weeks after infection, was observed upon transfer of spleen cells from chronically infected (16–24 week) mice into mice infected for 6 weeks. Adoptive suppression required transfer of histocompatible CD8+ cells [54, 55]. Second, adult thymectomy of infected mice results in almost complete abrogation of downregulation of granuloma size at 15 weeks and a loss in the ability of spleen cells to transfer suppression [56]. This observation suggests that maintenance of the suppressor cell population requires recent thymic emigrants, and that this population is characterized by high cellular turnover, which is consistent with their cyclophosphamide sensitivity [56].

Experimental work has provided evidence for the involvement of T suppressor cell circuits and idiotypic interactions in downregulating CD4+ Th reactivity to SEA. Modulation has been shown to involve Ia+ T suppressor inducers (Ts1)

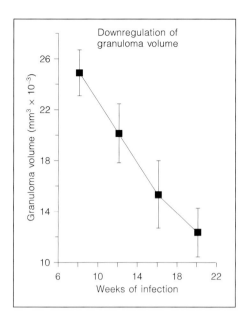

Fig. 1. C3H/HeN female mice were exposed to about 25 *S. mansoni* cercariae. Eggs are first laid at 5 weeks, and the maximal granulomatous response is seen at 8 weeks. Only the granulomas around live eggs containing a mature embryo were measured, i.e. those eggs laid 1–4 weeks before the mice were killed.

and I-J-restricted CD8+ suppressor effectors (Ts2) [50, 54; the genetic, molecular and biochemical identity of I-J remains mysterious; see ref. 57 and 58 for discussion]. Soluble T suppressor inducer factor (TsF1; derived from Ts1 cells) and soluble effector TsF2 (from Ts2 cells) have been described as being comprised of SEA-binding α-chains and I-J-determinant-bearing α-chains resembling T cell receptor (TCR) heterodimers [59]. An anti-idiotypic (anti-anti-SEA immunoglobulin) I-J restricted TsF2 has also been described [60]. CD8+ Ts2-derived TsF2 presumably acts directly, while CD4+ Ts2-derived TsF2 results in the release of TsF3 which acts nonspecifically to mediate suppression.

Putative Mechanisms of Immune Modulation: Utility of the T1/T2 Paradigm

Bloom et al. [57, 58] have recently integrated novel concepts generated by the T1/T2 paradigm to provide molecular mechanisms for the phenomenon of T cell suppression. They postulate that antigen-specific CD4+ cells (Ts1) shed their TCR (TsF1), against which an anti-idiotypic response is generated by CD4+ or CD8+ cells (Ts2). The TsF2 may be a shed anti-idiotypic receptor that may require clustering or multivalency on an antigen-presenting cell to clonally aner-gize a target T cell. TsF3 may be a lymphokine which suppresses the proliferation or cytokine production of the relevant CD4+ T helper cells. Indeed, production of IL-4 by CD8+ (type 2) cells was shown to mediate suppression of CD4+ (type 1) cells in a mycobacterial antigen-specific system [61].

Since the CD4+ cell lymphokine profile of acutely infected mice is character-ized by a predominance of IL-4, IL-5 and IL-10, it could be envisaged that the production of IFN-γ by CD8+ suppressor cells could suppress the proliferation of the Th2-type cells [62]. Indeed, analysis of the cytokine profile of several non-schistosome-antigen-related CD8+ murine Ts clones demonstrates that they secrete high levels of IFN-γ and IL-10, but not IL-2 or IL-4 [63, 64]. Suppression of Th1 and Th2 CD4+ clones by Ts clones was successfully neutralized by anti-IL-10 and anti-IFN-γ antibodies, respectively. Thus, production of this unique combination of lymphokines by Ts cells may account for the diminution of both Th1- and Th2-associated responses during chronic infection. The lack of IL-2 or IL-4 secretion by Ts cells may also help explain their apparent inability to self-renew in the periphery.

Several pieces of circumstantial evidence argue for the predominance of IFN-γ responses and their potential role in immune modulation during chronic infection. IFN-γ synthesis/secretion by explanted granulomas remains low and stable, while levels of IL-2 and IL-4 decrease precipitously during modulation [65]. Furthermore, polyclonally activated CD8+ populations from chronically infected mice show enhanced IFN-γ secretion [66]. Addition of anti-IFN-γ to an in vitro granuloma system increased the size of granulomas formed [67]. How-ever, recent experiments from this laboratory [Yap, G. et al., unpubl. results] demonstrated that mice genetically deficient in IFN-γ are nonetheless able to downregulate hepatic granuloma size.

An alternate model for cytokine-mediated modulation has been proposed by Stadecker [68]. It has been hypothesized that IL-10 induces a state of anergy by inhibiting the expression of costimulatory molecules on antigen presenting mac-rophages. IL-10 was shown to be responsible for the decreased expression of costi-mulatory B7 molecules by granuloma-derived macrophages and thereby decrease activation of an SEA-specific Th1 clone [69, 70]. It is not known whether IL-10-mediated anergy extends to Th2 clones as well. This question is of paramount importance since the predominant CD4+ lymphokine response to SEA is Th2-like, and it too becomes downregulated. In several systems, anergy has been most readily demonstrated in Th1 but not Th2-like responses [71–73]. Analysis of chronic infections in IL-10-deficient mice may help provide definitive evidence for the involvement or lack of this important counterregulatory cytokine in down-regulation. This may, however, be complicated by the autoimmune sequelae which beleaguer these mice.

Clearly, the molecules mediating modulation of CD4+-dependent granulomatous responses may involve one or more of many known or as yet unknown downregulatory cytokines. Identifying and understanding how these immunoregulatory factors operate to achieve a homeostatic balance between tissue protection and immunopathology remains an important challenge.

Properties of CD4+ T Helper Cells in the Chronic, Modulated Infection

From the discussion above, it is clear that the detailed mechanism for downregulation has not been elucidated. Because the population of SEA-reactive CD4+ Th cells is the primary effector for the granulomatous response and therefore the final target of any immunomodulatory mechanism, it is perhaps useful and informative to consider the state of SEA-reactive CD4+ T cells, as can be gathered from the in vivo and in vitro analyses. At various stages in the chronic phase, the size of circumoval granulomas decreases by a factor of 2–4. What accounts for this decrease in granuloma size? Is there a decrease in the frequency or recruitment of SEA-specific memory or effector cells? What happens to the lymphokine-secreting and proliferative potential of the memory/effector cells? While definitive frequency analysis of SEA-specific CD4+ precursors has not been carried out, it appears that there is a net decrease in the CD4+ helper activity in the chronic state [74]. It has been suggested that the CD4+ helper memory/effector cell pool is 'eroded' by the CD8+-regulatory cells. Since direct addition of chronic spleen cells did not decrease lymphokine secretion [74], it is reasonable to posit that regulation occurs at the level of proliferative recruitment/amplification of memory cells. This idea is consistent with a decreased density of lymphokine-positive cells in the lymph nodes and spleens of chronically infected mice [75]. Similarly, anergy-inducing regimens recently described in Th2 clones effect inhibition of proliferative responses, while IL-4 secretion is spared or unaffected [76]. Thus, it can be envisaged that during chronic infection, the generation of effectors in the lymph node and/or liver from memory cells could be decreased. The level of effector cell activity is best thought of as a function of the fractional events of effective versus ineffective memory/effector cell recruitment. This is presumably determined in part by the ratio of CD4+ to CD8+ regulators in the tissue site [77]. Systemic treatment with IL-2 could be thought of as increasing the fraction of effective recruitment events of memory T cells, thereby reversing diminished granulomatous responses in chronically infected mice [78].

Immune Downregulation of the Granulomatous Response during Chronic
Schistosoma japonicum *Infection*

S. japonicum-infected mice, in contrast to those infected with *S. mansoni*, showed only transient cell-mediated modulation, while regulatory cross-reactive idiotypes (CRI) were of major importance [79, 80]. Serum IgG1 from mice chronically infected with *S. japonicum* markedly decreased hepatic fibrosis in acutely infected mice, while transferred splenocytes were ineffective [81]. Regulatory CRI have also been described in humans infected with *S. japonicum* [82].

Clinical Disease Correlates with the Failure to Develop Downregulatory Mechanisms

The development of immune responses to egg antigens in humans infected with schistosomes resembles that in experimentally infected animals. Cross-sectional studies using antigen-induced in vitro proliferative responses as an index indicate that a great majority of acutely infected patients exhibit vigorous proliferative responses to SEA [83]. Asymptomatic chronically infected patients were predominantly low to moderate responders, while the proportion of high responders was greatly increased amongst ambulatory patients with hepatic and hepatosplenic disease [83]. Thus, it was hypothesized that during the course of infection immune responses to SEA are downregulated. Failure to modulate immune responsiveness correlated with the development of clinical disease and may be causally related to it. It is noteworthy that immuneresponsiveness is regained following curative chemotherapy [4]. Presumably, the removal of the inciting egg antigens led to termination of the relatively short-lived immunoregulatory constraints.

The elements of the immunoregulatory constraint operative on human immune responsiveness have been studied in some detail, at least in vitro. An idiotypically connected immunoregulatory circuit involving CRI expressed on anti-SEA antibodies and a series of anti-idiotypic T cells has been described [84]. The presence of autologous anti-idiotypic T cells reactive to anti-SEA antibodies from intestinal patients has been reported. Furthermore, similarly prepared anti-SEA antibodies from either acute or hepatosplenic patients did not induce an anti-idiotypic response [85]. Both CD4+ and CD8+ T cells are induced by the CRI in an MHC-unrestricted, antigen-presentation-independent manner [86]. CD8+ anti-idiotypic T cells can directly inhibit in vitro granuloma formation by CD4+ T helper clones, while CD4+ anti-idiotypic cells required CD8+ cells for suppressive activity. Thus, during the chronic phase of infection, regulatory CRI are represented in the anti-SEA IgG repertoire. How and why a subset of chronically infected patients fails to express this CRI is unknown. The relative influence of genetic and other host factors such as fetal exposure to antigens or idiotypes [87] and infection intensity on the development of immunoregulatory mechanisms remains unassessed.

The description of an apparently analogous situation in an animal model provides an opportunity to dissect these factors. Henderson et al. [88] have documented two distinct pathological syndromes in chronically infected male CBA/J mice. A majority of animals developed what was termed moderate splenomegaly syndrome (MSS), while 15–20% developed a hypersplenomegaly syndrome (HSS). HSS mice developed massive splenomegaly, ascites, thymic atrophy, cachexia and anemia. They exhibited extensive hepatic fibrosis morphologically analogous to that in humans with hepatosplenic disease. Importantly, the regulatory CRI defined in human populations was not well represented in the anti-SEA antibodies from HSS mice, while it was well represented in antibodies from acutely infected mice and in MSS mice. Thus, it was suggested that the MSS and HSS mice may represent models for asymptomatic and hepatosplenic patients, respectively [88].

The fact that an apparently homogeneous population of inbred mice with virtually equivalent infection intensities can exhibit distinct pathology and immunoregulation suggests that as yet unidentified factors or events act in a stochastic manner to influence the course of disease. Longitudinal studies of serologic markers in this population of mice may provide some clues to this enigma.

Fibrotic Reactions Induced by Schistosome Eggs

Fibrosis rather than granulomatous inflammation underlies most of the chronic pathology associated with schistosome infections. Fibrotic reactions in the liver are those most studied. In mice, most hepatic fibrosis is associated with the granulomas themselves [81, 89, 90]. In humans, the relation of hepatic fibrosis to granulomas is less clear, and most fibrosis surrounds portal veins. Hepatic portal fibrosis similar to that in humans (Symmers' fibrosis) has been described in infected chimpanzees [91], rabbits [92] and, on occasion, mice [88]. In both rabbits and chimpanzees, at least, the initial portal fibrosis is spatially independent of the granulomas themselves, although in the late stages eggs and granulomas crowd the fibrotic portal areas, perhaps directed there by vascular changes associated with the fibrosis and occlusion of distal portal venules.

Types I and III are the predominant collagen isotypes synthesized in both human and murine infections [81, 90, 93–96], and the in vitro synthetic rates and pathways are similar in the liver tissue from *S. mansoni*-infected mice and patients [89, 97]. The kinetics of collagen synthesis and degradation in *S. japonicum* and *S. mansoni* infection has been described [89, 90, 95]. Collagen biosynthesis and degradation are at their maximum a few weeks after the acute phase, when granulomatous responses are most florid. Biosynthetic and degradation rates are reduced during the chronic phase. A switch from a predominant type I to type III collagen profile has been reported to occur during the chronic phase [90, 95]. The spatial and temporal association between T-cell-mediated granulomatous responses and tissue fibrosis suggest parallel but not entirely concordant immunoregulation of both granuloma cell recruitment and fibrogenesis by T cells.

Thus, transfer of serum IgG1 from mice chronically infected with *S. japonicum* decreased both granuloma size and hepatic granuloma collagen biosynthesis and increased the type III:I collagen isotype ratio [81]. However, numerous observations have demonstrated differential regulatory effects on fibrosis and granuloma size. For instance, passive transfer of cells from mice infected for 10 weeks with *S. japonicum* decreased granuloma size, but increased collagen biosynthesis [81]. Hepatic hydroxyproline per egg decreases with increasing intensity in *S. mansoni* infections, while granuloma size changes little with infection intensity [98].

The fibrogenic process is regulated by a complex process involving T cell and macrophage interactions with cells of mesenchymal/fibroblastic lineage. T-cell-derived lymphokines regulate the fibrogenic process. Anti-IL-4 treatment [31, 99] and treatment with recombinant IFN-γ decreased fibrosis [35]. The profibrotic and antifibrotic effects of IL-4 and IFN-γ may at least in part be mediated by direct effects on the proliferation and collagen biosynthesis of fibroblasts [100].

A novel cytokine, fibrosin, associated with fibrosis in murine granulomas, has recently been cloned [101]. Fibrosin stimulates fibroblast proliferation as well as collagen and fibronectin production [102]. It has stimulatory effects on Ito cells, which are important in hepatic fibrogenesis [103]. TGF-1β synthesis was markedly increased in the livers of *S. mansoni*-infected mice [104], and TGF-β1 gene expression correlated with hepatic fibrosis [105]. Downregulation of fibrosin and TGF-β1 was associated with immune downregulation [41, 106].

When schistosome infections in mice are cured by chemotherapy in the acute stage, 8–10 weeks after infection, much of the fibrosis is rapidly reversible, and in the initial stages of collagen degradation, the extracellular collagen fragmented and was phagocytosed, as in other models of acute collagen degradation. Several months after the chemotherapy of these infections, the pattern of collagen breakdown changed. Collagen fragments were no longer found internalized by cells, lytic areas appeared, and fine granular or fibrillar material was found within collagen bundles [96]. Similar changes were noted in the livers of humans with schistosomal portal fibrosis [107]. Clinically, chronic hepatic fibrosis in *S. mansoni*-infected humans is often slowly reversible after treatment, and this process has been conveniently followed in the field by ultrasonography which demonstrated partial or complete resolution of portal fibrosis [108].

Conclusions

Most disease caused by schistosome infections is related to the host's immunological response to eggs laid in the veins of the host, rather than by the parasite itself. Detailed analyses of cellular and cytokine regulation of the granulomatous response to eggs indicate that it is a reaction predominantly mediated by CD4+

Th2 cells. The cellular and molecular linkages between granulomatous response and fibrosis are less well defined. Further studies to characterize direct and indirect effects of egg-reactive T cells on fibroblasts and their precursors should improve our understanding of these complex interactions.

A balance between tissue-protective and immunopathologic immune responses is manifested by active immunoregulatory mechanisms. The level of effective CD4+ Th cell activity is dynamically regulated by relatively short-lived regulatory suppressive mechanisms. Although a detailed picture of these various idiotype/anti-idiotype interactions involving antibodies and T cells is not as yet forthcoming, it is perhaps useful to consider the utility of the T1/T2 paradigm to explain the suppressor-effector functions of these immunoregulatory circuits.

Immunological studies of patient populations with different disease states have suggested a relationship between failure to downregulate anti-egg immune responses and severe hepatosplenic disease. These patients lack regulatory CRI on their anti-SEA immunoglobulin populations which are stimulatory to regulatory T cells. Further longitudinal and genetic characterization of this subpopulation may yield important information. Similarly, detailed longitudinal studies in the recently described murine model for hepatosplenic disease may allow for experimental approaches to questions which cannot be posed in studies of humans.

In addition to the intrinsic importance for the understanding of disease in patients, the immunopathology of schistosomiasis is important for the understanding of granulomatous inflammation and of Th2-mediated immunological reactions in general.

Acknowledgments

We are indebted to D. Jankovic and E. Pearce for permission to cite their unpublished data and to A. Sher, D. Jankovic, T. Wynn, F. Lewis and T. Kresina for reading the manuscript.

References

1   Hiatt RA, Sotomayor ZR, Sanchez G, Zambrana M, Knight WB: Factors in the pathogenesis of acute schistosomiasis mansoni. J Infect Dis 1979;139:659–666.
2   Hiatt RA, Ottesen EA, Sotomayor ZR, Lawley TJ: Serial observations of circulating immune complexes in patients with acute schistosomiasis. J Infect Dis 1980;142:665–670.
3   Ottesen EA, Hiatt RA, Cheever AW, Sotomayor ZR, Neva FA: The acquisition and loss of antigen-specific cellular immune responsiveness in human schistosomiasis. Clin Exp Immunol 1978;33: 38–47.
4   Gazzinelli G, Lambertucci JR, Katz N, Rocha RS, Marcôndes SL, Colley DG: Immune responses during human schistosomiasis mansoni. XI. Immunologic status of patients with acute infections and after treatment. J Immunol 1985;135:2121–2127.

5   Montesano MA, Lima RS, Correa-Oliviera R, Gazzinelli G, Colley DG: Immune responses during human *Schistosoma mansoni*. XVI. Idiotypic differences in antibody preparations from patients with different clinical forms of infection. J Immunol 1989;142:2501–2506.

6   Chen MG, Mott KE: Progress in assessment of morbidity to *Schistosoma mansoni* infection. A review of recent literature. Trop Dis Bull 1988;85:R1-R56.

7   Chen MG, Mott KE: Progress in assessment of morbidity due to *Schistosoma japonicum* infection. A review of recent literature. Trop Dis Bull 1988;85:R1-R45.

8   Barsoum RS: Schistosomal glomerulopathies. Kidney Int 1993;44:1–12.

9   von Lichtenberg F, Sadun EH, Cheever AW, Erickson DG, Johnson AJ, Boyce HW: Experimental infection with *Schistosoma japonicum* in chimpanzees. Parasitologic, clinical, serologic and pathological observations. Am J Trop Med Hyg 1971;20:850–893.

10   Chen MG, Mott KE: Progress in assessment of morbidity to *Schistosoma haematobium* infection. A review of recent literature. Trop Dis Bull 1989;86:R1-R36.

11   Cheever AW: Quantitative comparison of the intensity of *Schistosoma mansoni* infection in man and experimental animals. Trans R Soc Trop Med Hyg 1969;63:781–795.

12   Lichtenberg FV: Host response to eggs of *S. mansoni*. I. Granuloma formation in the unsensitized laboratory mouse. Am J Pathol 1962;41:711–731.

13   Eltoum IA, Wynn TA, Poindexter RW, Finkelman FD, Lewis FA, Sher A, Cheever AW: Suppressive effect of IL-4 neutralization differs for granulomas around *Schistosoma mansoni* eggs injected into mice compared to eggs laid in infected mice. Infect Immun 1995;69:2532–2536.

14   Warren KS, Domingo EO, Cowan RBT: Granuloma formation around schistosome eggs as a manifestation of delayed hypersensitivity. Am J Pathol 1967;51:735–756.

15   Buchanan RD, Fine DP, Colley DG: *Schistosoma mansoni* infection in mice depleted of thymus-dependent lymphocytes. II. Pathology and altered pathogenesis. Am J Pathol 1973;71:207–218.

16   Kassis AI, Warren KS, Mahmoud AAF: The *Schistosoma haematobium* egg granuloma. Cell Immunol 1978;38:310–318.

17   Mosmann TR, Coffman RL: TH1 and TH2 cells: Different patterns of lymphokine secretion lead to different functional properties. Ann Rev Immunol 1989;7:145–173.

18   Jankovic D, Sher A: Initiation and regulation of CD4+ T cell function in host-parasite models. Chem Immunol 1996;63:51–65.

19   Vella AT, Pearce EJ: CD4+ Th2 response induced by *Schistosoma mansoni* eggs develops rapidly through an early transient Th0-like stage. J Immunol 1992;148:2283–2290.

20   Henderson GS, Lu X, McCurley TL, Colley DG: In vivo molecular analysis of lymphokines involved in the murine immune response during *Schistosoma mansoni* infection. II. Quantification of IL-4 mRNA, IFN-γ mRNA, and IL-2 mRNA levels in the granulomatous livers, mesenteric lymph nodes, and spleens during the course of modulation. J Immunol 1992;148:2261–2269.

21   Wynn TA, Eltoum I, Cheever AW, Lewis FA, Gause WC, Sher A: Analysis of cytokine mRNA expression during primary granuloma formation induced by eggs of *Schistosoma mansoni*. J Immunol 1993;151:1430–1440.

22   Wynn TA, Cheever AW: Cytokine regulation of granuloma formation in schistosomiasis. Curr Opin Immunol 1995;7:505–511.

23   Lukacs NW, Boros DL: Lymphokine regulation of granuloma formation in murine schistosomiasis mansoni. Clin Immunol Immunopathol 1993;68:57–63.

24   Wynn TA, Eltoum I, Oswald IP, Cheever AW, Sher A: Endogenous interleukin 12 (IL-12) regulates granuloma formation induced by eggs of *Schistosoma mansoni* and exogenous IL-12 both inhibits and prophylactically immunizes against egg pathology. J Exp Med 1994;179:1551–1561.

25   Chensue SW, Warmington KS, Ruth J, Lincoln PM, Kunkel SL: Cross-regulatory role of interferon-gamma (IFN-γ), IL-4 and IL-10 in schistosome egg granuloma formation: In vivo regulation of Th activity and inflammation. Clin Exp Immunol 1994;98:395–400.

26   Chikunguwo SM, Kanazawa T, Dayal Y, Stadecker MJ: The cell-mediated response to schistosomal antigens at the clonal level: In vivo function of cloned murine egg antigen-specific CD4+ T helper type 1 lymphocytes. J Immunol 1991;147:3921–3925.

27   Zhu Y, Lukacs NW, Boros DL: Cloning of Th0 and Th2-type helper lymphocytes from liver granulomas of *Schistosoma mansoni*-infected mice. Infect Immun 1994;62:994–999.

28   Langley JG, Boros DL: T-lymphocyte responsiveness in murine schistosomiasis mansoni is dependent upon the adhesion molecules intercellular adhesion molecule-1, lymphocyte function-associated antigen-1 and very late antigen-4. Infect Immun 1995;63:3980–3986.

29   Lukacs NW, Chensue SW, Strieter RM, Warmington K, Kunkel SL: Inflammatory granuloma formation is mediated by TNF-α-inducible intercellular adhesion molecule-1. J Immunol 1994;152: 5883–5889.

30   Sher A, Coffman RL, Hieny S, Scott P, Cheever AW: Interleukin 5 is required for the blood and tissue eosinophilia but not granuloma formation induced by infection with Schistosoma mansoni. Proc Natl Acad Sci USA 1990;87:61–65.

31   Cheever AW, Williams ME, Wynn TA, Finkelman FD, Seder RA, Cox TM, Hieny S, Caspar P, Sher A: Anti-IL-4 treatment of Schistosoma mansoni-infected mice inhibits development of T cells and non-B, non-T cells expressing Th2 cytokines while decreasing egg-induced hepatic fibrosis. J Immunol 1994;153:753–759.

32   Pearce EJ, Cheever A, Leonard S, Covalesky M, Fernandez-Botran R, Kohler G, Kopft M: Schistosomiasis in IL-4 deficient mice. Int Immunol 1996;8:435–444.

33   Cheever AW, Finkelman FD, Caspar P, Heiny S, Macedonia JG, Sher A: Treatment with anti-IL-2 antibodies reduces hepatic pathology and eosinophilia in Schistosoma mansoni-infected mice while selectively inhibiting T cell IL-5 production. J Immunol 1992;148:3244–3248.

34   Ramadan MA, Gabr NS, Bacha P, Gunzler V, Phillips SM: Suppression of immunopathology in schistosomiasis by interleukin-2 targeted fusion toxin, $DAB_{389}IL-2$. Cell Immunol 1995;166:217–226.

35   Czaja MJ, Weiner FR, Takahashi S, Giambrone M-A, van der Meide PH, Schellekens H, Biempica L, Zern MA: γ-interferon treatment inhibits collagen deposition in murine schistosomiasis. Hepatology 1989;10:795–800.

36   Yamashita T, Boros DL: Changing patterns of lymphocyte proliferation. IL-2 production and utilization, and IL-2 receptor expression in mice infected with Schistosoma mansoni. J Immunol 1990; 145:724–731.

37   Yamashita T, Boros DL: IL-4 influences IL-2 production and granulomatous inflammation in murine schistosomiasis mansoni. J Immunol 1992;149:3659–3664.

38   Amiri P, Locksley RM, Parslow TG, Sadick M, Rector E, Ritter D, McKerrow JH: Tumor necrosis factor α restores granulomas and induces parasite egg-laying in schistosome-infected SCID mice. Nature 1992;356:604–607.

39   Joseph AL, Boros DL: Tumor necrosis factor plays a role in Schistosoma mansoni egg-induced granulomatous inflammation. J Immunol 1993;151:5461–5471.

40   Domingo EO, Warren KS: Endogenous desensitization: Changing host granulomatous response to schistosome eggs at different stages of infection with Schistosoma mansoni. Am J Pathol 1968;52: 369–379.

41   Wynn TA, Cheever AW, Jankovic D, Poindexter RW, Caspar P, Lewis FA, Sher A: An Il-12 based vaccination method for preventing fibrosis induced by schistosome infection. Nature 1995:376: 594–596.

42   Owhashi M, Horii Y, Ishii A: Eosinophil chemotactic factor in schistosome eggs: A comparative study of eosinophil chemotactic factors in the eggs of Schistosoma japonicum and S. mansoni in vitro. Am J Trop Med Hyg 1983;32:359–366.

43   Stavitsky AB: Immune regulation in schistosomiasis japonica. Immunol Today 1987;8:228–233.

44   Xu Y, Macedonia J, Sher A, Pearce E, Cheever AW: A dynamic analysis of splenic TH1 and TH2 lymphocyte functions in mice infected with Schistosoma japonicum. Infect Immun 1991;59:2934–2940.

45   Cheever AW, Xu Y, Macedonia JG: Analysis of egg granuloma formation in Schistosoma japonicum-infected mice treated with antibodies to interleukin-5 and gamma interferon. Infect Immun 1991;59:4071–4074.

46   Cheever AW, Xu Y, Sher A, Finkelman FD, Cox TM, Macedonia JG: Schistosoma japonicum-infected mice show reduced hepatic fibrosis and eosinophilia and selective inhibition of IL-5 secretion by CD4+ cells after treatment with anti-Il-2 antibodies. Infect Immun 1993;61:1288–1292.

47 Zwingenberger K, Hohmann A, Cadoso de Brito M, Ritter M: Impaired balance of interleukin-4 and interferon-γ production in infections with *Schistosoma mansoni* and intestinal nematodes. Scand J Immunol 1991:34:243–251.

48 Williams ME, Montenegro S, Domingues AL, Wynn TA, Teixeira K, Mahanty S, Coutinho A, Sher A: Leukocytes of patients with *Schistosoma mansoni* respond with a Th2 pattern of cytokine production to mitogen or egg antigens but with a Th0 pattern to worm antigens. J Infect Dis 1994;170: 946–954.

49 Colley DG: Immune response to a soluble schistosomal egg antigen preparation during chronic primary infection with *Schistosoma mansoni*. J Immunol 1975;115:150–156.

50 Chensue SW, Boros DL, David CS: Regulation of granulomatous inflammation in murine schistosomiasis. II. T suppressor cell-derived IC subregion encoded soluble suppressor factor mediates regulation of lymphokine production. J Exp Med 1983;157:219–230.

51 Grzych J-M, Pearce E, Cheever A, Caulada Z, Caspar P, Heiny S, Lewis F, Sher A: Egg deposition is the major stimulus for the production of TH2 cytokines in murine schistosomiasis mansoni. J Immunol 1991;146:1322–1327.

52 Lukacs N, Boros D: Utilization of fractionated soluble egg antigens reveals selectively modulated granulomatous and lymphokine responses during murine schistosomiasis mansoni. Infect Immun 1992;60:3209–3216.

53 Colley DG: Adoptive suppression of granuloma formation. J Exp Med 1976;143:696–700.

54 Chensue SW, Boros DL: Modulation of granulomatous hypersensitivity. I. Characterization of T lymphocytes involved in the adoptive suppression of granuloma formation in *Schistosoma mansoni*-infected mice. J Immunol 1979;123:1409–1414.

55 Green WF, Colley DG: Modulation of *Schistosoma mansoni* egg-induced granuloma formation: I-J restriction of T cell mediated suppression in a chronic parasitic infection. Proc Natl Acad Sci USA 1981;78:1151–1156.

56 Colley DG: T lymphocytes that contribute to the immunoregulation of granuloma formation in chronic murine schistosomiasis. J Immunol 1981:126:1465–1468.

57 Bloom BR, Modlin RL, Salgame P: Stigma variations: Observations on suppressor T cells and leprosy. Ann Rev Immunol 1992;10:453–488.

58 Bloom BR, Salgame P, Diamond B: Revisiting and revising suppressor T cells. Immunol Today 1992;13:131–136.

59 Perrin PJ, Phillips SM: The molecular basis of receptor mediated regulation of granulomatous hypersensitivity. in Yoshiada T, Torisu M (eds): Basic Mechanisms of Granulomatous Inflammation. London, Elsevier, 1989, pp 185–204.

60 Abe T, Colley DG: Modulation of *Schistosoma mansoni* egg-induced granuloma formation. III. Evidence for an anti-idiotypic, I-J-positive, I-J-restricted, soluble T suppressor factor. J Immunol 1984;132:2084–2088.

61 Salgame P, Abrams JS, Clayberger C, Goldstein H, Convit J, Modlin RI, Bloom BR: Different lymphokine profiles of functional subsets of human CD4+ and CD8+ T cell clones. Science 1991; 254:279–282.

62 Borojevic R: Experimental murine schistosomiasis mansoni: Establishment of the chronic phase of the disease. Mem Inst Oswaldo Cruz 1992;82:171–174.

63 Inoue T, Asano Y, Matsuoka S, Furutani-Seiki M, Aizawa S, Nishmura H, Shirai T, Tada T: Distinction of mouse CD8+ suppressor effector T cell clones from cytotoxic T cell clones by cytokine production and CD45 isoforms. J Immunol 1993;150:2121–2128.

64 Nanda NK, Sercarz E, Hsu D, Kronenberg M: A unique pattern of lymphokine synthesis is a characteristic of certain antigen-specific suppressor T cell clones. Int Immunol 1994;6:731–737.

65 Chensue SW, Terebuh PD, Warmington KS, Hershey SD, Evanoff HL, Kunkel SL, Higashi GI: Role of Il-4 and IFN-γ in *Schistosoma mansoni* egg-induced granuloma formation. Orchestration, relative contribution, and relationship to macrophage function. J Immunol 1992;148:900–906.

66 Vasconcellos JP, Pearce EJ: *Schistosoma mansoni* infection induces a type 1 CD8+ cell response. Mem Inst Oswaldo Cruz, in press.

67 Lammie PJ, Phillips SM, Linette GP, Michael AI, Bentley AG: In vitro granuloma formation using defined antigenic nidi. Ann NY Acad Sci 1986;465:340–350.

68   Stadecker MJ: The role of T-cell anergy in the immunomodulation of schistosomiasis. Parasitol Today 1992;8:199–204.
69   Villanueva FPO, Chikunguwo SM, Harris TS, Stadecker MJ: Macrophages from schistosomal egg granulomas induce unresponsiveness in specific cloned Th1 lymphocytes in vitro and downregulate schistosomal granulomatous disease in vivo. J Immunol 1994;152:1847–1852.
70   Villanueva FPO, Reiser H, Stadecker MJ: Regulation of T helper cell responses in experimental murine schistosomiasis by IL-10. Effect on expression of B7 and B7-2 costimulatory molecules by macrophages. J Immunol 1994;153:5190–5199.
71   Karpus WJ, Peterson JD, Miller SD: Anergy in vivo: Down-regulations of antigen specific CD4+ but not Th2 cytokine responses. Int Immunol 1994;6:721–730.
72   Gajewski TF, Lancki DW, Stack R, Fitch FW: 'Anergy' of Th0 helper T lymphocytes induces down-regulation of Th1 characteristics and a transition to a Th2-like phenotype. J Exp Med 1994;179:481–491.
73   Vidard L, Colarusso LJ, Benacerraf B: Specific T cell tolerance may reflect selective activation of lymphokine synthesis. Proc Natl Acad Sci USA 1995;92:2259–2262.
74   Chensue SW, Warmington KS, Hershey SD, Terebuh PD, Othman M, Kunkel SL: Evolving T cell responses in murine schistosomiasis. Th2 cells mediate secondary granulomatous hypersensitivity and are regulated by CD8+ T cells in vivo. J Immunol 1993;151:1391–1400.
75   Bogen SA, Villanueva POF, McCusker ME, Fogelman I, Garifallou M, El-Attar ER, Kwan P, Stadecker M: In situ analysis of cytokine responses in experimental murine schistosomiasis. Lab Invest 1995;73:252–258.
76   Sloan-Lancaster J, Evavold BD, Allen PM: Th2 cell clonal anergy as a consequence of partial activation. J Exp Med 1994;180:1195–1205.
77   Ragheb S, Boros DL: Characterization of granuloma T lymphocyte function from Schistosoma mansoni-infected mice. J Immunol 1989;142:3239–3246.
78   Mathew RC, Ragheb S, Boros DL: Recombinant IL-2 therapy reverses diminished granulomatous responsiveness in anti-L3T4-treated Schistosoma mansoni-infected mice. J Immunol 1990;144:4356–4361.
79   Olds GR, Stavitsky AB: Mechanisms of in vivo modulation of granulomatous inflammation in murine schistosomiasis japonicum. Infect Immun 1986:52:513–518.
80   Kresina TF, Olds GR: Concomitant cellular and humoral expression of a regulatory cross-reactive idiotype in acute Schistosoma japonicum infection. Infect Immun 1986;53:90–94.
81   Olds GR, Kresina TF: Immunoregulation of hepatic fibrosis in murine schistosomiasis japonica. J Infect Dis 1989;159:798–801.
82   Kresina TF, Cheever LW, Chireau M, Johnson J, Ramirez B, Peters P, Olds GR: Human EBV-transformed lymphocytes of patients with Schistosoma japonicum infection secrete idiotypically related immunoregulatory antibodies. Clin Immunol Immunopathol 1992;65:325–329.
83   Colley DG, Garcia AA, Lambertucci JR, Parra JC, Katz N, Rocha RS, Gazzinelli G: Immune responses during human schistosomiasis. XII. Differential responsiveness in patients with hepatosplenic disease. Am J Trop Med Hyg 1986;35:793–802.
84   Doughty BL, Goes AM, Parra JC, Rocha R, Cone JC, Colley DG, Gazzinelli G: Anti-idiotypic T cells in human schistosomiasis. Immunol Invest 1989;18:373–388.
85   Montesano MA, Freeman GL, Gazzinelli G, Colley DG: Immune responses during human Schistosoma mansoni. XVII. Recognition by monoclonal anti-idiotypic antibodies of several idiotypes on a monoclonal anti-soluble schistosomal egg antigen antibody and anti-soluble schistosomal egg antigen antibodies from patients with different clinical forms of infection. J Immunol 1990;145:3095–3099.
86   Parra JC, Lima MS, Gazzinelli G, Colley DG: Immune responses during human Schistosoma mansoni. XV. Antiidiotypic T cells can recognize and respond to anti-SEA idiotypes directly. J Immunol 1988;140:2401–2405.
87   Eloi-Santos SM, Novato-Silva E, Maselli VM, Gazzinelli G, Colley DG, Correa-Oliveira R: Idiotypic sensitization in utero of children born to mothers with schistosomiasis or Chagas' disease. J Clin Invest 1989;84:1028–1031.

88 Henderson GS, Nix NA, Montesano MA, Gold D, Freeman GL, McCurley TL, Colley DG: Two distinct pathologic syndromes in male CBA/J inbred mice with chronic *Schistosoma mansoni* infections. Am J Pathol 1993;142:703–714.

89 Dunn MA, Rojkind M, Warren KS, Hait PK, Rifas L, Seifter S: Liver collagen synthesis in murine schistosomiasis. J Clin Invest 1977;59:666–674.

90 Olds GR, Griffin A, Kresina TF: Dynamics of collagen accumulation and polymorphism in murine *Schistosoma japonicum*. Gastroenterology 1985;89:617–624.

91 Sadun EH, von Lichtenberg F, Cheever AW, Erickson DG: *Schistosoma mansoni* in the chimpanzee: The natural history of chronic infections following single and multiple exposures. Am J Trop Med Hyg 1970;19:258–277.

92 Cheever AW, Duvall RH, Minker R, Nash TE: Hepatic fibrosis in rabbits infected with Japanese and Philippine strains of *Schistosoma japonicum*. Am J Trop Med Hyg 1980;29:1327–1339.

93 Biempica L, Dunn MA, Kamel IA, Kamel R, Hait PK, Fleischner C, Biempica SL, Wu CH, Rojkind M: Liver collagen-type characterization in human schistosomiasis. A histological, ultrastructural, and immunocytochemical correlation. Am J Trop Med Hyg 1983;32:316–325.

94 Hu CH, Giambrone M-A, Howard DJ, Rojkind M, Wu GY: The nature of the collagen in hepatic fibrosis in advanced murine schistosomiasis. Hepatology 1982;2:366–371.

95 Meneza SE, Olds GR, Kresina TF, Mahmoud AAF: Dynamics of hepatic connective tissue matrix constituents during murine *Schistosoma mansoni* infection. Hepatology 1989;9:50–56.

96 Andrade ZA, Grimaud JA: Morphology of chronic collagen resorption. A study of the late stages of schistosomal granuloma involution. Am J Pathol 1988;132:389–399.

97 Dunn MA, Kamel R, Kamel IA, Biempica L, El Kholy A, Hait PK, Rojkind M, Warren KS, Mahmoud AAF: Liver collagen synthesis in schistosomiasis mansoni. Gastroenterology 1979;76:978–982.

98 Cheever AW: The intensity of experimental schistosome infections modulates hepatic pathology. Am J Trop Med Hyg 1986;35:124–133.

99 Cheever AW, Finkelman FD, Cox TM: Anti-interleukin-4 treatment diminishes secretion of Th2 cytokines and inhibits hepatic fibrosis in murine schistosomiasis japonica. Parasite Immunol 1995;17:103–109.

100 Kovacs EJ: Fibrogenic cytokines: The role of immune mediators in the development of scar tissue. Immunol Today 1991;12:17–23.

101 Prakash S, Robbins PW, Wyler DJ: Cloning and analysis of a murine cDNA that encodes a fibrogenic lymphokine, fibrosis. Proc Natl Acad Sci USA 1995;92:2154–2158.

102 Wyler DJ, Ehrlich HP, Postlethwaite AE, Raghow R, Murphy MM: Fibroblast stimulation in schistosomiasis. VII. Egg granulomas secrete factors that stimulate collagen and fibronectin synthesis. J Immunol 1987;138:1581–1586.

103 Greenwel P, Wyler DJ, Rojkind M, Prakash S: Fibroblast-stimulating factor 1, a novel lymphokine produced in schistosomal egg granulomas, stimulates liver fat-storing cells in vitro. Infect Immun 1993;61:3985–3987.

104 Czaja MJ, Weiner FR, Flanders KC, Giambrone M-A, Wind R, Biempica L, Zern MA: In vitro and in vivo association of transforming growth factor-β1 with hepatic fibrosis. J Cell Biol 1989;108:2477–2482.

105 Kresina TF, Qing HE, Delgi Esposti S, Zern MA: Hepatic fibrosis and gene expression changes induced by praziquantel treatment during immune modulation of *Schistosoma japonicum* infections. Parasitology 1993;107:374–404.

106 Prakash S, Postlethwaite AE, Wyler DJ: Alterations in influence of granuloma derived cytokines on fibrosis in the course of murine *Schistosoma mansoni* infection. Hepatology 1991;13:970–976.

107 Andrade ZA, Peixoto E, Guerret S, Grimaud JA: Hepatic connective tissue changes in hepatosplenic schistosomiasis. Hum Pathol 1992;23:566–573.

108 Homeida MA, Eltom I, Nash T, Bennett JL: Association of the therapeutic activity of praziquantel with the reversal of Symmers' fibrosis induced by *S. mansoni*. Am J Trop Med Hyg 1991;45:360–365.

Allen Cheever, Laboratory of Parasitic Diseases, NIAID, Building 4, Room 126,
Bethesda, MD 20892 (USA)

Freedman DO (ed): Immunopathogenetic Aspects of Disease Induced by Helminth Parasites.
Chem Immunol. Basel, Karger, 1997, vol 66, pp 177–208

....
Immunopathology of Echinococcosis

B. Gottstein, A. Hemphill

Institute of Parasitology, University of Bern, Switzerland

The Parasites

Echinococcus species are cestode parasites commonly known as small tape-worms of domesticated and wild carnivores. Their medical and economic relevance ows to their infection of humans and domesticated animals, where the parasitic larval stage may develop in various organs and thus may cause dramatic damage dependent upon lesion size and localisation within the organs. Two *Echinococcus* species are of medical and public health importance in that they may inflict severe disease in humans: *Echinococcus granulosus* is the causative agent of 'cystic echinococcosis' or 'cystic hydatid disease', whereas infection with *Echinococcus multilocularis* in man leads to 'alveolar echinococcosis' or 'alveolar hydatid disease'. Two other species of the genus *Echinococcus*, namely *Echinococcus vogeli* and *Echinococcus oligarthrus*, are mainly restricted to silvatic animals. Respective infection of humans is extremely rare, thus only little emphasis will be given to these two latter species.

E. granulosus is a small cestode tapeworm of 4–6 mm length when fully mature in the adult stage. The tapeworm lives as intestinal parasite firmly attached to the mucosa of the small intestine of dogs or occasionally other carnivores (life cycle, see fig. 1). The shedding of gravid proglottids (each containing several hundreds of eggs) or eggs passing in the feces of definitive hosts occurs within 4–5 weeks after infection. *E. granulosus* eggs are infective for intermediate hosts immediately after their release. Ingestion of *Echinococcus* eggs by susceptible intermediate animal hosts such as humans results in the release of an oncosphere within the gastrointestinal tract. Within a few minutes, this oncosphere penetrates the intestinal epithelium, and migrates into the lamina propria and the

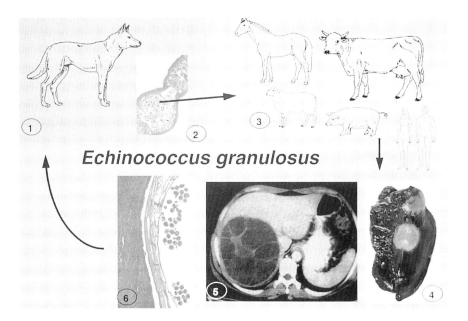

Fig. 1. Life cycle of *E. granulosus.* Adult tapeworms parasitize in the duodenum of carnivorous definitive hosts, mainly dogs *(1).* Parasite proglottids and eggs are shed with the feces *(2),* the latter being infectious for intermediate hosts *(3).* Hydatid cyst formation occurs predominantly in the liver *(4),* but also the lungs and other organs. Imaging techniques such as CT *(5)* demonstrate well delineated, fluid-filled, usually unilocular bladder-like lesions. Larger cysts may exhibit internal daughter cysts visible as septated segments within the primary cysts *(5).* The cyst itself consists of a very thin inner germinal and nucleated layer of predominantly syncytial structure *(6).* The germinal layer is externally protected by an acellular laminated layer of variable thickness. Endogenous formation of brood capsules and protoscoleces is a prerequisite for termination of the life cycle *(6),* which occurs when definitive hosts ingest protoscolex-containing hydatid cysts.

corresponding blood vessels. Subsequently, it is passively transported through blood or lymphatic vessels to primary target organs such as liver and lungs, less frequently to other organs. Here the oncosphere starts differentiation into a vesicle which will slowly expand by concentric enlargement. With time, usually within several months or years, a fully mature metacestode (= hydatid cyst) is formed, constituted by a fluid-filled, usually unilocular bladder. This cyst consists of an inner germinal and nucleated layer of predominantly syncytial structure. The germinal layer projects microtriches outwards into the externally supporting elastic laminated layer of variable thickness. This laminated layer, mainly consisting of carbohydrates, forms an acellular barrier separating the host and the parasite.

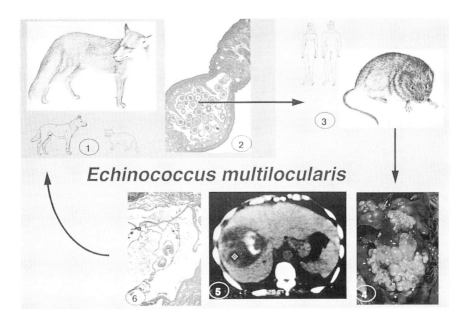

Fig. 2. The life cycle of *E. multilocularis* involves predominantly foxes as definitive hosts *(1)*, rarely other carnivores such as domestic dogs or house cats. Egg production by the tapeworm starts as early as 28 days after infection *(2)*. When ingested by a suitable intermediate host *(3)*, the parasite metacestode will primarily become established in the liver. Macroscopically, the typical lesion is characterised by a dispersed mass of fibrous tissue with a multitude of scattered cavities ranging from a few millimetres to centimetres in size *(4)*. The lesion often contains focal zones of calcification, as demonstrated by CT *(5)*. Histologically, a hepatic lesion consists of a conglomerate of small vesicles and cysts demarcated by a thin laminated layer with or without an inner germinative layer, and, predominantly in the rodent intermediate host, protoscolex formation *(6)*. The peroral uptake of protoscolex-containing metacestodes by definitive hosts terminates the life-cycle.

Surrounded by a host-produced fibrous adventitial layer, the laminated layer, despite its dense amorphous nature, allows the passage of host-derived macromolecules into the hydatid cysts. Particularly in humans, where unusually large cysts may develop, daughter cysts can form within the primary cyst. The endogenous formation of brood capsules and protoscoleces is a prerequisite for termination of the life cycle.

The natural life cycle of *E. multilocularis* involves predominantly red and arctic foxes as definitive hosts (fig. 2). Other carnivores such as the domestic dog or the house cat can occasionally be infected as well. As for *E. granulosus*, the adult-stage tapeworms attach to the mucosa of the small intestine. Egg production starts as early as 28 days after infection [1]. When ingested by a suitable intermediate host (small mammals such as microtine and arvicolid rodents, occasionally muskrats and others; accidentally also humans), digestive processes and other factors in the host gut result in hatching and release of the oncosphere. This becomes subsequently 'activated', most likely by the surface-active properties of bile components. The activated oncosphere penetrates the epithelial border of the intestinal villi, enters venous and lymphatic vessels to finally develop in the liver (very rarely, some may reach lungs or other organs). Maturation to the asexually proliferating metacestode within the liver tissue includes cellular proliferation, vesicularisation and formation of both a germinative and a syncytial tegumental layer, a central fluid-filled cavity, and synthesis of a peripheral laminated layer similar to the *E. granulosus* metacestode described above. In contrast to hydatid cysts, *E. multilocularis* metacestodes do not exhibit constant size growth of a single cyst, but proliferate by exogenous budding of metacestode tissue, thus progressively invading the surrounding tissue. These protrusions of the germinal layer of the metacestode grow into the host tissue, and thus may initiate parasite proliferation and metastasis formation [2]. There is strong evidence that these tissue-invading processes of the germinal layer are accompanied by continuous synthesis of the laminated layer, suggesting that this acellular structure protects the parasite from direct host effector immune mechanisms. Production of protoscoleces may take place within 2–4 months in susceptible hosts, but may also lack depending on the resistance status of the intermediate host species or strains (see below). For completion of the life cycle, definitive hosts must ingest protoscolex-containing metacestode tissue.

Echinococcus granulosus

Pathogenesis and Pathology

Cystic echinococcosis (hydatidosis) of humans refers to the disiease caused by infection with larval *E. granulosus*. Well-delineated spherical primary cysts are formed most frequently in the liver (approximately 65% of the cases), followed by the lungs (25%) and other organs such as kidney, spleen, brain, heart and bone [3]. Pathogenetic tissue damage is caused by replacement of host tissue by growing cysts and in some instances by vascular compromise (fig. 3, 4). Organ dysfunction results mainly from the gradual process of space-occupying repression or displacement of vital host tissue, vessels or organs. Consequently, clinical manifestations are primarily determined by the site, the size and the number of the cysts, and thus are markedly variable. Successful surgical removal of hydatid cysts is fortunately frequent, therefore fatality rates are low (varying between 1 and 4% for cases with first surgical intervention [3]), provided modern medical facilities are

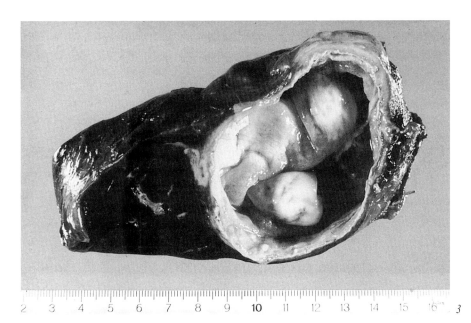

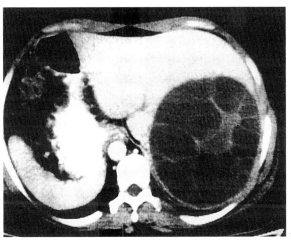

Fig. 3. Macrographic representation of an *E. granulosus* hydatid cyst (cross-section) in the liver of a patient with hepatic hydatid disease. Size bar in centimetres. The fully mature fluid-filled hydatid cyst is externally supported by an elastic laminated layer of variable thickness, and additionally surrounded by a host-produced fibrous adventitial layer, as shown in the picture (by courtesy of Prof. J. Eckert, University of Zürich).

Fig. 4. CT scan of an *E. granulosus* liver cyst segmented by the presence of inner daugthter cysts. Note the absence of peripheral calcifications which may occasionally characterize older cysts.

available. The histology of a typical hydatid cyst demonstrates the germinal layer as primary live parasite; it is surrounded by a parasite-derived thick laminated layer, rich in amino-carbohydrates, as shown by periodic acid-Schiff positivity. The germinal layer forms protoscoleces and brood capsules which are also found free in the cyst fluid (hydatid sand). Granulae, calcareous corpuscules and occasionally free daughter cysts are also often observed. Sometimes, only acid-fast-positive hooklets are demonstrable.

Cyst growth is expansive by a concentric increase in cyst size. The parasite evokes an immune response leading to formation of a host-derived collagenous capsule which often calcifies uniquely in the periphery of the cyst. Cholestasis may be present in the liver. There is often pressure atrophy of the surrounding parenchyma since these cysts can develop pressures of up to 80 cm H_2O. Accidental rupture of cysts can be followed by a massive release of cyst fluid and hematogenous dissemination of protoscolices, occasionally resulting in anaphylactic reactions and in multiple secondary cystic echinococcosis as protoscolices have the potential to develop into secondary cysts within the intermediate host [4, 5].

Immunology and Immunopathology

In any case, the primary site of host-parasite interaction is the mucosa of the host's gastrointestinal tract. Sparse information is available concerning the immune response to migrating and subsequently established oncospheres and their development to the metacestode of *Echinococcus* in humans. Diagnosis of echinococcosis is generally based upon a fully developed and still proliferating metacestode, which has already induced and potentially influenced a host immune response [reviewed in Heath, 6]. Cellular and humoral immune responses in man, in contrast to experimentally infected animals, can vary enormously, as evidenced, e.g., by the different patterns of parasite antigens recognized with respect to different patients and courses of disease [7, 8]. These disparities are likely to be related to human and/or parasite genetic diversity, unlike the uniform genetic background of most experimental animals [9]. Oncospheral antigens from *E. granulosus* can immunize mammals against further egg infection. However, already established cysts persist and seem not to be affected by anti-oncospheral immunity. Although a humoral and cellular anti-metacestode immune response occurs, permissiveness for hydatid growth is a common feature and may result from a capacity of the metacestode to vary, hide or disguise its antigens. Recently, evidence has been obtained that these parasites also alter the behaviour of leucocytes in ways compatible with local suspension of immunity [10].

Humoral Immune Responses/Antibodies. Antibody studies were primarily applied to follow up patients with cystic echinococcosis post-operatively, or to monitor patients after long-term chemotherapy. Up to now, such investigations have hardly been used to investigate potential immunopathological events which could be relevant for different courses of disease. Much emphasis was given to the specific determination of parasite-specific antibody isotypes [11, 12]. However, the low contribution of serology for monitoring the course of disease was accumulatively discussed [13].

Humoral immune parameters were investigated more recently in order to search for markers which could indicate the effectiveness of treatment with special respect to dividing the patients in full, partial, low and non-responders [14]. The authors postulated an adjuvant effect of a certain antibody class and subclass profile in connection with the efficient abortion of the metacestode. ELISA determination of the immunoglobulin production showed that the percentages of parasite-specific IgE antibody responses varied in the four clinical groups according to the success of benzoimidazole carbamate treatment (full responders 25%, partial responders 50%, low responders 65%, non-responders 100%). Conversely, the percentages of total IgG, IgG1 and IgG2 reactions in the four groups did not relate to the response to chemotherapy. Full responders had a higher percentage of IgG3 reactions than the other groups (full responders 75%, partial responders 67%, low responders 54%, non-responders 50%). In contrast to the findings for IgG3, and similarly to those for IgE, non-responders had the highest percentage of IgG4 reactions (full responders 75%, partial responders 67%, low responders 64%, non-responders 100%). Qualitative analysis of total IgG responses determined by immunoblotting showed that non-responders had the highest percentage of reactions to all subunits of antigens 5 and B, and full responders had the highest percentage of reactions to antigen 5 alone. The authors concluded that parasite-specific IgE concentrations combined with the Ig isotype banding pattern to antigens B and 5 could provide a useful marker for therapeutic success in hydatid patients. The demonstration of parasite-specific IgE has attracted particular attention due to its well-known relevance in helminthic diseases [11, 15, 16]. It is conceivable that parasite-specific IgE determination possesses a potential value in assessing risks with regard to anaphylactic reactions upon pre-operative or intra-operative cyst rupture [17]. Basophil-bound IgE could be demonstrated by provoking respective histamine release in vitro [18–20]. Strain variations of the parasite, as well as differences in the host-parasite relationship may significantly affect the serological response. For example, there were reports from Kenya of many cases of hepatic hydatid infection where conventional serological tests had not been able to detect any parasite-specific antibodies in the patient's serum [21, 22]. Patients with cystic echinococcosis (rarely in hepatic, relatively frequent in lung localisation of cysts) were repeatedly reported as seronegative prior to surgical intervention. However, rapid seroconversion could be observed in most of these patients already a few days after treatment. It appears very unlikely that antigen priming occurs at the time of infection. Thus it was postulated that the parasite activates one or several humoral immunosuppression mechanisms which are reverted following surgical removal of the cysts. A more detailed discussion on this topic will be presented below.

Occasionally, autoantibodies to both class I and class II major histocompatibility complex (MHC) gene products were demonstrated in patients with cystic echinococcosis. The particular respective interest views on the crucial role of these cell surface receptors during the induction of immune responses. It is tempting to speculate that these antibodies would subvert the host's immune responses in such a way as to promote the long-term survival of the parasite [23]. Another potential mechanism of *E. granulosus* antigens which may modulate immune response and host-parasite interplay was also discussed by Lightowlers et al. [23]. The parasite had been shown to express a gene encoding a protein which exhibits a high degree of amino acid sequence homology with the human protein cyclophilin [24], now known to be peptidyl prolyl cis-trans-isomerase [25]. The binding of cyclophilin to the fungal metabolite cyclosporin A was shown to have profound suppressive effects upon T cell function [26]. If the parasite contained a natural ligand for cyclophilin which would have some of the immunosuppressive activities of cyclosporin A, a role for such a ligand could exist in suppressing host immune responses and the survival of the parasite [23].

Cell-Mediated Immunity. The first approaches to study cell-mediated immunity in cystic echinococcosis included skin tests and basophil degranulation tests [reviewed by Schantz and Gottstein, 3]. The remarkable newer developments in basic cellular immunology have attracted the attention of parasite immunologists to parasite-specific host cellular immune responses, and implied the huge importance of the complex cytokine interplay at the site of the parasitic lesions, as well as at its periphery [28]. One of the first studies dealing with these topics assessed the in vitro lymphoproliferative response to *E. granulosus* antigen stimulation in 40 patients with cystic echinococcosis [29]. It demonstrated the absence of any correlation between serological and lymphoproliferative results. The diagnostic sensitivity of positive test reactions was 75% for both serology and lymphocyte proliferation. The fact that it was possible to find seronegative patients with a positive proliferation assay, and conversely proliferation-negative but seropositive patients, raised some basic questions about the mechanisms of induction, up- and down-regulation, and the different pathways of humoral and cell-mediated immune responses in different patients with cystic echinococcosis.

Investigations on the cell-mediated immune response in murine cystic echinococcosis resulted in the findings of (1) polyclonal B-cell activation [30]; (2) a marked reduction of the mean T cell percentage [31], combined with a significant increase in suppressor cell activity [32]; (3) direct splenic T lymphocyte cytotoxicity to the metacestode [33], and (4) impairment of the host defence potential by the formation of anti-HLA-reactive host antibodies [34]. The potential of the murine host to develop a parasite-specific cellular response which is able to eliminate the parasite was suggested to be modulated by parasite-derived effector substances [7, 35, 36]. In addition, local immune modulation by the parasite was shown to enhance susceptibility to mycobacterial infections close to the site of parasite lesions [37].

More recently, impairment in T cell subpopulations was documented during prolonged experimental secondary hydatid disease in mice [38]. Thus, intraperitoneally infected Balb/c mice were analysed, by means of flow cytometry, after 15 months of infection for the expression of the T cell markers CD3, CD4, and CD8 on T cells from peripheral blood, spleen, and thymus. These parameters were compared with those of age-matched controls. Infected mice had higher percentages of CD3+ and CD4+ cells in peripheral blood, and higher percentages of CD8+ cells in the spleen, when compared with control mice. In addition, CD4+ and CD8+ cells in peripheral blood, and CD8+ cells in the thymus, showed a higher expression of interleukin-2 (IL-2) receptors. These results indicate that interleukin-2 is very likely to play a significant role in experimental secondary echinococcosis, and they infer a link to putative macrophage activation and respective effector mechanisms.

Cytokines. Scarce information has been published yet on the cytokines synthesized during cystic echinococcosis in humans or animals. One of the few recent studies did address the question wether clinical differences in response to chemotherapy could be related to different immune response pathways and therefore different cytokine profiles [14].The search for markers indicating the effectiveness of treatment was concentrated on the relation of interferon-γ, (IFN-γ), IL-4, IL-10 synthesis. Cystic echinococcosis patients were divided into four clinical groups according to their response to albendazole/mebendazole therapy (full, partial, low and non-responders). Full responders stimulated in vitro were found to produce significantly more IFN-γ and significantly less IL-4 and IL-10 than peripheral blood mononuclear cells (PBMCs) from non-responders. PBMCs from partial and low responders produced intermediate values of cytokine concentrations. These results may potentially indicate an implementation of a Thl-cell activation in protective immunity and Th2 cell activation in susceptibility to hydatid disease. Related effector mechanisms may strongly depend upon macrophage activation in the periparasitic areas. Thus, IFN-γ synthesis in patients with predominant Th1 response pathway and a higher resistance degree following treatment fits basically to this hypothesis. On the other hand, in the presence of macrophages, hydatid cysts can induce non-specific mitotic reactions in certain subclasses of T cells. This is associated with the generation of suppressor T populations (and a potential switch to Th2) and is followed, after a period, by cellular depletion in thymus-dependent regions of local lymphoid tissues [10].

Survival Strategies

The mechanisms by which *E. granulosus* metacestodes evade host effector immune reactions are poorly understood. Thus this matter should be discussed on the basis of different working hypotheses (rather than on hard experimental data). It was postulated that the parasite modulates its molecular immunogenicity pattern by inducing a diversification of the host immune response, thus leading to the synthesis of 'useless' immunoglobulins. Parasite carbohydrates could play a major role also with respect to mitogenic exhaustion, thus eliciting a low-avidity host immune response [reviewed by Nieto et al., 39]. Some data supporting this hypothesis were recently provided by experimental anti-idiotype modulation in a murine model [40]. Other putative mechanisms were discussed by the same authors, including the consumption of complement components by molecular parasite factors in the vicinity of the hydatid cysts [41, 42]. Other potential immunomodulation pathways could be represented by cytotoxic parasite activities [35, 43]. With regard to immunosuppression phenomena including macrophage activity status, experimental evidence for parasite-induced mitogenesis and inhibition of macrophage activation was provided by Riley et al. [44] and Dixon et al. [36]. The apparently increased levels of autoantibodies against a variety of homologous antigens may have provided a clue to immune evasion mechanisms of *E. granulosus* metacestodes [34, 45, 46], however, more recent findings clearly suggest that there is no significant association between hydatid infection and the level of autoantibodies to a broad range of self-antigens [47]. With regard to cell-mediated autoimmunity, the peripheral autoreactive response was studied in patients with hydatid infection who showed a negative humoral response as compared to seropositive patients and healthy controls [48]. Using a limiting dilution analysis (LDA) of autologous mixed lymphocyte cultures, different LDA curves were observed for healthy controls and patients. All hydatid patients, independent of their humoral response, showed a higher number of autoreactive T cells than controls. These data showed that the increase of autoreactive T cells in hydatid patients correlates with the production of specific antibodies.

Echinococcus multilocularis

Pathogenesis/Pathology

Following infection of the intermediate host with *E. multilocularis* eggs, a metacestode (larva) develops primarily in the liver. Secondary lesions may be formed subsequently in the lungs, brain and other organs [3]. Macroscopically,

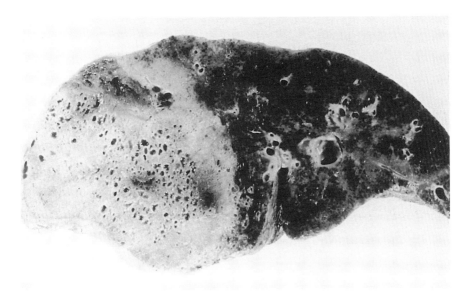

Fig. 5. Macrographic representation of the *E. multilocularis* metacestode (cross-section) in the liver of a patient highly susceptible to infection and disease. The metacestode mass consists of fibrous tissue encapsulating small parasite cysts as well as larger cysts filled with a jelly-like mass (by courtesy of Prof. J. Eckert, University of Zürich).

the typical lesion is characterised by a dispersed mass of fibrous tissue with a multitude of scattered cavities ranging from a few millimetres to centimetres in size [49] (fig. 5). In late chronic cases, a central necrotic cavity can be formed, containing a viscous, yellowish to brown fluid, which occasionally may be bacteriologically superinfected. The lesion often contains focal zones of calcification (fig. 6). Histologically, the hepatic lesion consists of a conglomerate of small vesicles and cysts demarcated by a thin laminated layer with or without an inner germinative layer. Metacestode proliferation is usually accompanied by a granulomatous host reaction. There is also evidence of vigorous augmentation of fibrous and germinative tissue on the periphery of the metacestode, but also of regressive changes centrally. In murine models of alveolar echinococcosis (AE), it was shown that experimental secondary AE induces an intense cellular inflammatory infiltration of the periparasitic hepatic area [50]. This inflammatory response may play a functional role in limiting or inhibiting the growth or even the fertility (= protoscolex formation) of the parasite in less permissive hosts [51, 52]. In contrast to infection in permissive rodent hosts, lesions from infected and thus susceptible humans rarely exhibit protoscoleces, brood capsules and calcareous cor-

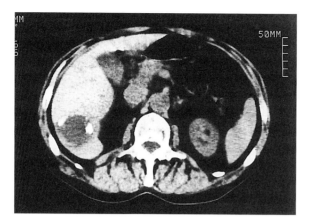

Fig. 6. Characateristic CT appearance of an active liver lesion induced by *E. multilocularis* metacestode. The large lesion is characterized by an irregular low-attenuation area and includes irregularly dispersed calcified areas.

puscles within vesicles and cysts. Metacestode development, and thus the either progressive or restrictive course of disease, seems also to be at least partially predetermined by the immunogenetic background of certain host mouse strains. However, susceptibility and resistance to infection with *E. multilocularis* metacestode in rodent intermediate hosts does probably not only depend upon immunogenetic factors but also upon mechanisms of innate resistance. Thus, cotton rats *(Sigmodon hispidus)* and jirds *(Meriones unguiculatus)* are generally more susceptible to infection with *E. multilocularis* than mice. Strains of mice that have been found to be particularly susceptible include AKR [53], CBA [54] Balb/c and C57BL/6J [55]. Relatively resistant inbred mouse strains include A/J [56], C57BL/10 [53] and C3H/HEJ [57, reviewed in Gottstein and Felleisen, 58]. However, multiple contradictory reports exist concerning the degree of susceptibility or resistance of the different mouse strains. Reasons for this could be significant variabilities in experimental infection techniques, and distinct differences between the parasite isolates used. Thus a complex situation concerning potential strain or isolate variation of the parasite was postulated [59]. Nevertheless, significant differences between individually infected inbred mice and the respective growth and fertilisation rates can be regularly observed. A similar situation was found in an outbred hyperendemic field study with naturally infected intermediate hosts such as *Arvicola terrestris*. This study demonstrated that in only 38% of naturally infected rodents protoscolex formation was possible, and that among the non-fertile group there was a large portion of calcified lesions which appeared to have died out [60] (fig. 7–10). Since inbred laboratory mice of the same H-2 haplotype differ signifi-

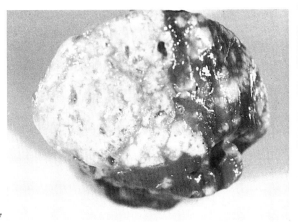

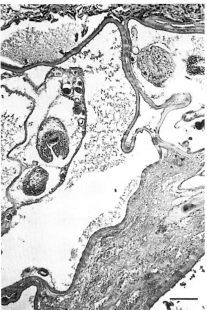

7

8

Fig. 7. Macrographic representation of the *E. multilocularis* metacestode (cross-section) in the liver of a highly susceptible mouse (naturally infected *A. terrestris* from Switzerland). The morphology is almost identical to lesions of human patients as shown in figure 5.

Fig. 8. Histological section of *E. multilocularis* lesions in the liver of a highly susceptible rodent. The cluster of microcysts includes the laminated layer and the inner germinal layer. Note the presence of protoscoleces developed in the cysts. Bar = 50 μm.

cantly in their susceptibility to *E. multilocularis*, it is probable that (at least part of) the control of susceptibility genetically maps outside the H-2 complex [61, 62].

Immunology and Immunopathology

Immune responses should, or must be, considered in dependence of different phases: reactions at the oncosphere penetration site within the host's intestinal tract, followed by migration, is often referred to as an 'early phase' immune response, while intrahepatic establishment of oncospheres followed by maturation to metacestode is considered as a 'late-phase' immune response. Antibody-mediated, complement-dependent destruction of oncospheres in the gut or at the tissue sites of migration is thought to be the most effective mechanism of host defence, although there is no experimental evidence for it in human AE [49]. It has been shown in the murine model that B lymphoblasts, eosinophils, neutro-

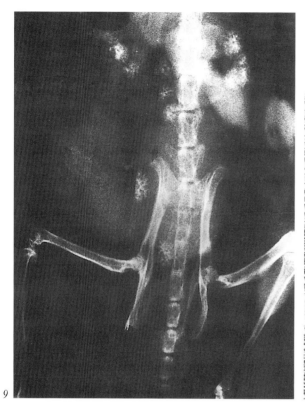
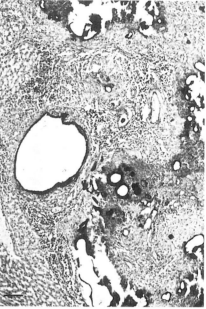

9

10

Fig. 9. X-ray image of a rodent *(A. terrestris)* naturally infected with *E. multilocularis* (infection proved later by post-mortem analysis; see corresponding fig. 10). Note the multiple calcified lesions, which proved later to consist of 'died-out' metacestode material as described below in figure 11.

Fig. 10. Histological section of *E. multilocularis* lesions in the liver of a relatively 'resistant' rodent. Abortive microcysts are embedded in the necrotic host tissue. The laminated layer may still remain; however, germinal cells are virtually absent. Note the high degree of calcification as also seen in corresponding X-ray images (see fig. 9). Bar = 100 μm.

phils and macrophages migrate to and concentrate in the vicinity of the developing oncosphere. In the early stages, at least, successful establishment of the parasite depends upon the competition between larval development and the establishment of a protective host immune response. The following sections will consider only immunological and immunopathological aspects concerning the established intrahepatic metacestode in humans and rodents.

Humoral Immune Responses/Antibodies. In most patients suffering from AE, parasite-specific antibodies, including all isotypes of immunoglobulins can be measured at diagnosis [63, 64]. The humoral immune response in AE may be associated with a characteristic hyperglobulinaemia, including other perturbations of serum proteins related to inflammatory reactions [65, 66]. However, protoscoleces and oncospheres of *E. multilocularis* can be lysed by antibody-mediated complement interaction. Increased levels of total IgE and parasite-specific serum IgE were detected in human AE [63, 67], as well as specific IgE bound to circulating basophils (shown by measuring of specific degranulation and histamine release in vitro [68]. However, clinical manifestations related to immediate-type hypersensitivity have never been reported, not even as a consequence of surgical manipulations or liver biopsies [65].

Although parasite-specific antibodies appear not to be directly controlling parasite proliferation, they seem to be involved in immunopathological mechanisms responsible for the occasional chronic granulomatous course of the disease, as described by Ali-Khan and Rausch [69], including histopathological changes related to the incidence of amyloid and immune-complex deposits in the liver of several Alaskan AE patients.

In the susceptible rodent model, a once established *E. multilocularis* metacestode appears well protected from the host immune response; the parasite proliferates progressively and metastasizes despite marked lymphoproliferative activity in the B and T cell areas of lymphoid tissues. In infected mice, a correlation was shown between parasitic mass and haematological parameters including anaemia, reticulocytosis, lymphocytopenia, neutrophilia, monocytosis and eosinopenia, i.e. all changes were directly proportional to the size of the metacestode. Specific and non-specific antibodies of various isotypes, as well as C3, were detected on the surface of metacestode structures as early as 4 weeks after intraperitoneal inoculation of *E. multilocularis* metacestode tissue [70–72]. The inability of parasite-specific antibodies alone to control parasite growth and host tissue infiltration may be due in part to 'complement-neutralizing' factors released by the metacestode causing complement depletion at the host-parasite interface [73] or to the inactivation of C3 as it enters the metacestode tissue [74, 75]. Various *E. multilocularis* antigens, their epitopes and respective genes have been characterized so far [reviewed in Lightowlers and Gottstein, 13]. Antibodies against surface structures and soluble molecules derived from protoscoleces, germinal layer, laminated layer and vesicular fluid respectively, can be demonstrated by IFAT. Some of these antigens were postulated to play a functional role in mechanisms modulating the host-parasite interplay. One antigenic protein called Em2 was characterized by using an anti-Em2 monoclonal antibody (MAb G11), which demonstrated a predominance of the Em2-epitope in the laminated layer formed within the metacestode tissue, synthesis starting approximately at day 12 after onco-

spheral development [76]. In view of determining a potential role of anti-lami-
nated layer antibodies in resistance to murine AE, the Em2-specific humoral
immune response in resistant C57BL/10-mice was found to be associated with the
ability of the host to synthesize antibodies to Em2 of the IgG3 and IgG1 isotype
[52]. In susceptible AKR and C57BL/6J mice, low levels of anti-Em2 antibodies
of the IgG2α isotype were detected. Anti-Em2 antibodies of the IgG3/IgG1 isotype, were absent, however. Due to its association to resistance, the anti-Em2-
IgG3 response in C57BL/10 mice deserves further consideration. In mice, antibodies directed against polysaccharides are predominantly of the IgG3 isotype
[77]. As discussed above, lectin-binding tests provided strong evidence for the
dominant carbohydrate nature of the Em2-antigen, thus establishing a correlative
link to the IgG3 subclass specificity developed by resistant C57BL/10 mice.

Cell-Mediated Immune Responses. It has been postulated that immunophy-
siopathological significance of the host's immune response to primary and secondary infection may be attributed primarily to T lymphocyte interactions. Basically, an infected host develops cell-mediated immunity, as exhibited by proliferation in vitro of PBMCs of AE patients upon parasite antigen stimulation [78,
79]. Parameters of cell-mediated immunity were used to study the in vitro lymphoproliferative response to *E. multilocularis* antigen stimulation in patients with
different courses of AE. Stimulation was very high in cured patients who had
radical surgery, or in patients with dead lesions. It was significantly lower in
patients who had partial surgical or no resection [79]. With regard to the functional role of cell-mediated immune response and lymphocyte activation in human
AE patients, a more detailed discussion on the matter will be provided below (see
'Cytokines' and 'Immunosuppression and T Cells').

Some very indicative findings were obtained in different murine models
reflecting susceptibility or resistance to AE. It was shown, that T lymphocytes
probably play the most important role in the immunological control of *E. multilocularis* infection. Baron and Tanner [80] reported that depletion of T cells
enhanced metastatic formation of *E. multilocularis*. In congenitally athymic nude
mice, *E. multilocularis* developed very rapidly, and the host tissue reaction was
minor compared to that of heterozygote mice [81]. Athymic nude BALB/cA *(nu/
nu)* mice were more susceptible to *E. multilocularis* than their heterozygous *nu/+*

Fig. 11. A Transmission electron micrographs of a piece peritoneal tissue originating
from a (per definition resistant) C57 Bl/10 mouse infected with *E. multilocularis*, embedded
in LR-White resin and processed for immunocytochemical staining with the MAb G11. The
region marked by arrowheads is shown at higher magnification in *B*. The parasite cyst is

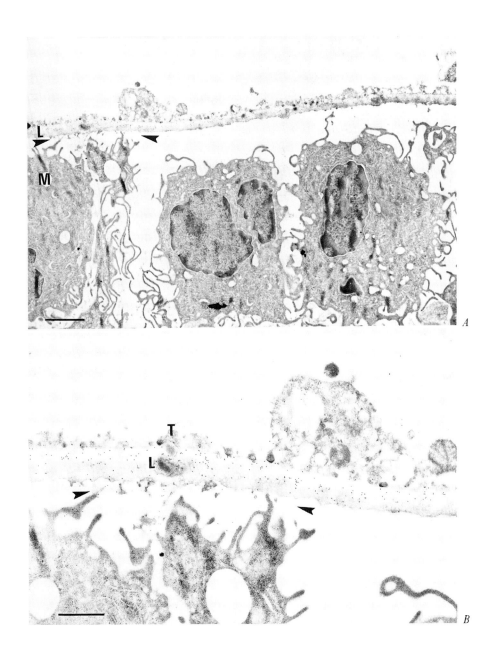

characterized by the laminated layer (L) and, characteristically for resistant hosts, the tegument (T) is very thin and has almost completely died out. Note the presence of macrophages (M) which are in direct contact with the laminated layer, and thus with the Em2 antigen. *A* bar = 2.6 μm. *B* Bar = 7.5 μm.

littermates [81, 82]. Experimental infection of SCID mice, and subsequently immunologically reconstituted mice, showed that lymphocytes were important in suppressing the growth of *E. multilocularis* metacestodes, and also indicated that protoscolex development was influenced by lymphocytes or their products [83].

E. multilocularis infection in permissive mouse strains resulted in the entire depletion of T-dependent zones of lymphoid organs and thymic involution during the period of rapid growth of the metacestode [51]. Baron and Tanner [84] concluded that activated macrophages may be included as key participants as they could be seen to adhere to the metacestode (fig. 14) and this adhesion was enhanced by opsonization. Alkarmi and Behbehani [85] suggested that the parasite survives by actively impairing cellular mechanisms of recognition and neutrophil chemotaxis in experimentally infected mice. This effect was attributed to phlogistic and chemotactic properties of *E. multilocularis* antigens, which furthermore may also modulate the intense inflammatory response and amyloidogenesis in AE [86].

Cytokines. The molecular basis of the cellular immunoregulation in patients with AE is poorly understood. The analysis of cytokine expression associated with lymphoid cell proliferation upon in vitro antigen stimulation has recently focused on the comparison of patients with active AE and healthy individuals [87]. Analysis of cytokine mRNA levels following *E. multilocularis* antigen stimulation of lymphocytes revealed the enhanced production of Th2 cell cytokine transcripts IL-3, IL-4 and IL-10 in patients (and to some degree in healthy individuals). Significantly, IL-5 mRNA was predominantly expressed in patients and was substantially absent in healthy control donors. The study provided evidence that a Th2 cell immune response is gradually activated during infection in patients susceptible to disease, with a still-unknown functional potential of IL-5, as there is presently no evidence for any relevant eosinophil interaction in AE. Still lacking are respective cytokine analyses in persons resistant to disease or infection. Another recent study focused on the analysis of the intrahepatic, periparasitic profile of expressed pro-inflammatory cytokine IL-1, IL-6 and tumour necrosis factor-α (TNF-α) mRNA, as well as the phenotypic characteristics of the cells on serial sections in immunohistochemistry [88]. In resistant patients with abortive liver lesions, IL-1, IL-6 and TNF-α mRNA were observed in macrophages located on the extreme periphery of the granuloma, between the lymphocytic ring and the liver parenchyma. TNF-α mRNA, located in the periparasitic area in cells morphologically identified as macrophages, were observed only in patients with active metacestodes, usually in association with centro-granulomatous necrosis. It was assumed that pro-inflammatory cytokines could be consistently produced by macrophages at the periphery of the periparasitic granuloma and could serve as mediators of acute-phase protein secretion and of fibrogenesis in that location.

The presence of isolated cytokine mRNA-expressing cells in the liver lobules and portal tracts could explain the spread of the fibrous process to the whole liver. In mice it was found that an IgG1-subclass-specific anti-Em2 response existed in resistant mice and an IgG2α-subclass-specific anti-Em2 response, albeit weak, in susceptible AKR mice. This observation raised the possibility that the differential induction of IgG subclasses may be regulated by different cytokines and could thus be Th2 or Th1 restricted [52]. Other indications on the potential role of cytokines pointed towards the T and natural killer (NK)-cell-derived cytokine IFN-γ. IFN-γ may be involved in the immunological control of AE because of its potent macrophage-stimulating effect, particularly in conjunction with TNF-α, a cytokine released mainly from cells of the monocyte line in response to stimuli from pathogens and cytokines. Treatment of *E. multilocularis*-infected SCID mice with recombinant human TNF-α had no effect on the growth of the larval cyst mass, but promoted the formation of granulomatous changes around the larval cyst [83]. SCID mice treated with TNF-α also appeared to have decreased numbers of protoscoleces [83]. The organization of the cytokine network in murine AE was experimentally approached by the analysis of spleen cells harvested at selected times from 1 to 26 weeks after infection and subsequently submitted to in vitro stimulation with Con A, LPS and a crude parasitic extract (EmAg) [89]. The study showed that infected mouse spleen cells stimulated in vitro with EmAg produced significantly higher levels of IFN-γ, IL-2, IL-5 and IL-10 over the first weeks of infection than those of uninfected mice. At 21 weeks after infection cytokine synthesis was almost fully suppressed. The complexicity of the response profile encountered may be related to the use of highly complex crude extract antigens. The investigation of stage-specific, purified antigens in the same kind of studies may provide clearer insights into immunopathogenic mechanisms responsible for the different courses and stages of disease in murine AE.

Survival Strategies

Immunosuppression and T Cells. Immunosuppression phenomena are likely to play a crucial role in murine AE at a more general level. Involution of the thymus and depletion of T cells in lymph nodes draining the metacestode lesion were observed [90]. Hinz and Domm [91] showed that progeny of infected NMRI female mice exhibited a reduced humoral immune response and were more susceptible to proliferation of *E. multilocularis* metacestode than the offspring of uninfected mothers. Malignant sarcomas were more likely to develop in A/J mice infected with *E. multilocularis*, indicating a potential depressive regulation of anti-tumour mechanisms by the parasite [56]. A decline of peritoneal lymphocyte, monocyte and eosinophil cell numbers replaced subsequently by neutrophils was observed during the phase of *E. multilocularis* proliferation [92]. This included splenomegaly, involution of the thymus and depletion of T cells in lymph nodes draining the metacestode lesion [50] although mechanisms responsible for these effects could not be elucidated. From a non-specific immunological point of view, Liance et al. [93] observed the delayed-type hypersensitivity response in vivo, after antigen challenge of infected resistant mice, to be significantly higher than in susceptible mice. Analysis of the phenotypic patterns of cells within the periparasitic granuloma in susceptible and resistant mice revealed an association between susceptibility and the persistence of numerous CD8+ T cells, together with a low macrophage number. In contrast, the periparasitic granuloma of resistant animals was characterised by a markedly elevated number of CD4+ T cells [94]. There was accumulating experimental evidence that the metacestode activates and also modifies lymphoid cell functions. Alkarmi and Behbehani [85] suggested that, in experimentally infected mice, the parasite survives by actively impairing cellular mechanisms of recognition and neutrophil chemotaxis. Recent reports showed that CD8+ T suppressor (Ts) cells with a low density of CD8 antigen (CD8[dull] cells) were detectable in spleens from mice infected with *E. multilocularis* [95] and in polyclonally activated lymphocytes from normal mice. Further analysis showed that *E. multilocularis* protoscoleces induced CD8+ Ts cells in vitro and were assumed to be responsible for immune suppression by inhibiting IL-2 production [96]. Another study focused on the parasite-specific humoral and cell-mediated immune responses investigated in AKR and C57BL/6J mice selected for susceptibility versus relatively resistant (C57BL/10) mice undergoing secondary AE [52]. The parasite-specific proliferative immune response of lymph node cells upon in vitro antigen stimulation remained weak in all three mouse strains. One month after infection, CD4+ lymphoblast cells dominated the total population of blast cells responding to *E. multilocularis* antigen stimulation in vitro in all three mouse strains. However, an unexpectedly high proportion of CD8+ T cells was included in blastogenesis. Three months after infection, a marked proportional increase in CD8+ T cells was seen in susceptible AKR and C57BL/6, but not in C57BL/10 mice. In parallel, the emergence of an immunosuppression phenomenon was demonstrated by significantly decreased responsiveness of lymph node cells to ConA stimulation in susceptible but not in resistant mice.

In human AE, Vuitton et al. [90] looked directly at the site of host-parasite interplay and found that the periparasitic granuloma, mainly composed of macrophages, myofibroblasts and T cells, contained a large number of CD4+ T cells in resistant patients with abortive or dead lesions. In susceptible patients with active metacestodes, the number of CD8+ T cells was increased, raising the question of an immunosuppressive process. Another study used the lymphoproliferative responsiveness investigated by in vitro lymphocyte stimulation to comparatively analyse patients grouped according to different courses of disease (spontaneous healers = resistant; patients cured by radical surgery = semi-resistant; patients with chronic course of disease = susceptible). Reduced responsiveness was demonstrated in patients with active lesions [79]. Resistant Alaskan patients harbouring a dead metacestode in their liver exhibited a high in vitro lymphoproliferative response to *E. multilocularis* crude antigen. The same was found for patients cured by complete surgical removal of the parasite. Consequently, it makes sense to postulate that the metacestode synthesises immunomodulating or immunosuppressing factors, which could be similar to those already known from *Taenia multiceps*, where the parasite can induce, for example, IL-2 receptor expression in naive T cells. Thus parasite mitogens may mimic antigen by supplying a first signal which primes the lymphocytes for mitosis in relation to a secondary signal such as IL-2 [10]. In this respect, modulating CD8+ suppressor T cells would offer explanations for some observations. The elevated CD8+ T cells in the periparasitic granulomatous area could locally suppress immune response by down-regulation of the lymphoid macrophage system. Indeed, one of the dominant immunopathological events in murine AE is lymphoproliferation associated with subsequent cellular depletion of local lymph nodes [32, 50] and local proliferation of macrophage-like cell types [50]. Then, AE in humans may run in parallel with T cell depletion in the circulation [90]. It became accumulatively evident that, with increasing parasitic mass and metacestode activity, the corresponding lymphoproliferative response becomes increasingly suppressed in human AE patients. Inactivated or surgically completely removed metacestodes are no longer able to induce immunosuppression. Therefore a strong cell-mediated immune response is restored. Reasons explaining the functional or baseline differences between resistance (no immunosuppression?) and susceptibility (immunosuppression?) may be immunogenetically related, i.e. the immunological predisposition to present certain parasitic antigens so as to induce secondarily either a suppressive or supportive cytokine profile may be dependent upon specific HLA types. In human AE, the question was strategically approached by determining the gene frequency (typed by PCR-SSO) of lymphoid HLA-DR antigens in patients with different forms of disease, i.e. patients healed by radical surgery, patients with a regressive course, and patients with a progressive course of disease despite continuous benzimidazole therapy. Preliminary investigations showed that, compared to controls or patients with progressive AE, the frequency of the HLA-DR13 antigen was increased in patients with complete surgical resection or a regressive course of disease, thus reflecting a relative good prognosis for such AE patients [97]. Further analyses on larger groups of patients will allow to dissect more precisely HLA profiles in relation to resistance or susceptibility phenomena. The aim would be to identify class I or class II MHC-restricted T cell epitopes of *E. multilocularis* which may be directly or indirectly responsible for the induction or inhibition of immunosuppression phenomena.

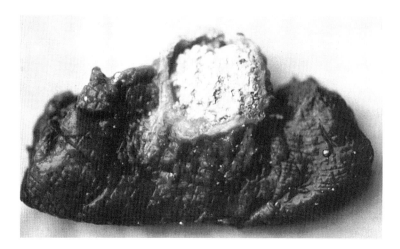

Fig. 12. Macrographic representation of the first inactive 'died-out' lesion of *E. multi-locularis* metacestode removed surgically from the liver of a healthy person resistant to metacestode proliferation and thus to disease. The encapsulated necrotic mass consists of calcified fibrous tissue without living parasite. However, the lesion still contains Em2-positive laminated layer (by courtesy of Dr. R. L. Rausch, University of Washington).

Immune Segregation by the Laminated Layer. Preliminary experiments in vivo and in vitro indicated that the laminated layer may play an important role in protecting the developing *E. multilocularis* oncosphere from host immune reactions [98, 99]. Recently, using the murine monoclonal antibody MAb G11 [76] which specifically reacts with an epitope present on the previously characterized Em2-antigen of *E. multilocularis* metacestodes [100], it was shown, by immuno-fluorescence and immuno-electron microscopy, that the corresponding parasite antigenic molecule was primarily expressed in the laminated layer adjacent to the germinal layer of the metacestode [101], as well as in oncospheres that had developed for 13 days in vitro [58, 99]. In field studies, upon screening of human patients, it became evident that the laminated layer can remain within the infected but resistant host tissue for a long time, even after spontaneous dying-out of the larval parasite [102] (fig. 12–13). This was indirectly proven by demonstrating a remarkably long persistence of anti-Em2 antibodies in serum from patients with so-called 'aborted' or 'died-out' lesions. Complete surgical removal of those lesions was immediately followed by a rapid decrease of anti-Em2 antibody concentrations to 'negative' levels [103]. Although aborted metacestode lesions no longer contained living parasitic material [104], the Em-2-positive laminated layer alone appeared to serve as a potent and permanent immunostimulant for an

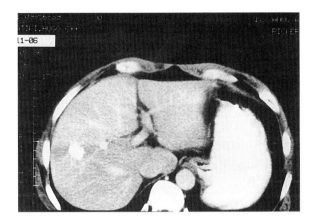

Fig. 13. Characteristic CT appearance of an abortive liver lesion reflecting a 'died-out' *E. multilocularis* metacestode as shown in figure 11. The small lesion is characterized by a small high-attenuation area with complete calcification (by courtesy of Dr. R.L. Rausch, University of Washington).

indefinite period until surgery. Even a resistant host seems not to be able to remove the remaining Em2-positive material, either immunologically or physiologically, thus providing an indication for the functionally protective role of this laminated structure. Preliminary biochemical investigations elucidated the substantial nature of the immunodominant Em2 molecule within the laminated layer [52]. The accessibility of this metacestode antigen for the host cells appears to be restricted to the laminated layer of the metacestode (fig. 14). This laminated layer was shown to consist predominantly of carbohydrates, including galactose, galactosamine and glucosamine [105]. The Em2 antigen itself was also shown to be largely composed of carbohydrates by its resistance to proteinase K digestion and chloroform extraction and by the strong lectin-binding activity, demonstrating the presence of β-D-galactose, (α)-D-galNAc, β-D-gal(1-3)-D-galNAc, (D-glcNAc)2 and NeuNAc. Furthermore, the protective role of the laminated layer was supported by the experimental evidence that only those *E. multilocularis* metacestode were able to survive and proliferate in the rodent host that were able to synthesize an Em2-positive laminated layer [99]. It was shown that oncospheres started to synthesize the laminated layer within 2 weeks after egg-hatching (a period corresponding approximately to that required for a host to generate a specific systemic immune response). A pre-existing immune response to the oncosphere surface can indeed prevent, or at least suppress the development of a secondary infection [106]. However, no protection is achieved against established

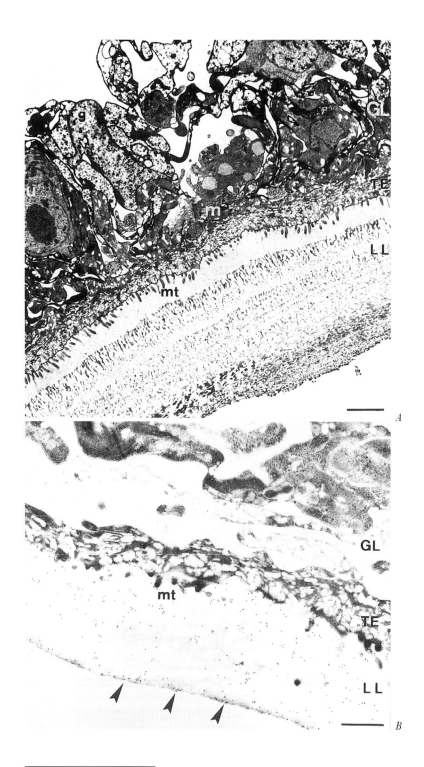

A

B

metacestodes already carrying the laminated layer. This suggests that the laminated layer masks and protects the developing parasite organism, as indicated by the finding that even single oncospheres and vesicular cysts surrounded by a laminated layer are capable of surviving in an intermediate host and inducing experimental secondary AE, but not protoscoleces lacking the laminated layer [99]. Non-surviving protoscoleces are probably killed by activated macrophages based upon arginine-dependent generation of reactive nitrogen intermediates [107]. In permissive rodent hosts, mature vesicles appeared not to be affected by these, or similar, mechanisms, which may be dependent upon suppression of macrophage activation as discussed above.In hosts, predetermined to resistance by establishing an appropriate cellular and cytokine profile, the destructive effect imposed upon the laminated layer by activated macrophages may be the key factor for restriction, and thus definitively deserves more intensive studies.

Other Forms of Hydatid Disease

Echinococcus vogeli

E. vogeli is maintained primarily in a silvatic predator-prey cycle including mainly the bush dog and occasionally domestic dogs as definitive hosts. Predominantly, pacas serve as intermediate hosts, although humans rarely also become infected. However, the growth pattern of the larva was found to differ in pacas

Fig. 14. A Transmission electron micrograph of the wall of an *E. multilocularis* metacestode. The metacestode consists of an inner, germinal layer (GL) which is largely composed of connective tissue, muscle cells (m), glycogen storage cells (g), and undifferentiated cells (u, characterized by a large nucleus and nucleolus). The germinal layer is followed by the tegument (TE), a syncytial layer which surrounds the entire metacestode, and which plays an important role with respect to uptake of nutrients and excretion of waste material. Originating from the tegument, microtriches (mt) protrude outwards well into the acellular laminated layer (LL) whose components are synthesized within the tegument and secreted via these structures. Due to the microtriches, the surface area of the parasite is enhanced severalfold. Note that the specimen was fixed in the presence of tannic acid and embedded in Epon 812 resin to demonstrate the ultrastructural architecture of the carbohydrate-rich laminated layer. Bar = 2.1 μm. *B* Transmission electron micrograph of the wall of an *E. multilocularis* metacestode embedded in LR-White. Sections were labeled with the MAb G11 which specifically reacts with the Em2 antigen, and a secondary goat-anti-mouse antibody conjugated to 10-nm gold particles. Labeling is found exclusively on the laminated layer (LL), and is particularly enriched around the microtriches (mt). Gold particles are also found on the outer surface of the laminated layer (arrowheads). The Em2 antigen is absent from the tegument (TE) and the germinal layer (GL). Bar = 1.2 μm.

and in man [108]. The metacestode of *E. vogeli* is polycystic and fluid-filled, with a tendency to form multi-chambered conglomerates. The predilection site in the intermediate host is the liver. Endogenous proliferation and convolution of both germinal and laminated layers lead to the formation of secondary subdivisions of the primary vesicle, including the production of brood capsules and protoscoleces. The geographical distribution of *E. vogeli* is roughly restricted to the the northern half of South America, with human cases identified in Brazil, Colombia, Venezuela, Panama and Ecuador [109, 110].

Echinococcus oligarthrus

E. oligarthrus includes only felids (mainly the cougar, the jaguar, the ocelot, the jaguarondi and Geoffroyi's cat) as definitive hosts, with the larval stage occurring in subcutaneous muscles of large South American rodents such as agoutis and pacas. The metacestode is, like *E. vogeli*, polycystic and fluid-filled. There is less subdivision into secondary chambers and the laminated layer is significantly thinner than that of *E. vogeli*. So far, two cases of infection with larval *E. oligarthrus* have been reported in human patients in Venezuela and Brazil [111, 112].

Immunopathology of *E. vogeli and* E. oligarthrus

Clinically, the metacestode of *E. vogeli* is represented by a primary, polycystic, hepatic abscess visible on the liver surface, often extending deep into the parenchyma. Some foci of hepatic calcification can also be present. The organs such as mesentery, omentum, intercostal muscles, diaphragm, lungs, pleura, pericardium and heart can occasionally also be affected due to extension of the primary liver cyst. The cyst can be of enormous size, composed of aggregation of smaller cysts (from 0.2 to 8 cm in diameter) The clinical and histological features of *E. vogeli* metacestodes are considered to be intermediate to those of *E. granulosus* and *E. multilocularis*; indications have also been provided by immunological antigen profile analyses [113]. Growth of these cyst takes place by both endogenous and exogenous proliferation. Endogenous proliferation results in a large, polycystic metacestode, with multiple cavities. Each cavity is surrounded by a thin, acellular, laminated layer, the germinal parasite tissue, and is filled with the vesicle fluid. The internal surface of the germinal layer forms the brood capsules in which the protoscoleces develop. *E. vogeli* cysts are normally surrounded by a fibrous capsule similar to the adventitia found around hydatid cysts of *E. granulosus*. However, in terms of pathogenicity, exogenous proliferation is more important because it is invasive, like in *E. multilocularis*. However, the *E. vogeli* polycystic metacestodes exhibit a more controlled spread, and thus are less pathogenic. Due to the very small number of human cases of *E. vogeli* infections reported so far, there is only little information with regard to the immunopathology of this species. Pulmonary cysts may present with expectoration, fever and chills. A humoral immunoresponse takes place, since serological tests for hydatid cysts are usually positive with patients infected by *E. vogeli* [113]. Peripheral eosinophilia is present only rarely. In some areas of the fibrous capsule surrounding the parasite, a granulomatous reaction may be seen, especially around degenerated vesicles. The hooklets, if found in fluid or tissues, have characteristic sizes which allow the discrimination from other species of *Echinococcus* [114].

In the first reported case of *E. oligarthrus* infection [111], a computed tomography revealed a single orbital, retroocular cyst approximatively the same size as the eye. Diagnosis was possible only upon surgery, where cyst fluid containing protoscoleces and hooklets and internal tissues were taken. The second case published so far [112] demonstrated clear wall features of cysts, thus resembling very much those of *E. vogeli*. However, discrimination of both species is unambiguous based upon significant morphological differences of parasite hooklets. No studies have been published so far on the immunopathology of *E. oligarthrus*.

References

1 Thompson RCA, Eckert J: Observations on *Echinococcus multilocularis* in the definitive host. Parasitol Res 1983;69:335–345.
2 Eckert J, Thompson RCA, Mehlhorn H: Proliferation and metastases formation of larval *Echinococcus multilocularis*. Parasitol Res 1983;69:737–748.
3 Schantz PM, Gottstein B: Echinococcosis (hydatidosis); in Walls KM, Schantz PM (eds): Immunodiagnosis of Parasitic Diseases. Orlando, Academic Press, 1986, vol 1, pp 69–107.
4 Smyth JD, Davies Z: Occurrence of physiological strains of *Echinococcus granulosus* demonstrated by in vitro culture of protoscoleces from sheep and horse hydatid cysts. Int J Parasitol 1974;4: 443–445.
5 Gottstein B, Reichen J: Echinococcosis/hydatidosis; in Cook GC (ed): Manson's Tropical Diseases, ed 20. London, Saunders, 1996, pp 1486–1508.
6 Heath DD: Immunobiology of Echinococcus infections; in Thompson RCA (ed): The Biology of *Echinococcus* and Hydatid Disease. London, Allen & Unwin, pp 164–188.
7 Lightowlers MW, Haralambous A, Rickard MD: Amino acid sequence homology between cyclophilin and a cDNA-cloned antigen of *Echinococcus granulosus*. Mol Biochem Parasitol 1989;36: 287–294.
8 Furuya K, Nishizuka M, Honma H, Kumagai M, Sato N, Takahashi M, Uchino J: Prevalence of human alveolar echinococcosis in Hokkaido as evaluated by Western blotting. Jap J Med Sci Biol 1990;43:43–49.
9 Smyth JD, McManus D: The physiology and biochemistry of cestodes. Cambridge, Cambridge University Press, 1989.
10 Dixon J: Host-parasite relations in echinococcosis: Recent evidence for immunoregulation by metacestodes. XVII Int Congr of Hydatidology, Limassol, Nov 6–10, 1995.
11 Pinon JM, Poirriez J, Lepan H, Geers R, Penna R, Fernandez D: Value of isotypic characterization of antibodies to *Echinococcus granulosus* by enzyme-linked immuno-filtration assay. Eur J Clin Microbiol 1987;6:291–295.
12 Baldelli F, Papili R, Francisci D, Tassi C, Stagni G, Pauluzzi S: Post-operative surveillance of human hydatidosis: Evaluation of immunodiagnostic tests. Pathology 1992;24:75–79.
13 Lightowlers M, Gottstein B: Immunodiagnosis of echinococcosis; in Thompson RCA, Lymbery AJ (eds): *Echinococcus* and Hydatid Disease. Wallingford, CAB International, pp 355–410.

14   Rigano R, Profumo E, Ioppolo S, Notargiacomo S, Ortona E, Teggi A, Siracusano A: Immunological markers indicating the effectiveness of pharmacological treatment in human hydatid disease. Clin Exp Immunol 1995;102:281–185.

15   Matossian RM, Kane GJ, Chantler SN, Batty I, Sarhadian HJ: The specific immunoglobulin in hydatid disease. Immunology 1972;22:423–430.

16   Wattal C, Mohan C, Agarwal SC: Evaluation of specific immunoglobulin E by enzyme-linked immunosorbent assay in hydatid disease. Int Arch All Appl Immunol 1987;87:98–100.

17   Blasco Navalpotro MA, Corrales Rodriguez de Tembleque M, Poza Jimenez A, Sanchez Gomez Navarro J: Anaphylactic shock caused by spontaneous rupture of hepatic hydatid cyst into inferior vena cava. Rev Clin Esp 1993;192:49–50.

18   Lynardier F, Luce H, Abrego A, Huguier M, Dry J: Human basophil degranulation test in diagnosis of hydatidosis. Br Med J 1980;280:1251–1252.

19   Sacdpraseuth JS, Meunier J, Spagnol F: Application du test de dégranulation des basophiles humains au diagnostic de l'hydatidose. Lyon Méd 1981;245:141–146.

20   Aceti A, Celestino D, Teggi A, Caferro M: Spontaneous in vitro generation of histamine releasing factor from mononuclear cells of patients with hydatidosis. Int Arch Allergy Immunol 1992;98: 247–251.

21   Eckert J, Gemmell MA, Soulsby EJL (eds): Immunodiagnosis of hydatid disease in man. FAO/ UNEP/WHO Guidelines for Surveillance, Prevention and Control of Echinococcosis/hydatidosis. Geneva, WHO, 1981, pp 46–65.

22   Chemtai AK, Okelo GBA, Kyobe J: Application of immunoelectrophoresis (IEIP 5) test in the diagnosis of human hydatid disease in Kenya. E Afr Med J 1981;58:583–586.

23   Lightowlers MW, Mitchell GF, Rickard MD: Cestodes; in Warren KS (ed): Immunology and Molecular Biology of Parasitic Infections. Boston, Blackwell Scientific, pp 438–472.

24   Lightowlers MW, Liu D, Haralambous A, Rickard MD: Subunit composition and specificity of the major cyst fluid antigens of *Echinococcus granulosus*. Mol Biochem Parasitol 1989;37:171–182.

25   Takahashi N, Hayano T, Suzuki M: Peptidyl-prolyl cis-trans isomerase is the cyclosporin A-binding protein cyclophilin. Nature 1989;337:473–475.

26   Hess AD, Esa AH, Colombani PM: Mechanisms of action of cyclosporine: Effects on cells of the immune system and on subcellular events in T cell activation. Transplant Proc 20, 29–40.

27   Lightowlers MW, Mitchell GF, Rickard MD: Cestodes; in Warren KS (ed): Immunology and Molecular Biology of Parasitic Infections. Boston, Blackwell Scientific, pp 438–472.

28   De Rycke PH, Janssen D, Osuna A, Lazuen J: Immunohomeostasis in hydatidosis *(Echinococcus granulosus)*; in Ehrlich R, Nieto A, Yarzabal L (eds): Basic Research in Helminthiases. Montevideo, Ediciones Logos, 1990, pp 217–228.

29   Siracuso A, Teggi A, Quintieri F, Notargiacomo S, De Rosa F, Vicari G: Cellular immune response of hydatid patients to *Echinococcus granulosus* antigens. Clin Exp Immunol 1988;72:400–405.

30   Cox DA, Marshall-Clarke S, Dixon JB: Activation of normal murine B cells by *Echinococcus granulosus*. Immunology 1989;67:16–20.

31   Wangoo A, Ganguly NK, Mahajan RC: Lymphocyte subpopulations and blast transformation studies in experimental hydatidosis. Ind J Med Res 1987;85:149–153.

32   Riley EM, Dixon JB: Experimental *Echinococcus granulosus* infection in mice: Immunocytochemical analysis of lymphocyte populations in local lymphoid infections during early infection. Parasitology 1987;94:523–532.

33   Wangoo A, Ganguly NK, Mahajan RC: Specific T cell cytotoxicity in experimental *Echinococcus granulosus* infected mice. Ind J Med Res 1987;86:588–590.

34   Ameglio F, Saba F, Bitti A, Aceti A, Tanigaki N, Sorrentino R, Dolei A, Tosi R: Antibody reactivity to HLA classes I and II in sera from patients with hydatidosis. J Infect Dis 1987;156:673–676.

35   Annen J, Köhler P, Eckert J: Cytotoxicity of *Echinococcus granulosus* cyst fluid in vitro. Parasitol Res 1981;65:79–88.

36   Dixon JB, Jenkins P, Allan D: Immune recognition of *Echinococcus granulosus*. I. Parasite-activated, primary transformation by normal murine lymph node cells. Parasite Immunol 1982;4:33–45.

37   Ellis ME, Sinner W, Asraf Ali M, Hussain Qadri SM: Echinococcal disease and mycobacterial infection. Ann Trop Med Parasitol 1991;85:243–251.

38   Rueda MC, Osuna A, Derycke PH, Janssen D: Changes in T-Cell subpopulations in mice during prolonged experimental secondary infection with *Echinococcus granulosus*. Biosci Rep 1995;15: 201–208.

39   Nieto A, Fernandez C, Ferreira AM, Diaz A, Baz A, Bentancor A, Casabo L, Dematteis S, Irigoin F, Marco M, Miguez M: Mechanisms of evasion of host immune response by *E. granulosus*; in Ehrlich R, Nieto A (eds): Biology of Parasitism. Montevideo, Ediciones Trilce, 1994.

40   Baz A, Hernandez A, Dematteis S, CArol H, Nieto A: Idiotypic modulation of the antibody response of mice to *Echinococcus granulosus* antigens. Immunology 1995;84:350–354.

41   Ferreira AM, Würzner R, Hobart MJ, Lachmann P: Study of the in vitro activation of the complement alternative pathway by *Echinococcus granulosus* hydatid cyst fluid. Parasite Immunology 1995;17:245–251.

42   Diaz A, Ferreira AM, Nieto A: *Echinococcus granulosus:* Interactions with host complement in secondary infection in mice. Exp Parasitol 1995;80:473–482.

43   Janssen D, Osuna A, Lazuen L, de Rycke PH: Comparative cytotoxicity of secondary hydatid cysts, protoscoleces, and in vitro developed microcysts of *Echinococcus granulosus*. J Helminthol 1992; 66:124–131.

44   Riley EM, Dixon JB: Experimental *Echinococcus granulosus* infection in mice: Immunocytochemical analysis of lymphocyte populations in local lymphoid infections during early infection. Parasitology 1987;94:523–532.

45   Pini C, Pastore R, Valesini G: Circulating immune complexes in sera of patients infected with *Echinococcus granulosus*. Clin Exp Immunol 1983;51:572–578.

46   Mori H, Wernli B, Weiss N, Franklin RM: Auto-antibodies in humans with cystic or alveolar echinococcosis. Trans R Soc Trop Med Hyg 1986;81:978–990.

47   Colebrook AL, Lightowlers MW: Lack of an association between hydatid disease and autoimmunity. Parasite Immunol 1995;17:219–222.

48   Quintieri F, Rigano R, Pugliese O, Teggi A, Siracusano A: Further evaluation of autoreactive T cells in hydatid patients. Immunol Lett 1994;40:59–63.

49   Gottstein B: *Echinococcus multilocularis* infection: Immunology and immunodiagnosis. Adv Parasitol 1992;31:321–380.

50   Ali-Khan Z, Siboo R: Pathogenesis and host response in subcutaneous alveolar hydatidosis. I. Histogenesis of alveolar cyst and a qualitative analysis of the inflammatory infiltrates. Parasitol Res 1980;62:241–254.

51   Ali-Khan Z: Host-parasite relationship in echinococcosis. I. Parasite biomass and antibody response in three strains of inbred mice against graded doses of *Echinococcus multilocularis* cysts. II. Cyst weight, hematologic alterations, and gross changes in the spleen and lymph nodes of C57L mice against graded doses of *Echinococcus multilocularis* cysts. J Parasitol 1974;60:231–235 (pt I), 236–242 (pt II).

52   Gottstein B, Wunderlin E, Tanner I: *Echinococcus multilocularis*: Parasite-specific humoral and cellular immune response subsets in mouse strains susceptible (AKR, C57BL/6J) or 'resistant' (C57BL/10) to secondary alveolar echinococcosis. Clin Exp Immunol 1994;96:245–252.

53   Liance M, Vuitton DA, Guerret-Stocker S, Carbillet JP, Grimaud JA, Houin R: Experimental alveolar echinococcosis. Suitability of a murine model of intrahepatic infection by *Echinococcus multilocularis* for immunological studies. Experientia 1984;40:1436–1439.

54   Lukashenko NP: Comparative study of the genesis of the cysts of *Alveococcus multilocularis* (Leuckart, 1863) Abuladze, 1959 in some mammals and man from a consideration of host-parasite relationship. Med Parazitol (Mosk) 1966;35:474–481.

55   Alkarmi TO, Ali-Khan Z: Chronic alveolar hydatidosis and secondary amyloidosis: Pathological aspects of the disease in four strains of mice. Br J Exp Pathol 1984;65:405–417.

56   Lubinski G, Desser SS: Growth of the vegetatively propagated strain of larval *Echinococcus multilocularis* in C57L/J, B6AF1 and A/J mice. Can J Zool 1963;42:1213–1216.

57   Yamashita J, Ohbayashi M, Kitamura Y, Suzuki K, Okugi M: Studies on echinococcosis. VIII. Experimental *Echinococcus multilocularis* in various rodents; especially on the difference of susceptibility among uniform strains of the mouse. Jap J Vet Res 1958;6:135–155.

58   Gottstein B, Felleisen R: Protective immune mechanisms against the metacestode of *Echinococcus multilocularis*. Parasitol Today 1995;11:320–326.

---

59 Thompson RCA, Lymbery A: The nature, extent and significance of variation within the genus *Echinococcus*. Adv Parasitol 1988;27:209–258.

60 Gottstein B, Saucy F, Wyss C, Siegenthaler M, Jacquier P, Schmitt M, Brossard M, Demierre G: Investigations on a Swiss area highly endemic for *Echinococcus multilocularis*. Appl Parasitol, in press.

61 Kroeze WK, Tanner CE: Studies on the genetics of host responses to infections with *Echinococcus multilocularis* in rodents; in Skamene E (ed): Genetic Control of Host Resistance to Infection and Malignancy. New York, Liss, 1985, pp 477–481.

62 Kroeze WK, Tanner CE: *Echinococcus multilocularis:* Susceptibility and responses to infection in inbred mice. Int J Parasitol 1987;17:878–883.

63 Gottstein B, Eckert J, Woodtli W: Determination of parasite-specific immunoglobulins using the ELISA in patients with echinococcosis treated with mebendazole. Z Parasitenkd 1984;70:385–389.

64 Vuitton DA, Lassegue A, Miguet JP, Herve P, Barale T, Seilles E, and Capron A: Humoral and cellular immunity in patients with hepatic alveolar echinococcosis. A 2-year follow-up with and without flubendazole treatment. Parasite Immunol 1984;6:329–340.

65 Miguet JP, Monange C, Carbillet JP, Bernard F, Pageaut G, Camelot G, Gillet M, Carayon P, Gisselbrecht H: L'échinococcose alvéolaire du foie. A propos de 20 cas observés en Franche-Comté. II. Etude anatomo-pathologique. Arch Fr Mal App Dig 1976;65:23–32.

66 Engler R, Jayle MF: Glycoprotéines plasmatiques et processus granulomateux. Ann Anatom Pathol 1976;21:45–58.

67 Ito A, Smyth JD: Adult cestodes; in Soulsby EJL (ed): Immune Responses in Parasitic Infections. Immunology, Immunopathology and Immunoprophylaxis. Boca Raton, CRC Press, pp 115–163.

68 Vuitton DA, Bresson-Hadni S, Lenys D, Flausse F, Liance M, Wattre P, Miguet JP, Capron A: IgE-dependent humoral immune response in *Echinococcus multilocularis* infection: Circulating and basophil bound specific IgE against *Echinococcus* antigens in patients with alveolar echinococcosis. Clin Exp Immunol 1988;71:247–252.

69 Ali-Khan Z, Rausch RL: Demonstration of amyloid and immune complex deposits in renal and hepatic parenchyma of Alaskan alveolar hydatid disease patients. Ann Trop Med Parasitol 1987;81:381–392.

70 Ali-Khan Z, Siboo R: *Echinococcus multilocularis*: Distribution and persistence of specific host immunoglobulins on cyst membranes. Exp Parasitol 1981;51:159–168.

71 Kroeze WK, Tanner CE: *Echinococcus multilocularis*: Responses to infection in Mongolian gerbils. Exp Parasitol 1986;17:1–9.

72 Alkarmi TO, Alshakarchi Z, Behbahani K: *Echinococcus multilocularis:* The non-specific binding of different species of immunoglobulins to alveolar hydatid cysts grown in vivo and in vitro. Parasite Immunol 1988;10:443–457.

73 Hammerberg B, Musoke AJ, Williams JF: Activation of complement by hydatid cyst fluid of *Echinococcus granulosus*. J Parasitol 1977;63:327–331.

74 Kassis AI, Tanner CE: The role of complement in hydatid disease: In vitro studies. Int J Parasitol 1976;6:25–35.

75 Kassis AI, Tanner CE: *Echinococcus multilocularis*: Complement's role in vivo in hydatid disease. Exp Parasitol 1977;43:390–395.

76 Deplazes P, Gottstein B: A monoclonal antibody against *Echinococcus multilocularis* Em2 antigen. Parasitology 1991;103:41–49.

77 Callard RE, Turner MW: Cytokines and Ig switching: Evolutionary divergence between mice and humans. Parasitol Today 1990;11:200–203.

78 Bresson-Hadni S, Vuitton DA, Lenys D, Liance M, Racadot E, Miguet JP: Cellular immune response in *Echinococcus multilocularis* infection in humans. I. Lymphocyte reactivity to *Echinococcus* antigens in patients with alveolar echinococcosis. Clin Exp Immunol 1989;78:61–66.

79 Gottstein B, Mesarina B, Tanner I, Ammann RW, Eckert J, Wilson JF, Lanier A, Parkinson A: Specific cellular and humoral immune responses in patients with different long-term courses of alveolar echinococcosis (infection with *Echinococcus multilocularis*). Am J Trop Med Hyg 1991;45:734–742.

80 Baron RW, Tanner CE: The effect of immunosuppression on secondary *Echinococcus multilocularis* infections in mice. Int J Parasitol 1976;6:37–42.

81 Kamiya H, Kamiya M, Ohbayashi M, Nomura T: Studies on the host resistance to infection with *Echinococcus multilocularis*. 1. Difference of susceptibility of various rodents, especially of congenitally athymic nude mice. J Parasitol Jpn 1980;29:87–100.

82 Kamiya H, Kamiya M, Ohbayashi M: Studies on the host resistance to infection with *Echinococcus multilocularis*. 2. Lytic effect of complement and its mechanism. J Jpn Parasitol 1980;29:169–179.

83 Playford MC, Ooi HK, Ito M, Kamiya M: Lymphocyte engraftment conveys immunity and alters parasite development in scid mice infected with *Echinococcus multilocularis*. Parasitol Res 1993; 79:261–268.

84 Baron RW, Tanner CE: *Echinococcus multilocularis* in the mouse: The in vitro protoscolicidal activity of peritoneal macrophages. Int J Parasitol 1977;7:489–495.

85 Alkarmi T, Behbehani K: *Echinococcus multilocularis*: Inhibition of murine neutrophil and macrophage chemotaxis. Exp Parasitol 1989;69:16–22.

86 Alkarmi TO, Ali-Khan Z: Phlogistic and chemotactic activities of alveolar hydatid cyst antigen. J Parasitol 1989;74:711–719.

87 Sturm D, Menzel J, Gottstein B, Kern P: Interleukin-5 is the predominant cytokine produced by peripheral blood mononuclear cells in alveolar echinococcosis. Infect Immun 1995;63:1688–1697.

88 Vuitton DA, Bresson-Hadni S, Godot V, Deschaseaux M, Racadot E: Expression of proinflammatory cytokine mRNA in the periparasitic granuloma of human alveolar echinococcosis. Int Congr of Hydatidology, Limassol Nov 6–10, 1995.

89 Vuitton DE, Emery, I Godot V, Bresson-Hadni S, Leclerc C, Liance M, Houin R (1995b) Cytokines in the host-E.multilocularis relationship. Experimental and human data. Abstract A1 of the XVII Int. Congr. of Hydatidology, Limassol/Cyprus, November 6–10, 1995.

90 Vuitton DA, Bresson-Hadni S, Laroche L, Kaiserlian D, Guerret-Stocker S, Bresson JL, Gillet M: Cellular immune response in *Echinococcus multilocularis* infection in humans. II. Natural killer cell activity and cell subpopulations in the blood and in the periparasitic granuloma of patients with alveolar echinococcosis. Clin Exp Immunol 1989;78:67–74.

91 Hinz E, Domm S: Die experimentelle *Echinococcus multilocularis*-Infektion von Muttermäusen und ihre Bedeutung für die Nachkommen. Tropenmed Parasitol 1980;31:135–142.

92 Devouge M, Ali-Khan Z: Intraperitoneal murine alveolar hydatidosis: Relationship between the size of the larval cyst mass, immigrant inflammatory cells, splenomegaly and thymus involution. Tropenmed Parasitol 1983;34:15–20.

93 Liance M, Bresson-Hadni S, Meyer JP, Houin R, Vuitton DA (1990) Cellular immunity in experimental *Echinococcus multilocularis* infection. I. Sequential and comparative study of specific in vivo delayed-type hypersensitivity against *E. multilocularis* antigens in resistant and sensitive mice. Clin Exp Immunol 82, 373–377.

94 Bresson-Hadni S, Liance M, Meyer JP, Houin R, Bresson JL, Vuitton DA: Cellular immunity in experimental *Echinococcus multilocularis* infection. II. Sequential and comparative phenotypic study of the periparasitic mononuclear cells in resistant and sensitive mice. Clin Exp Immunol 1990;82:378–383.

95 Kizaki T, Kobayashi S, Ogasawara K, Good RA, Day NK, Onoé K: Immune suppression induced by protoscoleces of *Echinococcus multilocularis* in mice: Evidence for the presence of CD8dull supressor cells in spleens of mice intraperitoneally infected with *E. multilocularis*. J Immunol 1991; 147:1659–1666.

96 Kizaki T, Ishige M, Kobayashi S, Bingyan W, Kumagai M, Day NK, Good RA, Onoe K: Suppression of T-cell proliferation by CD8+ T cells induced in the presence of protoscolices of *Echinococcus multilocularis* in vitro. Inf Imm 1993;61:525–533.

97 Gottstein B, Bettens F: Association between HLA-DR13 and susceptibility to alveolar echinococcosis. J Infect Dis 1994;169:1416–1417.

98 Sakamoto T, Sugimura M: Studies on echinococcosis. XXIII. Electron microscopical observations on histogenesis of larval *Echinococcus multilocularis*. Jap J Vet Res 1970;18:131–144.

99 Gottstein B, Deplazes P, Aubert M: *Echinococcus multilocularis*: Immunological study on the 'Em2-positive' laminated layer during in vitro and in vivo post-oncospheral and larval development. Parasitol Res 1992;78:291–297.

100 Gottstein B: Purification and characterization of a specific antigen from *Echinococcus multilocularis*. Parasite Immunol 1985;7:201–212.

101 Hemphill A, Gottstein B: Immunology and morphology studies on the proliferation of in vitro cultivated *Echinococcus multilocularis* metacestodes. Parasitol Res 1995;81:605–614.

102 Rausch RL, Wilson JF, Schantz PM, McMahon BJ: Spontaneous death of *Echinococcus multilocularis*: Cases diagnosed serologically by Em2-ELISA and clinical significance. Am J Trop Med Hyg 1987;36:576–585.

103 Lanier AP, Trujillo DE, Schantz PM, Wilson JF, Gottstein B, McMahon BJ: Comparison of serologic tests for the diagnosis and follow-up of alveolar hydatid disease. Am J Trop Med Hyg 1987;37:609–615.

104 Condon J, Rausch RL, Wilson JF: Application of the avidin-biotin immunohistochemical method for the diagnosis of alveolar hydatid disease from tissue sections. Trans R Soc Trop Med Hyg 1988;82:731–735.

105 Kilejian A, Schwabe CW: Studies on the polysaccharides of the *Echinococcus granulosus* cyst, with observations on a possible mechanism for laminated membrane formation. Comp Biochem Physiol 1971;40B:25–36.

106 Lloyd S: Progress in immunization against parasitic helminths. Parasitology 1981;83:225–242.

107 Kanazawa T, Asahi H, Hata H, Mochida K, Kagei N, Stadecker MJ: Arginine-dependent generation of reactive nitrogen intermediates is instrumental in the in vitro killing of protoscoleces of *Echinococcus multilocularis* by activated macrophages. Parasite Immunol 1993;15:619–623.

108 Rausch RL, D'Alessandro, A, Rausch VR: Characteristics of the larval *Echinococcus vogeli* Rausch and Bernstein 1972 in the natural intermediate host, the paca, *Cuniculus paca* L. (Rodentia: Dasyproctidae). Am J Trop Med Hyg 1981;30:1043–1052.

109 D'Alessandro A, Rausch RL, Cuello C: *Echinococcus vogeli* in man, with a review of polycystic hydatid disease in Colombia and neighbouring countries. Am J Trop Med Hyg 1979;28:303–317.

110 Ferreira AM, Nishioka SA, Rocha A, D'Alessandro A: *Echinococcus vogeli* polycystic hydatid disease: Report of two Brazilian cases outside the Amazon region. Trans R Soc Trop Med Hyg 1995;89:286–287.

111 Lopera RD, Melendez RD, Fernandez I, Sirit J, Perera MP: Orbital hydatid cyst of *Echinococcus oligarthrus* in a human in Venezuela. J Parasitol 1989;75:467–470.

112 D'Alessandro A, Ramirez LE, Chapadeiro E, Lopes ER, De Mesquita PM: Second recorded case of human infection by *Echinococcus oligarthrus*. Am J Trop Med Hyg 1995;52:29–33.

113 Gottstein B, D'Alessandro A, Rausch RL: Immunodiagnosis of polycystic hydatid disease/polycystic echinococcosis due to *Echinococcus vogeli*. Am J Trop Med Hyg 1995;53:558–563.

114 Rausch RL, Rausch VR, D'Alessandro A: Discrimination of the larval stages of *Echinococcus oligarthrus* (Diesing, 1863) and E. vogeli Rausch and Bernstein, 1972 (Cestoda: Taeniidae). Am J Trop Med Hyg 1978;29:1195–1202.

Prof. Dr. Bruno Gottstein, Institute of Parasitology, University of Bern, Länggass-Strasse 122, CH–3001 Bern (Switzerland)

Freedman DO (ed): Immunopathogenetic Aspects of Disease Induced by Helminth Parasites.
Chem Immunol. Basel, Karger, 1997, vol 66, pp 209–230

....

Taenia solium Cysticercosis: Host-Parasite Interactions and the Immune Response

A. Clinton White, Jr., Prema Robinson, Raymond Kuhn

Departments of Medicine, Microbiology and Immunology, Baylor College of
Medicine, Houston, Tex., and the Department of Biology, Wake-Forest University,
Winston-Salem, N.C., USA

Introduction

Infection of the human central nervous system with the metacestode form
(tissue cyst) of *Taenia solium* causes neurocysticercosis (NCC). To complete its
life cycle, the metacestode must persist in the tissues of the intermediate host for
months to years. The cysts have developed mechanisms to avoid the host inflammatory and immune response and to provide for their own nutrition. Experimental models suggest that active infection is associated with stimulation of T helper 2
cytokines and immunoglobulin production. In contrast, dying parasites are associated with granulomatous inflammation and T helper 1 cytokines. Our hypothesis is that disease (e.g. human NCC) results when the parasite can no longer modulate the host response. In this review, we will examine the mechanisms involved
in host-parasite interactions, discuss the implications of these data for the pathogenesis of human NCC, and review data on protective vaccines for *Taenia* infections.

Epidemiology, Life Cycle and Clinical Manifestations

Prevalence of Cysticercosis

Prior to the 1990s, reliable epidemiologic data on the prevalence of NCC
were limited. Confirmation of infection required the use of neuroimaging, biopsy,
or autopsy studies, which were not readily available in endemic areas [1]. Serologic assays using crude antigens were both insensitive and nonspecific [2, 3]. The

development of the enzyme-linked immunotransfer blot assay (EITB) using parasite glycoproteins provided the first specific assay of infection which could be used in large field studies [4]. Subsequently, with the increasing availability of neuroimaging studies and the application of the EITB assay, cysticercosis was recognized as a major cause of neurologic disease worldwide [5, 6].

It is estimated that 4 million people worldwide harbor the porcine tapeworm, and the prevalence appears to be increasing [7, 8]. For each patient with a tapeworm, there are thought to be 10 or more people infected with the cyst stage. The prevalence of infection with the cyst stage is now estimated to be approximately 50 million persons [9]. However, data from recent epidemiologic studies suggest that this figure may underestimate the true prevalence [6].

There is a wide geographic distribution of cysticercosis, with areas of high prevalence in Mexico, Central and South America, India, and Subsaharan Africa [1, 8, 10]. NCC is also endemic in Korea, China, Indonesia, and Southeast Asia [6, 11, 12]. Studies from Mexico, South America, India, and Subsaharan Africa have revealed that up to half of all cases of adult-onset seizures are due to NCC [6, 13–16]. Thus, NCC is thought to be the major reason that epilepsy is twice as common in developing countries as compared to developed countries [5].

In the United States, with the recent influx of immigrants, cysticercosis is being increasingly recognized [17–20]. Most of the cases are imported. However, locally acquired cases have been clearly documented in New York, Chicago, Los Angeles, and elsewhere in the US [21–24]. For example, 1.3% of the members of an orthodox Jewish community in New York City were found to be EITB positive [25]. Seropositivity was associated with domestic employees from endemic regions. NCC was common in Europe during the 19th century, but with improved animal husbandry, locally acquired disease has been eliminated in Western Europe. Until recently, NCC was common in Eastern Europe. At present, few locally acquired cases are described. NCC continues to be prevalent in Portugal [26].

In Mexico, studies have found a prevalence rate of at least one cysticercus in the central nervous system in approximately 2% of unselected autopsies (ranging from 0.4 to 3.5%) [27]. Recent studies employing the EITB assay have identified seroprevalence rates of 4.9–22.6% among inhabitants of endemic villages in Latin America [2, 6, 28, 29]. In contrast to these studies from rural areas, only 1.5% of patients in Lima referred for endoscopy had evidence of cysticercosis [30]. Furthermore, studies from Mexico, Ecuador, and Peru have all demonstrated that up to half of all NCC patients will have negative EITB tests [2, 31, 32]. Medina et al. [14] identified evidence of NCC in 50 of 100 consecutive patients in Mexico City with adult-onset seizures. Similarly, NCC was the most common cause of adult-onset seizures in a study from Ecuador [13]. Eighteen percent of neurological referral patients in Lima had positive EITB tests [33]. Up to half of all pigs from endemic villages are infected [6]. Most studies from Latin America demonstrate higher prevalence rates among residents of rural areas, especially areas where pigs are raised [33].

The prevalence of NCC in Africa is similar to that in Latin America. Between 0.45 and 7% of the autopsies of patients from pig raising areas reveal evidence of NCC [10, 16]. In a large epidemiologic study from Togo (West Africa), 2.4% of the population had evidence of cysticercosis, including 39% of patients with epilepsy [15]. In large case series of black South African patients with epilepsy, 28–38% had evidence of NCC on CT scan [34, 35]. Twenty-one percent of epileptics in Rwanda were EITB positive [6]. Furthermore, there is a high prevalence of cysticercosis in pigs in all pig-raising areas [16].

In India, NCC is also a common cause of neurologic disease. Up to half of the patients with seizure disorders have serologic evidence of NCC [6, 10]. Gulati et al. [36] demonstrated that 24% of 361 epileptic patients in Delhi had unequivocal evidence of NCC by MRI. Additional patients had evidence of disappearing lesions on their scans. Brain biopsies of similar patients elsewhere in India have shown that nearly all of these disappearing lesions are due to NCC [37, 38].

Few data are available on the prevalence of cysticercosis in China. Large case series of patients with NCC continue to be described with seroprevalence rates of up to 16% in selected populations [39]. Nearly 10% of neurologic patients in Beijing were found to be EITB positive [6]. A nationwide survey of parasitic infections identified a high prevalence of cysticercosis in 27 of 30 provinces/autonomous zones/municipalities, but some areas were apparently spared [40]. NCC was felt to be among the more common serious parasitic diseases in that survey, with nearly 9,000 cases identified [40]. NCC is also common elsewhere in Asia. For example, 14% of epileptics in Bali were EITB positive. Similarly, NCC is common among epileptic patients in Korea [12].

Life Cycle of Taenia

In the usual cycle of transmission, man acquires intestinal infection with pork tapeworms by ingestion of undercooked pork infected with *T. solium* cysticerci. In the intestine, the protoscolex evaginates and attaches to the intestinal wall by means of suckers. The intestinal parasite develops by forming segments termed proglottids from the caudal end of the scolex. The proglottids gradually mature as they are separated from the scolex by newly produced segments. As they mature, the proglottids form testes and ovaries. The eggs are fertilized within the proglottids. The terminal proglottids contain approximately 50,000 eggs each and are shed intermittently in the feces. The intermediate host, normally the pig, is infected by ingestion of parasite eggs or proglottids from human feces. The eggs are induced to hatch and activate by the action of gastric and intestinal fluids. The hatched larvae, also called the oncospheres, escape from the eggs and penetrate the intestinal mucosa. Little is known about how the oncospheres invade. We have demonstrated that *Taenia* oncospheres produce excretory/secretory peptidases, which may facilitate invasion [41].

After invasion, the oncospheres migrate via the blood stream throughout the body of the intermediate host. It is not known whether the oncospheres actively migrate to specific tissues or merely passively lodge in the tissues with high blood flow (e.g. muscles, brain). However, over a period of 3 weeks to 2 months, the oncospheres enlarge and mature into cysticerci. During this period, the external surface changes from the folded surface of the oncosphere to numerous microvilli on the postoncosphere larvae to numerous microtriches on the surface of the mature cyst. The life cycle is completed when humans consume undercooked pork containing the cysts.

Human Cysticercosis

Man can also act as an intermediate host for *T. solium* when ova are ingested. The oncospheres are released, penetrate the intestinal mucosa, and migrate throughout the body to produce human cysticercosis. Larval cysts can develop in almost any tissue, but most cysts are found in the central nervous system, skeletal muscle, the subcutaneous tissue, and the eye. The clinical manifestations are varied and nonspecific. They depend to a great extent on the location and number of cysts and on the host response. If lesions are few and reside in nonstrategic areas of the body such as the muscle or even certain portions of the brain, infection may be asymptomatic. Even with neurologic disease, there is usually an asymptomatic period (typically 4–5 years, but up to 30 years) before the onset of disease [42]. This incubation period approximates the estimated life span of the tissue cyst [43, 44]. During this asymptomatic period, there is little inflammation surrounding the cysts (fig. 1). Thus, disease may result primarily from host inflammatory response to dying cysts.

The most common clinical manifestation of cysticercosis is seizures [1, 17, 18, 20, 45]. The seizures are usually described as generalized, but focal seizures, and secondary generalization is also common. In our experience, patients with seizures invariably have evidence of inflammation on neuroimaging studies (e.g. contrast enhancement, edema, or calcifications) [20, 46]. Typically, CT or MRI scans will either show enhancing lesions, often with a central hypodense area, or calcified lesions (fig. 2). In some cases, scans only reveal focal areas of enhancement (fig. 3), which often resolve without treatment. Patients with only parenchymal disease have a good prognosis, whether or not they receive antiparasitic agents [45, 47–50]. In a recent controlled trial, patients with parenchymal NCC were randomized to corticosteroids plus either albendazole, praziquantel, or placebo. While the cysts disappeared somewhat faster in the groups treated with antiparasitic drugs, the only clinical differences were a slightly higher rate of

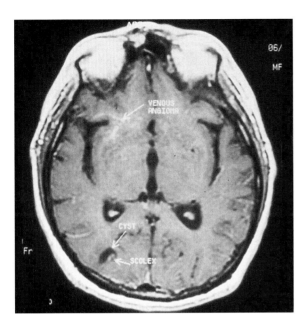

Fig. 1. Magnetic resonance imaging study with gadolinum contrast of the brain of a patient with AIDS and asymptomatic NCC. The arrows point to the cyst in the occipital lobe showing a visible scolex. Since there is no inflammation, the walls of the cyst cannot be distinguished from surrounding brain tissue. Originally published in White et al. [46] with permission from the publisher.

hydrocephalus in those randomized to antiparasitic drugs [51]. The recent literature has increasingly identified NCC as a major cause of self-limited neurologic disease (e.g. focal enhancing lesions on CT scan in patients presenting with seizures) [37, 38].

About 20% of cases of NCC present with cysts in the ventricles [17, 20, 45, 52] (fig. 4). Ventricular NCC typically presents with hydrocephalus from mechanical obstruction of cerebrospinal fluid [52–54]. In contrast to the generally favorable prognosis of parenchymal disease, extraparenchymal NCC usually requires surgical intervention and may be fatal [52, 54]. Less common manifestations of NCC include cysts in the basilar meninges (with chronic meningitis or communicating hydrocephalus), spinal cord lesions, and localized infarction [1, 17, 20, 52]. Cysts can also cause symptoms in the eyes, subcutaneous tissues, and muscle [1, 17, 55].

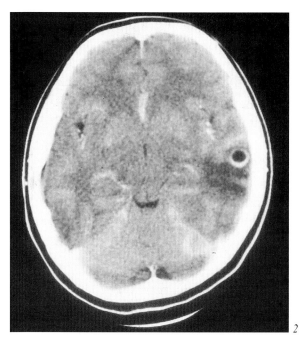

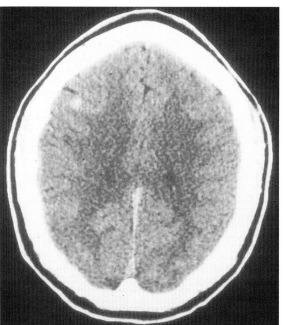

Pathology

T. solium lives in tissues as a fluid-filled cyst (or metacestode). The cyst has a thin, semitransparent wall. The scolex is invaginated and appears as an opaque 4- to 5-mm nodule on one side of the cyst. The cyst fluid is a complex mixture of parasite molecules and host serum components. The size and shape of the cyst vary with pressure from surrounding tissue. In the brain, the cysts are round with a diameter of approximately 1 cm [56]. There may be a surrounding capsule of variable thickness consisting of astrocytes and collagen fibers, but the capsule is usually minimal in the central nervous system and eye. The bladder wall consists of three layers – a cuticle layer containing microtriches (which are in turn coated by a carbohydrate glycocalyx), a layer of pseudoepithelium and muscularis, and a loose layer of connective tissue containing a network of canaliculi. The mural nodule contains the invaginated scolex and an associated spiral canal, also with a

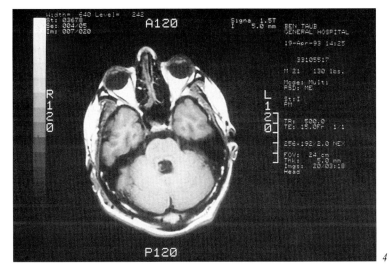

Fig. 2. Computer axial tomography scan with contrast of the brain of a patient with NCC, who presented with recurrent seizures showing a single cystic lesion in the right parietal love with associated ring enhancement and edema. Originally published in Shandera et al. [20] and used with permission from the publisher.

Fig. 3. Computer axial tomography scan with contrast of the brain of a patient with NCC, who presented with seizures showing a single area of enhancement in the right frontal lobe.

Fig. 4. Magnetic resonance imaging study with gadolinum contrast of the brain of a patient who presented with hydrocephalus showing a cyst with visible scolex in the 4th ventricle.

trilaminar membrane. A small excretory pore near the end of the spiral canal connects the digestive canal to the surrounding tissue. Viable cysticerci (from pig muscle) have little surrounding host inflammation, usually only a few mononuclear cells and variable numbers of eosinophils near the excretory pore [57]. A similar pathologic picture is found for cysts at autopsy in humans who died without symptoms of cysticercosis [56, 58]. In contrast, most cysts from patients with active disease display a prominent inflammatory response, including lymphocytes, eosinophils, granulocytes, and plasma cells [56]. The inflammatory process progresses through a series of discrete stages [44]. In the colloidal stage, the appearance of the cyst is similar to a colloid cyst with gelatinous material in the cyst fluid and hyaline degeneration of the larva. In the granular nodular stage, the cyst begins to contract and the walls are replaced by focal lymphoid nodules and necrosis. Finally, the granulation tissue is replaced by collagenous structures and calcification in the nodular calcified stage [44].

Host-Parasite Interactions

The metacestode must survive in the tissues of the intermediate host to complete its life cycle. Since the cysts actually enlarge within the tissues, they must acquire amino acids from the host to produce structural proteins. The bladder walls of *Taenia crassiceps* cysts contain pinocytotic vesicles that appear to transport host proteins across the tegument [59, 60]. After being discharged below the tegument, host proteins can diffuse into the cyst fluid. Some of these vesicles fuse with lysosomes, suggesting that acid proteases could be involved in digesting host material [59]. Markers of fluid endocytosis (lucifer yellow, colloidal gold, and dextran) were not internalized, but markers for adsorptive endocytosis (ruthenium red, ferritin, and protein-A peroxidase) were readily absorbed [60].

Host macromolecules are the most potent stimulus for cyst pinocytosis. Uptake of host molecules is inhibited by low temperature [60, 61]. Uptake is saturable, but only at protein concentrations similar to those of serum [60]. Kalinna and McManus [62] claim to have isolated an Fc-like receptor by IgG affinity chromatography, but formal receptor-ligand-binding studies were not reported. The receptor was identified as paramyosin by amino-terminal sequencing. Others found no correlation between the presence or type of Fc component and the uptake of proteins in vitro [60]. One interpretation of the data is that paramyosin, which is highly charged, may bind with low affinity to a number of host proteins and facilitate adsorptive endocytosis.

After uptake into the vesicular fluid, host proteins are slowly degraded [60, 63, 64]. Several investigators failed to identify proteolytic activity within the cyst fluid [60, 64]. In contrast, we have identified several proteases, which are found primarily in the cyst wall [65]. IgG degradation appears to be mediated primarily by a cysteine proteinase, which we have purified from *T. crassiceps* cysts [White, C., submitted]. The sequence of the 50 terminal amino acids includes a single cysteine at position 23, similar to the position of the active-site cysteine of proteinases of the papain family. The surrounding amino acids show homology to the active site of other cysteine proteinases, but diverge sufficiently to suggest that this enzyme may represent a new family of cysteine proteinase.

Metacestodes and the Host Gonadal Function

Female mice are more susceptible to *T. crassiceps* infections and develop more intense infections than their male littermates. Gonadectomy increases the parasite burden in male mice, but decreases the parasite burden in the females [66, 67]. The effects of gonadectomy can be reversed by treatment with 17β-estradiol or 5α-dihydrotestosterone [67]. The effect of androgens or estrogens on the parasites is not direct since hormone supplementation did not affect growth of the parasites in vitro [66]. The effects of testosterone appear to be immune mediated, since sublethal irradiation increases intensity of infection in male mice or oophorectomized female mice, but not in intact females or orchiectomized males [66]. Similarly, neonatal thymectomy equalizes the intensity of infection in the sexes [68]. In male mice, there is a 200-fold increase in estrogen level, but 90% suppression of testosterone levels. The increased estrogens and decreased androgens correlate with the parasite burden [69]. In contrast, female mice have slightly increased levels of estrogens [69]. Interestingly, the increase in estrogens paralleled the production of IL-6, which has been shown to stimulate aromatase activity [69].

Taenia and Complement

There is a complex interaction between taeniid parasites and host complement. Destruction of oncospheres in immune animals is mediated by the classical complement pathway [70, 71]. Similarly, *T. solium* oncospheres can be killed in vitro by heat-inactivated sera from patients with cysticercosis when complement activity is restored [72]. Resistance to infection with *Taenia taeniaeformis* oncospheres in naive mice also requires complement [73]. Since these naive animals lack specific antibody, the alternative pathway is also important in determining susceptibility. Davis and Hammerberg [74] have demonstrated deposition of C3b on the surface of oncospheres and postoncosphere larvae in vitro for both sensitive and resistant strains. However, only the resistant mice produced C5a. Thus, in susceptible hosts, oncospheres may be able to modulate complement activation.

Complement has little effect on viable metacestodes. Tissue cysts actually contain hemolytically active host complement within the cyst fluid [75]. There is

---

only limited deposition of complement on the parasite membrane in vivo and no apparent ill effects [76, 77]. Complement deposition correlates with areas of leukocyte attachment in vitro. Studies with metacestodes in vitro suggest that excretory products from the parasites activate and consume complement in the space surrounding the cysts [78]. Others have noted, however, that some morphologically intact parasites may have C3b on their membranes [79].

Metacestodes and Granulocytes

In experimental infection, an infiltrate of neutrophils and eosinophils envelops the developing metacestode [80]. However, there is no evidence of any detrimental effect on the parasite, perhaps due to inhibition of neutrophil function [81]. Eosinophil chemotactic activity has been identified in *T. taeniaeformis* infection [82]. Potter and Leid [83] isolated a protein with eosinophil chemotactic activity with a molecular weight of 91 kD by gel filtration chromatography, but of 10.4 kD by SDS-PAGE. There is also evidence that arachidonic acid metabolites from the parasites have eosinophil chemotactic activity [82, 84]. Seifert and Geyer [85] reported inhibition of mast cell degranulation by *T. crassiceps* excretory products.

The Metacestode and Immunoglobulin

Antibody is thought to play a critical role in the immune response to *Taenia* oncospheres. Infected or immunized animals are partially or totally immune to challenge with eggs [86–89]. While T cells are involved in the generation of this immune response [71], passive immunization studies have shown that protection can be transferred with antibody alone [70, 71]. Studies with cobra venom factor have demonstrated that protective immunity requires complement [71]. Recent studies have used antibody to identify and clone protective antigens [90, 91].

In contrast, there appears to be little role for antibody in the immune response to the metacestode stage [86]. For example, Musoke and Williams [92] found no evidence for antibody-mediated destruction of *T. taeniaeformis* metacestodes in rats. Other groups have shown that immune serum, especially with complement, can affect metacestodes. However, the dissociation between viability of cysticerci noted histologically and the presence or type of antibody response suggests that antibody has little effect on the established metacestode.

Viable cysticerci in tissues contain host immunoglobulin in the cyst fluid [75, 93]. Similarly, most viable parasites also contain immunoglobulin on their external surface [94–97]. While some of the antibody is likely to recognize cyst antigens, the majority is not specific for parasite antigens [96, 97]. In some studies, an association was noted between the presence of surface immunoglobulin and parasite survival [97, 98]. Harris et al. [99] noted increased growth of *Taenia ovis* in vitro when incubated with immune serum. For *T. taeniaeformis*, the immunoglobulin binds to the bladder wall and not to the scolex [77]. Several groups have suggested that the parasites have Fc receptors for host immunoglobulins [64]. However, formal receptor-ligand-binding studies have not been reported.

Several groups have noted mitogenic responses of host lymphocytes to parasite extracts. Sealy et al. [100] noted stimulation of naive human B cells with material from *T. solium*. Judson et al. [101] identified mitogenic activity from cyst fluid and parasite extracts of a number of cestodes. The activity from *Taenia multiceps* cyst fluid adhered to carbohydrate polymers, suggesting lectin-like activity. Subsequent studies suggest that this material primarily stimulates T cells [102]. If in fact immunoglobulin is the primary protein source for the parasite, these mitogens might stimulate the host to generate immunoglobulins, which could be taken up by the parasites and digested.

Interactions with the Host Cellular Immune Response

Acute infection with taeniid oncospheres is associated with depression of the host immune response. For example, pigs infected with *T. solium* eggs had decreased numbers of T cells and CD4 cells in the peripheral blood [103]. There was an inverse correlation between the number of CD4 cells and the number of cysts found after sacrificing the animals. Similarly, during acute infection with *T. taeniaeformis*, spleen cells from rats displayed a decreased proliferative response to mitogens [104].

There is also evidence of immunosuppression by the cyst stage. Pathologic studies have shown minimal inflammation surrounding viable cysts in vitro. Similarly, patients with cysticercosis do not display a proliferative response in vitro or a skin test response in vivo to cysticercal antigens [105]. When cysts were implanted in the peritoneal cavity of mice, there was a decrease in the mitogenic response of splenic lymphocytes to concanavalin A [106]. The immunosuppression, however, faded as the larvae died. The supernatants of *T. solium* cysts cultured in vitro suppressed the mitogenic response of human peripheral blood mononuclear cells [107]. Similarly, supernatants of *T. taeniaeformis* can decrease the proliferative response and the production of IL-2 by rat spleen cells [108]. Mice infected with *T. crassiceps* displayed suppressed proliferative responses [109]. These effects seem to be mediated, at least in part, by modulation of the role of macrophages as antigen-presenting cells [102, 110].

Depressed immune response is not a reflection of inability to respond to the parasites. Pigs experimentally infected with *T. solium* can clear their infection if stimulated with a vaccine prepared from extracts of metacestodes [111]. Similarly, both pigs and humans develop a prominent inflammatory response to dying cysts. This granulomatous inflammatory response sometimes coexists with viable cysts that elicit no inflammation. Furthermore, there is no clinical evidence of increased susceptibility to *Taenia* infections in patients with cysticercosis. Thus, the effects on the immune response are likely to be localized to the area immediately surrounding the parasite.

Taenia *Infection and Cytokines*

There are at present few data published on cytokine responses in *Taenia* infections. Infection with *Taenia* species is associated with elevated immunoglobulin. In mice infected with *T. crassiceps*, levels of IgG1 and IgE are elevated, a pattern associated with T helper 2 cytokine levels [112, 113]. Infected patients also have elevated parasite-specific immunoglobulin, but primarily within the central nervous system [114]. Increased production of IL-6 has been documented both in serum and in stimulated spleen cells of infected mice [69]. In other cestode infections, IL-6 has been documented to drive production of IgG1 and IgE [115]. There is also increased production of the T helper 2 cytokines IL-4 and IL-10 [113]. Active infection is also associated with suppression of proinflammatory and T helper 1 cytokines [113]. *Taenia* excretory products downregulate IL-2 production [108]. In addition, parasite molecules have been shown to decrease IL-1 and IL-2 production [116].

The death of the parasite is associated with a granulomatous inflammatory response. The IgG isotypes, in response to dead parasites, switch to a predominance of IgG2a, a pattern associated with interferon gamma production [112]. In humans, parasite death is associated with elevations of neopterin (a marker for macrophage activation) and soluble IL-2 receptor within the spinal fluid [114]. Preliminary data from a few human biopsies also noted IL-12, interferon gamma, and IL-6 associated with a degenerating cysticercus [117]. Similarly, we have documented production of IL-2 and interferon gamma message in granulomas surrounding dying *T. crassiceps* cysts [Robinson et al., submitted]. Thus, viable parasites appear to induce T helper 2 cytokines and suppress the host T helper 1 response. In contrast, death of the metacestodes is predominantly associated with T helper 1 cytokines.

Parasite Molecules that Modulate Host Responses

Table 1 lists purified parasite molecules that have been implicated in the interaction of *Taenia* metacestodes and the intermediate host.

Metacestodes and Oxidative Metabolites

The ability to detoxify reactive oxygen intermediates is essential for the survival of tissue-dwelling parasites. Leid et al. [118, 119] have examined in detail the oxygen-metabolizing enzymes of *T. taeniaeformis*. They purified a superoxide dismutase from *T. taeniaeformis* larvae [120]. This enzyme is a tetramer with a

Table 1. Parasite molecules that interfere with the host response to *Taenia* metacestodes

Parasite molecules	Effect on the host
Taeniaestatin	inhibits complement proteins
	decreases IL-1 and IL-2 production and lymphocyte proliferation
	inhibits granulocyte chemotaxis and aggregation
Paramyosin	inhibits the classical complement pathway
Sulfated polysaccharides	activate, consume complement
Glutathione-S-transferase, glutathione peroxidase, glutathione reductase and superoxide dismutase	detoxify reactive oxygen intermediates
Cysteine proteinase	digests host immunoglobulin
PGE$_2$	induces T helper 2 response and suppress the inflammation
Parasite factors that have not been well defined	downregulate macrophage function
	decrease lymphocyte proliferation and IL-2 and interferon-γ production
	increase IL-4 and IL-10 production

native M_r of 64 kD, containing copper and zinc. A glutathione-S-transferase (GST) was purified from *T. taeniaeformis* metacestodes [118, 119]. The enzyme has a molecular weight of 26–28 kD by SDS-PAGE. Parasites were shown to actively secrete both enzymes, and the secreted GST is recognized by antibody from infected rats. Glutathione reductase and glutathione peroxidase activities have also been identified from *T. taeniaeformis* [118, 119].

Paramyosin

T. solium paramyosin was first identified in studies of parasite antigens recognized by serum from patients with NCC. When parasite extracts were separated by counterimmunoelectrophoresis, only a single band, termed antigen B, was recognized by a majority of sera [86]. Antigen B was purified and found to consist of multimers of a 95-kD protein that bound tightly to collagen [121]. Studies of the amino acid sequence and antigenicity have demonstrated that antigen B is a paramyosin [122]. While paramyosins are usually thought of as intracellular proteins associated with cellular myosin, antigen B was found to be localized both within the parasite and excreted into the surrounding tissue [123]. Paramyosin binds to C1 and inhibits classical pathway complement activation [124]. No effects were noted on C4 activation, decay of the C3 convertase, or efficiency of C3–9 in lysing sheep red blood cells [124]. Paramyosin was implicated as an IgG Fc receptor in one study, but formal receptor-binding studies were not performed [62].

Taeniaestatin

Suquet et al. [125] have identified and purified a protease inhibitor in the excretory/secretory material of *T. taeniaeformis* metacestodes. The purified inhibitor, also called taeniaestatin, is a glycoprotein with a molecular weight of 9.5 kD by gel filtration, but 19.5 kD by SDS-PAGE [125]. This enzyme inhibited host proteases, including trypsin and chymotrypsin. Taeniaestatin inhibited both classical and alternative pathway activation of complement in vitro [118]. Alternative pathway inhibition seemed to be primarily due to inhibition of factor D, since lysis of unsensitized rabbit red blood cells by both normal human serum (supplemented with EGTA and magnesium) and factor D-deficient serum supplemented with bovine factor D were inhibited [118]. When sheep red cells coated with IgG and complement components C1, C4, and C2 were incubated with taeniaestatin, cleavage of C3 was totally inhibited [118]. In the presence of taeniaestatin, mitogen-stimulated proliferation and IL-2 production of rat spleen cells and IL-1 stimulation of mouse thymocytes were markedly impaired [116, 126]. In addition, taeniaestatin interfered with C5a-stimulated equine neutrophil chemotaxis and aggregation in vitro [81, 127].

Sulfated Polysaccharides

Intact *Taenia* metacestodes are surrounded by a halo of material that stains with alcian blue. When this layer is intact, there are only few inflammatory cells surrounding the parasites [128]. Hammerberg et al. [129] detected anticomplementary activity excreted by *T. taeniaeformis* in vitro. Further characterization of the fractions that inhibited complement showed that they consist of polysulfated mucopolysaccharide-like material containing galactose, glucose, and glucosamine in a ratio of 4:1:4, as well as amino acids. This glycosaminoglycan was associated with activation of complement and consumption of complement either in vitro or when injected into experimental animals [78]. Similar polysulfated glycosaminoglycans can interfere with the lytic activities of complement [130].

Prostaglandins

Prostaglandin E_2 has been isolated from the secretory/excretory fluid of *Taenia* metacestodes [131]. Prostaglandins, and PGE_2 in particular, may play an important role in the modulation of the host response by parasites [132]. For example, PGE_2, when present at priming of T cells, inhibits the generation of T helper 1 cytokines [133].

Control and Prevention of *Taenia* Infection

The International Task Force for Disease Eradication has identified NCC as one of a limited number of infections for which eradication is both feasible and important [9, 134]. The main focus of earlier control efforts was the eradication of porcine cysticercosis through improved animal husbandry and meat inspection. This approach resulted in the near eradication of *T. solium* infection in the United States and other developed countries. In contrast, similar approaches have had almost no impact in Third World Countries for several reasons. First, pigs are typically used as scavengers to clean areas of waste, and are not provided with food. Raising animals in pens or areas where they cannot scavenge for food requires that the farmers provide them with food, which is typically an economic impossibility. Second, farmers are often able to recognize infected pigs (e.g. by observing cysts in the tongue). Rather than suffer the economic loss from having the animals condemned, poor farmers will often sell them informally rather than in abattoirs, where the meat is inspected [135, 136]. Even intense educational efforts have had minimal impact on the prevalence of infection [137].

In an attempt to eradicate human tapeworm carriage, mass chemotherapy of endemic populations has been tried as a second approach to control [138]. In a pilot study in Ecuador, mass chemotherapy with praziquantel resulted in elimination of intestinal tapeworm carriage and marked reduction in the rate of porcine cysticercosis [138]. The results of a similar approach in Mexico were less successful. Furthermore, mass chemotherapy of canine tapeworm carriers has not been an effective control measure [139].

Population studies of ovine cysticercosis have suggested that the immune response in the intermediate host is critically important in limiting infection [139]. Since this immunity is largely mediated by antibody along with complement and is directed at the oncosphere stage, Johnson et al. [90] took advantage of this response by using antibody to screen an oncosphere stage *T. ovis* λgt11 cDNA expression library. Immune serum identified a prominent 47- to 52-kD band. Rabbit antisera to that antigen was affinity-purified and used to screen the library. A single clone (termed 45W) was identified that provided a high degree of protection when cloned into pGEX-1 and expressed as a GST fusion protein (GST-45W). This antigen has now been developed as a commercial vaccine by modification of the carboxy-terminal amino acids (GST-45B/X). This modified recombinant protein, along with saponin, provided 92–98% protection in field studies. In subsequent large-scale field studies in 19 farms in New Zealand and Australia, when animals were vaccinated at 6–7 weeks of age, the vaccine was 85–100% effective in Australia and 83% effective in New Zealand [140]. This vaccine is now available commercially for veterinary use in New Zealand [140].

Subsequently, two other *T. ovis*-oncosphere protective antigens (M_r 16 and 18 kD) have been cloned which could potentially be developed into a multicomponent vaccine. There are also some data on vaccine directed at the metacestode stage. Molinari et al. [111] demonstrated that pigs immunized with crude preparations prepared from *Taenia solium* cysts were immune to challenge with eggs. The immune response resulted in granulomatous inflammation surrounding the few parasites that were found in tissues [111, 141].

Summary

Taenia parasites have developed elaborate mechanisms of interacting with their intermediate hosts. The oncospheres which invade the intermediate host are susceptible to antibody and complement. However, by the time the host has generated an antibody response, the parasites have begun to transform to the more resistant metacestode. The metacestodes have elaborate means of evading complement-mediated destruction, including paramyosin which inhibits C1q, taeniaestatin which inhibits both classical and alternate pathways, and sulfated polysaccharides which activate complement away from the parasite. Similarly, antibody does not seem to be able to kill the mature metacestode. In fact, the parasites may even stimulate the host to produce antibody, which could be bound via Fc receptors and used as a source of protein. Finally, taeniaestatin and other poorly defined factors may interfere with lymphocyte proliferation and macrophage function, thus paralyzing the cellular immune response. Since the symptoms of NCC are typically associated with a brisk inflammatory response, we hypothesize that disease is primarily caused by injured or dying parasites. This hypothesis raises important questions in assessing the role of chemotherapy in the management of NCC, as well as in the evaluation of clinical trials, most of which were uncontrolled.

References

1   Del Brutto OH, Sotelo J: Neurocysticercosis: An update. Rev Infect Dis 1988;10:1075–1087.
2   Schantz PM, Sarti E, Plancarte A, Wilson M, Criales JL, Roberts J, Flisser A: Community-based epidemiological investigation of cysticercosis due to *Taenia solium*: Comparison of serological screening tests and clinical findings in two populations in Mexico. Clin Infect Dis 1994;18:879–885.
3   Ramos-Kuri M, Montoya RS, Padilla A, Gevensky T, Diaz ML, Sciutto E, Sotelo J, Larralde C: Immunodiagnosis of NCC: Disappointing performance of serology (ELISA) in an unbiased sample of neurologic patients. Arch Neurol 1992;49:633–636.
4   Tsang VCW, Brand JA, Boyer AE: An enzyme-linked immunoelectrotransfer blot assay and glycoprotein antigens for diagnosing human cysticercosis *(Taenia solium)*. J Infect Dis 1989;159:50–59.
5   International League against Epilepsy: Relationship between epilepsy and tropical diseases. Epilepsia 1994;35:89–93.
6   Tsang VCW, Wilson M: *Taenia solium* cysticercosis: An under-recognized but serious public health problem. Parasitol Today 1995;11:124–126.

7   Ito A, Smyth JD: Adult cestodes – immunology of the lumen-dwelling cestode infections; in Soulsby EJL (ed): Immune Responses in Parasitic Infections: Immunology, Immunopathology, and Immunoprophylaxis. Boca Raton, CRC Press, 1987, pp 115–163.

8   Schantz PM: Surveillance and control programs for cestode diseases: in Miller MJ, Love EJ eds): Parasitic Diseases: Treatment and Control. Boca Raton, Florida, CRC Press, 1989, pp 275–290.

9   Centers for Disease Control: Update: International task force for disease eradication. MMWR 1992;41:691, 697–698.

10 Mahajan RC: Geographical distribution of human cysticercosis; in Flisser A, Willms K, LaClette JP, Larralde C (eds): Cysticercosis: Present State of Knowledge and Perspectives. New York, Academic Press, 1982, pp 39–46.

11 Theis JH, Goldsmith RS, Flisser A, Koss J, Chioino C, Plancarte A, Segura A, Widjana D, Sutisna P: Detection by immunoblot assay of antibody to *Taenia solium* cysticerci in sera from residents of rural communities and from epileptic patients in Bali, Indonesia. Southeast Asian J Trop Med Public Health 1994;25:464–468.

12 Kong Y, Cho SY, Cho MS, Kwon OS, Kang WS: Seroepidemiological observation of *Taenia solium* cysticercosis in epileptic patients in Korea. J Korean Med Sci 1993;82:145–152.

13 Del Brutto OH, Santibañez R, Noboa CA, Aguirre R, Diaz E, Alarcón TA: Epilepsy due to neurocysticercosis: Analysis of 203 patients. Neurology 1992;42:389–392.

14 Medina MT, Rosas E, Rubio-Donnadieu F, Sotelo J: Neurocysticercosis as the main cause of late-onset epilepsy in Mexico. Arch Intern Med 1990;150:325–327.

15 Dumas M, Grunitzky E, Deniau M, Dabis F, Bouteille B, Belo M, Pestre-Alexandre M, Catanzano G, Darde ML, D'Almeida M: Epidemiological study of neurocysticercosis in Northern Togo (West Africa). Acta Leiden 1989;57:191–196.

16 Geerts S: Cysticercosis in Africa. Parasitol Today 1995;11:389.

17 McCormick GF: Cysticercosis: Review of 230 patients. Bull Clin Neurosci 1985;50:76–101.

18 Earnest MP, Reller LB, Filley CM, Grek AJ: Neurocysticercosis in the United States: 35 cases and a review. Rev Infect Dis 1987;9:961–979.

19 Scharf D: Neurocysticercosis. Arch Neurol 1988;45:777–780.

20 Shandera WX, White AC, Jr, Chen J, Diaz P, Armstrong R: Cysticercosis in Houston, Texas: A report of 112 cases. Medicine 1994;73:37–52.

21 Schantz PM, Moore AC, Muñoz JL, Hartman BJ, Schaefer JA, Aron AM, Persaud D, Sarti E, Wilson M, Flisser A: Neurocysticercosis in an orthodox Jewish community in New York City. N Engl J Med 1992;327:692–695.

22 Sorvillo FJ, Waterman SH, Richards FO, Schantz PM: Cysticercosis surveillance: Locally acquired and travel-related infection and detection of intestinal tapeworm carriers in Los Angeles. Am J Trop Med Hyg 1992;47:365–371.

23 Centers for Disease Control: Locally acquired neurocysticercosis – North Carolina, Massachusetts, and South Carolina, 1989–1991. MMWR 1992;41:1–4.

24 Stamos JK, Chadwick EG, Hahn YS, Schantz PM, Wilson M, Rowley AH: New onset seizures due to cysticercosis in low-risk children in Chicago, 1988–1993 (abstract M15). Abstracts of the 34th Interscience Conference on Animicrobial Agents and Chemotherapy. Orlando, American Society for Microbiology, 1994, p 198.

25 Moore AC, Lutwick LI, Schantz PM, Pilcher JB, Wilson M, Hightower AW, Chapnick EK, Abster EIM, Grossman JR, Fried JA, Ware DA, Haichou X, Hyon SS, Barbour RL, Antar R, Hakim A: Seroprevalence of cysticercosis in an orthodox Jewish community. Am J Trop Med Hyg 1995;53:439–442.

26 Monteiro L, Coelho T, Stocker A: Neurocysticercosis – a review of 231 cases. Infection 1992;20:61–65.

27 Flisser A: Neurocysticercosis in Mexico. Parasitol Today 1988;4:131–137.

28 Sarti E, Schantz PM, Plancarte A, Wilson M, Gutierrez I, Aguilera J, Roberts J, Flisser A: Epidemiological investigation of *Taenia solium* taeniasis and cysticercosis in a rural village of Michoacan state, Mexico. Trans Soc Trop Med Hyg 1994;88:49–52.

29 Diaz F, Garcia HH, Gilman RH, Gonzalex AE, Castro M, Tsang VCW, Pilcher JB, Vasquez LE, Lescano M, Carcamo C, Madico G, Miranda E, the Cysticercosis Working Group in Peru: Epidemiology of taeniasis and cysticercosis in a Peruvian village. Am J Epidemiol 1992;135:875–882.

Cysticercosis

30   Garcia HH, Martinez M, Gilman R, Herrera G, Tsang VCW, Pilcher JB, Diaz F, Verastegui M, Gallo C, Porras M, Alvarado M, Naranjo J, Miranda E: Diagnosis of cysticercosis in endemic regions. Lancet 1991;338:549–551.

31   Cruz ME, Cruz I, Preux P-M, Schantz P, Dumas M: Headaches and cysticercosis in Ecuador, South America. Headache 1995;35:93–97.

32   Garcia HH, Herrera G, Gilman RH, Tsang VCW, Pilcher JB, Diaz JF, Candy EJ, Miranda E, Naranjo J, the Cysticercosis Working Group in Peru: Discrepancies between cerebral computed tomography and western blot in the diagnosis of neurocysticercosis. Am J Trop Med Hyg 1994;50: 152–157.

33   Garcia HH, Gilman RH, Tovar MA, Flores E, Jo R, Tsang VCW, Diaz F, Torres P, Miranda E, the Cysticercosis Working Group in Peru: Factors associated with *Taenia solium* cysticercosis: Analysis of nine hundred fourty-six Peruvian neurologic patients. Am J Trop Med Hyg 1995;52:145–148.

34   van As AD, Joubert J: Neurocysticercosis in 578 black epileptic patients. S Afr Med J 1991;80: 327–328.

35   Dansey RD, Hay M, Cowie RL: Seizures and NCC in black men. S Afr Med J 1992;81:424–425.

36   Gulati P, Jena AN, Tripathi RP, Puri V, Sanchetee PC: MRI (magnetic resonance imaging) spectrum of epilepsy. J Indian Med Assoc 1994;92:110–112.

37   Chandy MJ, Rajshekhar V, Prakash S, Ghosh S, Joseph T, Abraham J, Chandi SM: Cysticercosis causing single, small CT lesions in Indian patients with seizures. Lancet 1989;i:390–391.

38   Rajshekhar V: Etiology and management of single CT lesions in patients with seizures: Understanding a controversy. Acta Neurol Scand 1991;84:465–470.

39   Wei G-Z, Li C-J, Meng J-M, Ding M-C: Cysticercosis of the central nervous system: A clinical study of 1,400 cases. Chin Med J 1988;101:493–500.

40   Yu SH, Xu LQ, Jiang ZX, Han JJ, Zhu YG, Chang J, Lin JX, Xu FN: Nationwide survey of human parasite in China. Southeast Asian J Trop Med Public Health 1994;25:4–10.

41   White AC, Jr, Baig S, Robinson P: *Taenia saginata* oncosphere excretory/secretory peptidases. J Parasitol 1996;82:7–10.

42   Dixon HBF, Lipscomb FM: Cysticercosis: An analysis and follow-up of 450 cases. Med Res Counc Spec Rep Ser 1961;299:1–58.

43   Itabashi HH: Pathology of CNS cysticercosis. Bull Clin Neurosci 1983;48:6–17.

44   Escobar A: The pathology of neurocysticercosis; in Palacios E, Rodriguez-Carbajal J, Taveras J (eds): Cysticercosis of the Central Nervous System. Springfield, Thomas, 1983, pp 27–54.

45   Carpio A, Placencia M, Santillán F, Escobar A: A proposal for classification of neurocysticercosis. Can J Neurol Sci 1994;21:43–47.

46   White AC, Jr, Dakik H, Diaz P: Asymptomatic neurocysticercosis in a patient with AIDS and cryptococcal meningitis. Am J Med 1995;99:101–102.

47   Mitchell WG, Crawford TO: Intraparenchymal cerebral cysticercosis in children: Diagnosis and treatment. Pediatrics 1988;82:76–82.

48   Kramer LD, Locke GE, Byrd SE: Cerebral cysticercosis: Documentation of natural history by CT. Radiology 1989;171:459–462.

49   Estañol B, Corona T, Abad P: A prognostic classification of cerebral cysticercosis: Therapeutic implications. J Neurol Neurosurg Psychiatry 1986;49:1131–1134.

50   Gardner B, Goldberg M, Heiner D: The natural history of parenchymal central nervous system cysticercosis (abstract). Neurology 1984;34(suppl 1):90.

51   Carpio A, Santillán F, León P, Flores C, Hauser WA: Is the course of neurocysticercosis modified by treatment with antihelminthic agents? Arch Intern Med 1995;155:1982–1988.

52   Bandres J, White AC, Jr, Samo T, Murphy E, Harris R: Extraparenchymal neurocysticercosis: Report of five cases and review of the literature on management. Clin Infect Dis 1992;15:799–822.

53   Lobato R, Lamas E, Portillo JM, Roger R, Esparza J, Rivas JJ, Muñoz MJ: Hydrocephalus in cerebral cysticercosis. J Neurosurg 1981;55:786–793.

54   Estañol B, Kleriga E, Loyo M, Mateos H, Lombardo L, Gordon F, Saguchi AF: Mechanisms of hydrocephalus in cerebral cysticercosis: Implications for therapy. Neurosurgery 1983;13:119–123.

55   Cardenas F, Quiroz H, Plancarte A, Meza A, Dalma A, Flisser A: *Taenia solium* ocular cysticercosis: Findings in 30 cases. Ann Ophthalmol 1992;24:25–28.

56   Gutierrez Y: Cysticercosis, Coenurosis, and Sparganosis: Diagnostic Pathology of Parasitic Infection with Clinical Correlation. Philadelphia, Lea & Febiger, 1990, pp 432–459.
57   Aluja AS, Vargas G: The histopathology of porcine cysticercosis. Vet Parasitol 1988;28:65–77.
58   Ridaura Sanz C: Host response in childhood neurocysticercosis. Child's Nerv Syst 1987;3:206–207.
59   Threadgold LT, Dunn J: *Taenia crassiceps*: Regional variation in ultrastructure and evidence of endocytosis in the cysticercus tegument. Exp Parasitol 1983;55:121–131.
60   Ambrosio J, Landa A, Merchant MT, LaClette JP: Protein uptake by cysticerci of *Taenia crassiceps*. Arch Med Res1994;25:3235–3330.
61   Threadgold LT, Dunn J: *Taenia crassiceps*: Basic mechanisms of endocytosis in the cysticercus. Exp Parasitol 1984;58:263–269.
62   Kalinna B, McManus DP: An IgG (Fc gamma)-binding protein of *Taenia crassiceps* (Cestoda) exhibits sequence homology and antigenic similarity with schistosome paramyosin. Parasitology 1993;106:289–296.
63   Damian RT: The exploitation of host immune responses by parasites. J Parasitol 1987;73:3–13.
64   Hayunga EG, Sumner MP, Letonja T: Evidence for selective incorporation of host immunoglobulin by strobilocerci of *Taenia taeniaeformis*. J Parasitol 1989;75:638–642.
65   White AC, Jr, Molinari JL, Pillai AV, Rege AA: Detection and preliminary characterization of *Taenia solium* metacestode proteases. J Parasitol 1992;78:281–287.
66   Huerta L, Terrazas LI, Sciutto E, Larralde C: Immunologic mediation of gonadal effects on experimental murine cysticercosis caused by *Taenia crassiceps*. J Parasitol 1992;87:471–476.
67   Terrazas LI, Bojalil R, Gevezensky T, Larralde C: A role for 17-beta-estradiol in immunoendocrine regulation of murine cysticercosis *(Taenia crassiceps)*. J Parasitol 1994;80:563–568.
68   Bojalil R, Terrazas LI, Govensky T, Sciutto E, Larralde C: Thymus-related cellular immune response in sex-associated resistance to experimental murine cysticercosis *(Taenia crassiceps)*. J Parasitol 1993;79:384–389.
69   Larralde C, Morales J, Terrazas I, Govensky T, Romano MC: Sex hormone changes induced by the parasites lead to feminization of the male host in murine *Taenia crassiceps* cysticercosis. J Steroid Biochem Mol Biol 1995;52:575–580.
70   Musoke AJ, Williams JF: The immunologic response of the rat to infection with *Taenia taeniaeformis*. V. Sequence of appearance of protective immunoglobulins and the mechanism of action of 7S2a antibodies. Immunology 1975;29:855–866.
71   Mitchell GF, Goding JW, Rickard MD: Studies on immune responses to larval cestodes in mice. Increased susceptibility of certain mouse strains and hypothymic mice to *Taenia taeniaeformis* and analysis of passive transfer of resistance with serum. Austr J Exp Biol Med Sci 1977;55:165–186.
72   Molinari JL, Tato P, Lara-Aguilera R, White AC, Jr: Effects of serum from neurocysticercosis patients on the structure and viability of *Taenia solium* oncospheres. J Parasitol 1993;79:124–127.
73   Davis SW, Hammerberg B: Activation of the alternative pathway of complement by larval *Taenia taeniaeformis* in resistant and susceptible strains of mice. Int J Parasitol 1988;18:591–597.
74   Davis SW, Hammerberg B: *Taenia taeniaeformis*: Evasion of complement-mediated lysis by early larval stages following activation of the alternative pathway. Int J Parasitol 1990;20:587–593.
75   Machnicka B, Grzybowski J: Host serum proteins in *Taenia saginata* metacestode fluid. Vet Parasitol 1986;19:47–54.
76   Conder GA, Picone J, Geary AM, DeHoog J, Williams JF: Lytic effects of normal serum on isolated postoncospheral and metacestode stages of *Taenia taeniaeformis*. J Parasitol 1983;69:465–472.
77   Letonja T, Hammerberg B: Third component of complement, immunoglobulin deposition, and leukocyte attachment related to surface sulfate on larval *Taenia taeniaeformis*. J Parasitol 1983;69:637–644.
78   Hammerberg B, Williams JF: Interaction between *Taenia taeniaeformis* and the complement system. J Immunol 1978;120:1033–1038.
79   Correa D, Dalma D, Espinoza B, Plancarte A, Rabiela T, Madrazo I, Gorodezky C, Flisser A: Heterogeneity of humoral immune components in human cysticercosis. J Parasitol 1985;71:535–541.
80   Englekirk PG, Williams JF: *Taenia taeniaeformis* (Cestoda) in the rat: Ultrastructure of the host-parasite interface on days 8 to 22 postinfection. J Parasitol 1983;69:828–837.

Cysticercosis

81   Leid RW, Grant RF, Suquet CM: Inhibition of equine neutrophil chemotaxis and chemokinesis by a *Taenia taeniaeformis* proteinase inhibitor, taeniaestatin. Parasit Immunol 1987;9:195–204.
82   Potter K, Leid RW: A review of eosinophil chemotaxis and function in *Taenia taeniaeformis* infections in the laboratory rat. Vet Parasitol 1986;20:103–116.
83   Potter KA, Leid RW: Isolation and partial characterization of an eosinophil chemotactic factor from metacestodes of *Taenia taeniaeformis* (ECF-Tt). J Immunol 1986;136:1712–1717.
84   Potter K, Leid RW, Kolattukudy PE, Espelie KE: Stimulation of equine eosinophil migration by hydroxyacid metabolites of arachidonic acid. Am J Pathol 1985;21:361–368.
85   Seifert B, Geyer E: Inhibition of in vitro and in vivo mast cell degranulation by *Taenia crassiceps* metacestode in vitro incubation products. Int J Microbiol 1989;271:521–531.
86   Flisser A, Perez-Monfort R, Larralde C: The immunology of human and animal cysticercosis. Bull World Health Organ 1979;57:839–856.
87   Rickard MD, Williams JF: Hydatidosis/cysticercosis: Immune mechanisms and immunization against infection. Adv Parasitol 1982;21:229–296.
88   Rickard MD: Immunization against infection with larval cestodes using oncospheral antigens; in Flisser A, Willms K, LaClette JP, Larralde C (eds): Cysticercosis: Present State of Knowledge and Perspectives. New York, Academic Press, 1982, pp 633–646.
89   Rickard MD, Howell MJ: Helminth vaccines; in Taylor AER, Baker JR (eds): In vitro Methods for Parasite Cultivation. New York, Academic Press, 1987, pp 407–451.
90   Johnson KS, Harrison GBL, Lightowlers MW, O'Hoy KL, Cougle WG, Dempster RP, Lawrence SB, Vinton JG, Heath DD, Rickard MD: Vaccination against ovine cysticercosis using a defined recombinant antigen. Lancet 1989;338:585–587.
91   Ito A, Bogh HO, Lightowlers MW, Mitchell GF, Takami T, Kamiya M, Onitake K, Rickard MD: Vaccination against *Taenia taeniaeformis* infection in rats using a recombinant protein and preliminary analysis of the induced antibody response. Mol Biochem Parasitol 1991;44:43–52.
92   Musoke AJ, Williams JF: Immunological responses of the rat to infection with *Taenia taeniaformis:* Protective antibody response to implanted parasites. Int J Parasitol 1976;62:265–269.
93   Hustead ST, Williams JF: Permeability studies of taeniid metacestodes. 1. Uptake of proteins by larval stages of *Taenia taeniaformis, T. crassiceps,* and *Echinococcus granulosus.* J Parasitol 1977; 63:314–321.
94   Willms K, Arcos L: *Taenia solium:* Host serum proteins on the cysticercus surface identified by an ultrastructural immunoenzyme technique. Exp Parasitol 1977;43:396–406.
95   Siebert AE, Good AH: *Taenia crassiceps:* Effects of normal and immune serum on metacestodes in vitro. Exp Parasitol 1979;48:164–174.
96   Craig PS: Surface-associated proteins and host IgG on early and late metacestode stages of *Taenia pisiformis.* Parasite Immunol 1988;10:243–254.
97   McManus DP, Lamsam S: *Taenia crassiceps* surface immunoglobulin: Parasite- or host-derived. Parasitology 1990;101:127–137.
98   Kwa BH, Liew FY: Studies on the mechanism of long-term survival of *Taenia taeniaformis* in rats. J Helminthol 1978;52:1–6.
99   Harris A, Heath DD, Lawrence SB, Shaw RJ: Ultrastructure of changes at the surface during early development of *Taenia ovis* cysticerci in vitro. Int J Parasitol 1987;17:903–910.
100   Sealy M, Ramos C, Willms K, Ortiz-Ortiz L: *Taenia solium:* Mitogenic effect of larval extracts on murine B lymphocytes. Parasite Immunol 1981;3:299–307.
101   Judson DG, Dixon JB, Skerritt GC: Occurrence and biochemical characterization of cestode lymphocyte mitogens. Parasitology 1987;94:151–160.
102   Rakha NK, Dixon JB, Jenkins P, Carter SD, Skerritt GC, Marshall-Clarke S: Modification of cellular immunity by *Taenia multiceps* (Cestoda): Accessory macrophages and CD4+ lymphocytes are affected by two different coenurus factors. Parasitology 1991;103:139–147.
103   Molinari JL, Tato P, Valles Y: Inmunodepresion de linfocitos T en cerdos, modulada por *Cysticercus cellulosae.* Rev Latinoam Microbiol 1987;29:293–300.
104   Letonja T, Hammmerverg C, Schurig G: Evaluation of spleen lymphocyte responsiveness to a T-cell mitogen during early infection with larval *Taenia taeniaformis.* Parasitol Res 1987;73:265–270.

105 Flisser A, Rivera L, Trueba J, Espinoza B, Yadoleff-Greenhouse V, Sierra A, Larralde C: Immunology of human neurocysticercosis; in Flisser A, Willms K, LaClette JP, Larralde C (eds): Cysticercosis: Present State of Knowledge and Perspectives. New York, Academic Press, 1982, pp 549–563.

106 Willms K, Merchant MT, Arcos L, Sealey M, Díaz de León L: Immunopathology of cysticercosis; in Larralde C, Willms K, Ortiz L, Seal Mol (eds): Molecules, Cells, and Parasites in Immunology. New York, Academic Press, 1980, pp 145–162.

107 Molinari JL, Tato P, Reynoso OA, Cazares JML: Depressive effect of a *Taenia solium* cysticercus factor on cultured human lymphocytes stimulated with phytohaemoglutinin. Ann Trop Med Parasitol 1990;84:205–208.

108 Burger CJ, Rikihisa Y, Lin YC: *Taenia taeniaformis* inhibition of mitogen induced proliferation and interleukin 2 production in rat splenocytes by larval in vitro product. Exp Parasitol 1986;62: 216–222.

109 Sciutto E, Fragoso G, Baca M, de la Cruz V, Lemus L, Lamoyi E: Depressed T-cell proliferation associated with susceptibility to experimental infection with *Taenia crassiceps* infection. Infect Immun 1995;63:2277–2281.

110 Rakha NK, Dixon JB, Skerritt GC, Carter SD, Jenkins P, Marshall-Clarke S: Lymphoreticular responses to metacestodes: *Taenia multiceps* (Cestoda) can modify interaction between accessory cells and responder cells during lymphocyte activation. Parasitology 1991;102:133–140.

111 Molinari JL, Meza R, Suarez B, Palacios S, Tato P, Retana A: *Taenia solium:* Immunity in hogs to the cysticercus. Exp Parasitol 1983;55:340–357.

112 Zakroff SGH, Beck L, Platzer EG, Spiegelberg HL: The IgE and IgG subclass responses of mice to four helminth parasites. Cell Immunol 1989;119:103–201.

113 Villa OF, Kuhn RE: Mice infected with the larvae of *Taenia crassiceps* exhibit a Th2-like immune response with concomitant energy and downregulation of Th1-associated phenomena. Parasitology 1996;112:561–570.

114 Rolfs A, Muhlschlegel F, Jansen-Rosseck R, Martins AR, Bedaque EA, Tamburus WM, Pedretti L, Schulte G, Feldmeier H, Kremsner P: Clinical and immunologic follow-up study of patients with neurocysticercosis after treatment with praziquantel. Neurology 1995;45:532–538.

115 Estes DM, Teale JM: In vivo effects of anticytokine antibodies on isotype restriction in *Mesocestoides corti*-infected BALB/c mice. Infect Immun 1991;59:836–842.

116 Leid RW, Suquet CM, Bouwer HGA, Hinrichs DJ: Interleukin inhibition by a parasite proteinase inhibitor, taeniaestatin. J Immunol 1986;137:2700–2702.

117 Restrepo B, Llaguno P, Ma S, Encisco J, Teale J: Characterization of the inflammatory response in the human brain infected by the cysticercus of the flatworm *Taenia solium* (abstract 65). 44th Annual Meeting of the American Society of Tropical Medicine and Hygiene. San Antonio, American Society of Tropical Medicine and Hygiene, 1995.

118 Leid RW, Suquet CM, Tanigoshi L: Parasite defense mechanisms for evasion of host attack: A review. Vet Parasitol 1987;25:147–162.

119 Leid RW, Suquet CM, Tanigoshi L: Oxygen detoxifying enzymes in parasites: A review. Acta Leiden 1989;57:107–114.

120 Leid RW, Suquet CM: A superoxide dismutase of metacestodes of *Taenia taeniaeformis*. Molec Biochem Parasitol 1986;18:301–311.

121 Plancarte A, Flisser A, Larralde C: Fibronectin-like properties of antigen B from cysticerci of *Taenia solium:* in Flisser A, Willms K, LaClette JP, Larralde C, Ridaura C, Beltrán F (eds): Cysticercosis: Present State of Knowledge and Perspectives. New York, Academic Press, 1982, pp 453–463.

122 LaClette JP, Lnada A, Arcos L, Willms K, Davis AE, Shoemaker CB: Paramyosin is the *Schistosoma mansoni* (Trematoda) homologue of antigen B from *Taenia solium* (Cestoda). Molec Biochem Parasitol 1991;44:287–295.

123 LaClette JP, Merchant M, Willms K: Histological and ultrastructural localization of antigen B in the metacestode of *Taenia solium*. J Immunol 1987;73:121–129.

124 LaClette JP, Shoemaker CB, Richter D, Arcos L, Pante N, Cohen C, Bing D, Nicholson-Weller A: Paramyosin inhibits complement C1. J Immunol 1992;148:124–128.

125 Suquet C, Green-Edwards C, Leid RW: Isolation and partial characterization of a *Taenia taeniaeformis* metacestode proteinase inhibitor. Int J Parasitol 1984;14:165–172.

126 Leid RW, Suquet CM, Perryman LE: Inhibition of antigen- and lectin-induced proliferation of rat spleen cells by a *Taenia taeniaeformis* proteinase inhibitor. Clin Exp Immunol 1984;57:187–194.

127 Leid RW, Grant RF, Suquet CM: Inhibition of neutrophil aggregation by taeniaestatin, a cestode proteinase inhibitor. Int J Parasitol 1987;17:1349–1353.

128 Bogh HO, Lightowlers MW, Sullivan ND, Mitchell GF, Rickard MD: Stage-specific immunity to *Taenia taeniaeformis* infection in mice. A histological study of the course of infection in mice vaccinated with either oncosphere or metacestode antigens. Parasit Immunol 1990;12:153–162.

129 Hammerberg B, Dangler C, Williams JF: *Taenia taeniaeformis:* Chemical composition of parasite factors affecting coagulation and complement cascades. J Parasitol 1980;66:569–576.

130 Tschopp J, Masson D: Inhibition of the lytic activity of perforin (cytolysin) and of late complement components by proteoglycans. Molec Immunol 1987;24:907–913.

131 Leid RW, McConnell LA: PGE$_2$ generation and release by the larval stage of the cestode, *Taenia taeniaeformis.* Prostaglandins Leukotrienes Med 1983;11:317–323.

132 Belley A, Chadee K: Eicosanoid production by parasites: From pathogenesis to immunomodulation? Parasitol Today 1995;11:327–334.

133 Katamura K, Yamauchi T, Fudui T, Ohshima Y, Mayumi M, Furushi K: Prostaglandin E$_2$ at priming of naive CD4+ T cells inhibits acquisition of ability to produce IFN-gamma and IL-2, but not IL-4 and IL-5. J Immunol 1995;155:4604–4612.

134 Schantz PM, Cruz M, Sarti E, Pawlowski Z: Potential eradicability of taeniasis and cysticercosis. Bull Pan Am Health Organ 1993;27:397–401.

135 The Cysticercosis Working Group in Peru: The marketing of cysticercotic pigs in the sierra of Peru. Bull World Health Organ 1993;71:223–228.

136 Gemmel M, Matyas Z, Pawlowski Z, Soulsby EJL (eds): Guidelines for the Surveillance, Prevention, and Control of Taeniasis/Cysticercosis. Geneva, World Health Organization, 1983.

137 Bronfman M, Flisser A, Sarti E, Schantz PM, Gleizer M, Loya M, Plancarte A, Avila G, Allan J, Fineblum W: Evaluation of health education for control of *Taenia solium* in a rural community in Mexico (abstract 272). Programs and Abstracts of the 44th Meeting of the American Society of Tropical Medicine and Hygiene. San Antonio, American Society of Tropical Medicine and Hygiene, 1995.

138 Cruz M, Davis A, Dixon H, Pawlowski ZS, Proana J: Operational studies on the control of *Taenia solium* taeniasis/cysticercosis in Ecuador. Bull World Health Organ 1989;67:401–407.

139 Gemmell MA, Lawson JR, Roberts MG, Kerin BR, Mason CJ: Population dynamics in echinococcosis and cysticercosis: Comparison of the response on *Echinococcus granulosus, Taenia hydatigena* and *T. ovis* to control. Parasitology 1986;93:357–369.

140 Rickard MD, Harrison GBL, Heath DD, Lightowlers MW: *Taenia ovis* recombinant vaccine – 'quo vadis'. Parasitology 1995;110(suppl):S5–S9.

141 Molinari JL, Meza R, Tato P: *Taenia solium:* Cell reactions to the larvae *(Cysticercus cellulosae)* in naturally parasitized immunized hogs. Exp Parasitol 1983;56:327–338.

A. Clinton White, MD, Department of Medicine, Room 561E, Baylor College of Medicine, 1 Baylor Plaza, Houston, TX 77030 (USA)

Subject Index

CD1, intestinal infection response 54
Collagen, synthesis, schistosomiasis 169, 170
Complement, *Taenia solium* interactions 217, 218
Cystic echinococcus, *see Echinococcus granulosus*

Der proteases, role, immunoglobulin E response 10
Dva-1
  antibody specificity 6
  structure 8, 9

Echinococcus granulosus
  immune response
    antibodies 182–184
    cell-mediated immunity 184, 185
    cytokines 185, 186
  life cycle 177–179
  morphology 177
  pathogenesis 180, 182
  survival strategies 186
Echinococcus multilocularis
  antigens 191, 192, 198, 199
  course of disease 196, 197
  immune response
    antibodies 191, 192
    cell-mediated immunity 192, 194
    cytokines 194, 195
    phases 189, 190
  life cycle 179, 180
  pathogenesis 186–189
  survival strategies
    immune segregation by laminated layer 198, 199, 201
    immunosuppression, T cells 195–197
  susceptibility of mice strains 188, 189
Echinococcus oligarthrus
  hosts 202
  immunopathology 202, 203
Echinococcus vogeli
  hosts 201
  immunopathology 202, 203
  life cycle 201, 202

Eosinophil
  cytotoxic properties 28
  hookworm response 76, 77
  immunoglobulin E, helminth response 109, 110
  interleukin-5, development 28, 30
  myocardial effects 112, 113
  neurocysticercosis response 218
  onchocerciasis
    chemotaxis 35, 36
    degranulation 36, 37
    granulation effect on corneal clarity 37
    role
      dermatitis 28–31
      keratitis 31–33
  pulmonary effects 113, 114
  Toxocara canis response 105, 107, 109–116
Eosinophilic enteritis
  etiology 62, 63
  individual susceptibility 83, 84
  tolerance 88, 89

γ-Glutamyl transpeptidase
  autoimmunity induction 17, 18
  sequence homology
    Bm2325 14, 15
    species 16
  tropical pulmonary eosinophilia syndrome role 17–19
Goblet cell, nematode removal 53
gp15/400
  antibody specificity 6, 9
  processing 8

Heligmosomoides polygyrus
  gastrointestinal infection, rodents 42, 43
  immune response 51, 52
Hookworm, *see* individual species
  adult worm secretion
    acetylcholinesterase 82
    anticoagulants 80
    hyaluronidase 82
    neutrophil inhibitory factor 83
    proteases 80, 81
  anemia mechanisms 77
  burden, host response 84, 85

cytokine response 85, 86
diagnosis 90
immune stimulation 72, 73
immunopathology 85–87
individual susceptibility 83, 84
intestinal interactions 79, 80
invasion 77, 78
larva development 78, 79
neuroendocrine involvement, infection 87
protective immunity 73, 74
tolerance 88, 89
treatment 90, 91
Hyaluronidase, hookworm secretion 82

Immunoglobulin E
antigens
ABA-1 6–8
Bm2325 13–15, 17
Dva-1 6, 8, 9
gp15/400 6, 8, 9
paramyosin 12, 13
echinococcosis response 183, 191
interleukin-4, production 2
protease role, response 9–12
receptors 1
role, helminth infection
animal models 3, 4
humans 4, 5
intestinal infection 46, 47
serum concentration 1
Immunoglobulin G4, protease role, response 10–12
Interferon-γ
echinococcosis response 185, 194, 195
schistosomiasis role 162, 164, 166, 170
Interleukin-1, neurocysticercosis response 220
Interleukin-2
deficient mice, nematode infection 56
neurocysticercosis response 220
schistosomiasis role 162, 163, 166
Interleukin-4
echinococcosis response 184
immunoglobulin E, role, production 2
intestinal infection response 53, 54
protective immunity, intestine 45

schistosomiasis role 162, 166, 170
T cell differentiation role 3
Interleukin-5
echinococcosis response 194, 195
role, eosinophil development 28, 30
Interleukin-10
deficient mice, nematode infection 56
echinococcosis response 184
schistosomiasis role 166
Interleukin-12
protective immunity, intestine 46
schistosomiasis role 163

Lymphatic filariasis, see also Brugia malayi, Wuchereria bancrofti
age dynamics 137, 138
animal models 145
bacterial infection risk 142
clinical manifestations
asymptomatic amicrofilaremics 140, 141
filarial fever, adeno-lymphangitis 141–143
lesion sites 144
lymphedema 143, 144
onset 138, 139
tropical pulmonary eosinophilia 143
concomitant immunity 150, 151
cuticle composition 133, 134, 152
demographics, endemic areas 136, 137
gender effects on incidence 137
geographic distribution 125, 136
histopathology 144, 145
history of study 126
immune response
antibodies 146
cytokines 147
T helper cells 145–147, 152
natural history 149, 150
parasites 125, 127, 131, 132
periodicity 127, 130, 131
protective immunity 151
susceptibility, maternal influence 148
tolerance 148
transmission 139
treatment 133, 152
vaccination 134–136

Major basic protein, deposition in onchocerciasis 28, 29, 37
Mast cell
    cytokine production 48
    growth factors 47–49
    hyperplasia, nematode infection 50
    mucosal mast cell maturation 47, 48
    nematode removal, gut 51, 52
    proteases, nematode infection 50, 51

Necator americanus, see also Hookworm
    cutaneous manifestations 64
    immune response 75–77
    intestinal histopathology 72
    life cycle 63
    pulmonary manifestations 65, 66
    symptoms of infection 69, 70
Neurocysticercosis, see also Taenia solium
    clinical manifestations 212, 213
    pathology 215, 216
    prevalence 209–211
    serologic assay 209, 210
    treatment 223
    vaccination 223, 224
Neutrophil inhibitory factor, hookworm
    secretion 83
Nippostrongylus brasiliensis
    gastrointestinal infection, rodents 42,
        43, 51
    intestinal pathology, infection 44

Onchocerciasis
    animal models 31, 34, 35
    clinical manifestations 26
    cytokine response 34, 35
    eosinophil
        chemotaxis 35, 36
        degranulation 36, 37
        granulation effect on corneal clarity
            37
        role
            dermatitis 28–31
            keratitis 31–33
    microfilariae antigens 26–29
    treatment 31

Paramyosin
    immunoglobulin E binding 12, 13, 19
    modulation of host response 221, 222
Platelet-activating factor, hookworm
    defense 86, 87
Prostaglandin E_2, modulation of host
    response 222

River blindness, see Onchocerciasis

Schistosoma haematobium
    host localization 159
    life cycle 159
Schistosoma japonicum
    granuloma formation
        cytokine role 163, 164
        immune downregulation 167, 168
    host localization 159
    life cycle 159
Schistosoma mansoni
    granuloma formation
        cytokine role 161–163
        immune downregulation 164
    host localization 159
    life cycle 159
Schistosomiasis
    acute toxemic disease 160
    animal models 161, 168, 169
    circumoval granulomas
        immune downregulation 164–169
        immunopathogenesis 161–164
    fibrotic reactions induced by eggs 169,
        170
    pathology of chronic disease 160, 161
Serpin
    role in immunoglobulin E response 11,
        12
    structure in helminths 11, 12
Smw32, role in immunoglobulin E
    response 10
Stem cell factor
    mast cell production role 47, 48
    role, intestinal nematode infection 48,
        49
Strongyloides venezuelensis, gastrointes-
    tinal infection in rodents 42, 43